Practical Guide to Common Clinical Procedures and Emergencies

Practical Guide to Common Clinical Procedures and Emergencies

Professor Chandra M. Kumar, MBBS, DA, FFARCS, FRCA, MSc
Professor of Anaesthesia,
School of Health, University of Teeside
The James Cook University Hospital
Middlesbrough TS4 3BW, UK

Professor Chris Dodds, MB, MRCGP, FRCA
Professor of Anaesthesia,
School of Health, University of Teeside
The James Cook University Hospital
Middlesbrough TS4 3BW, UK

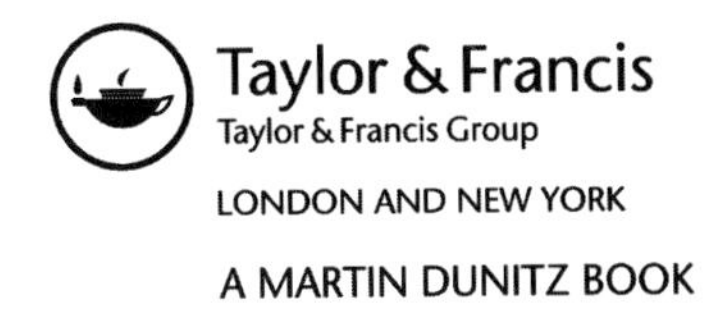

LONDON AND NEW YORK

A MARTIN DUNITZ BOOK

First published in the United Kingdom in 2005
by Taylor & Francis, an imprint of the Taylor & Francis Group, 2 Park Square, Milton Park, Abingdon, Oxon OX14 4RN

Tel.: +44 (0)20 7017 6000
Fax.: +44 (0)20 7017 6699
E-mail: info@dunitz.co.uk
Website: http://www.dunitz.co.uk

A CIP record for this book is available from the British Library.

Library of Congress Cataloging-in-Publication Data

Data available on application

ISBN 90 265 1971 0

Distributed in North and South America by

Taylor & Francis
2000 NW Corporate Blvd
Boca Raton, FL 33431, USA

Within Continental USA
Tel: 800 272 7737; Fax: 800 374 3401
Outside Continental USA
Tel: 561 994 0555; Fax: 561 361 6018
E-mail: orders@crcpress.com

Distributed in the rest of the world by
Thomson Publishing Services
Cheriton House
North Way
Andover, Hampshire SP10 5BE, UK
Tel.: +44 (0)1264 332424
E-mail: salesorder.tandf@thomsonpublishingservices.co.uk

Typesetting: Charon Tec Pvt. Ltd, Chennai, India
Printed by: Kyodo Printing Co. (Singapore) Pte. Ltd.

Contents

Contributors xi

Preface xxi

Section 1 Basic Skills 1

1. Setting up an intravenous infusion 3
   Gerry Appleton
2. Intravenous drugs 7
   Gerry Appleton
3. How to perform a venous cannulation 12
   Chris Dodds
4. Cannulation of peripheral arteries 17
   Fiona L. Clarke
5. Maintaining an airway 21
   Tim Meek
6. Intubation skills 28
   Tim Meek
7. Assessment of consciousness 34
   Roger Strachan
8. Taking consent 40
   Barry Nicholls
9. Taking an ECG 49
   Chandrika Roysam
10. Interpreting the ECG 53
    Chandrika Roysam
11. Simple local anaesthetic techniques 60
    Dave Murray
12. Basic suturing techniques 70
    Philip A. Corbett and William A. Corbett
13. Scrub/sterile techniques 78
    Gillian Davies
14. Simple patient monitoring 86
    Nigel Puttick
15. Urinary catheterisation 94
    David Chadwick
16. Using a medical simulator 102
    Ronnie J. Glavin

17. How to prepare to speak at an educational meeting 108
J. David Greaves
18. Using audio-visual material in presentations 114
J. David Greaves
19. Electrical safety 123
Steve Graham
20. Writing a discharge letter 131
Philip A. Corbett and William A. Corbett

Section 2 Higher Skills **137**

21. Sedation 139
Mike G. Bramble
22. Intravenous regional anaesthesia (Bier's Block) 145
Chandra M. Kumar
23. Central venous access 151
Fiona L. Clarke
24. Ultrasound and its application in venous access 157
Oliver Weldon
25. Acute pain assessment and patient controlled analgesia 164
Christine Sinclair
26. Inserting a naso-gastric tube 172
Ian Conacher
27. Paediatric vascular access 177
Christopher J. Vallis
28. Removing a foreign body from the eye 184
John R. Clarke

Section 3 Respiratory Skills **193**

29. Oxygen therapy 195
Praveen Kalia
30. Airway assessment 203
Simon Gardner and Dave Ryall
31. Drainage of a pleural effusion 208
Ian Conacher
32. Insertion of a chest drain 211
Kyee H. Han
33. CPAP therapy 219
Chris Dodds
34. Practical guide to non-invasive ventilation 223
E. Sowden and Stephen Murphy

35. Pulmonary function tests 228
Mark Weatherhead and George Antunes
36. Lumbar puncture 235
Roger Strachan

Section 4 Cardiovascular Skills **243**

37. Drainage of a pericardial effusion 245
Robert J.R. Meikle
38. Pulmonary artery catheterization 250
Emilio Garcia
39. Cardiac output measurement 256
Khalid J. Khan
40. Intra-aortic balloon counter-pulsation 264
James Park
41. Temporary pacing 274
Deepak Kejariwal and Basant K. Chaudhury

Section 5 Anaesthetic Skills **281**

42. Checking an anaesthesia machine 283
Nigel Puttick
43. Monitoring and anaesthesia 292
Stephen Bonner
44. Difficult intubation 302
Simon Gardner and David Ryall
45. Spinal anaesthesia 308
Tim Meek and John Hughes
46. Epidural anaesthesia 315
Tim Meek and John Hughes
47. Major peripheral nerve blocks 322
Martin Herrick

Section 6 Critical Care Skills **333**

48. Ventilators 335
Fiona L. Clarke
49. Conventional tracheostomy 341
Derek A. Bosman
50. Percutaneous dilatational tracheostomy 348
Stephen Chay
51. Bronchoscopy 355
Harry Gribbin

52. Intracranial pressure measurement 362
Kathryn A. Price
53. Intravenous feeding lines and total parenteral nutrition 368
Judith C. Wright
54. Diagnostic peritoneal lavage 374
Jonathan R. Easterbrook and Robert Wilson
55. Haemodialysis and haemofiltration 378
David Reaich
56. Brain stem death testing 383
Stephen Bonner

Section 7 Specific Advanced Skills 389

57. Echocardiography—requesting an echocardiogram 391
Mike J. Stewart
58. Neonatal resuscitation 401
Samir Gupta and Sunil Sinha
59. Fetal heart rate monitoring in labour 409
Helen R. Simpson

Section 8 Emergencies 417

60. Hypovolaemia 419
L. Jeyaraj and Gerard Danjoux
61. Acute asthma 426
Harry Gribbin
62. Anaphylaxis 432
Jacqui Gedney
63. Epilepsy 440
Peter Newman and Maureen Pearce
64. The management of near-drowning 446
Jason Easby
65. Hypothermia 451
Diane Monkhouse
66. Overdose 456
Samit Mitra and Gaynor Creaby
67. Stridor 463
Mike Tremlett
68. The immediate management of head injuries 471
Roger Strachan
69. Adult cardio-respiratory resuscitation 477
Carol Tennant

Section 9 Algorithms **487**

Appendix 1: Adult basic life support 489
Appendix 2: Advanced life support algorithm for the management of cardiac arrest in adults 490
Appendix 3: Paediatric basic life support 491
Appendix 4: Paediatric advanced life support 492
Appendix 5: Newborn life support 493
Appendix 6: Consent 494
Appendix 7: Adverse reaction form 495

Index **497**

Contributors

Dr George Antunes
Consultant Chest Physician
The James Cook University Hospital
Marton Road
Middlesbrough TS4 3BW, UK

Mrs Gerry Appleton
Director of Nursing
Freeman Hospital
Freeman Road
Newcastle upon Tyne, NE7 7DN, UK

Dr Stephen Bonner
Consultant in Anaesthesia and Intensive Care Medicine
The James Cook University Hospital
Marton Road
Middlesbrough TS4 3BW, UK

Mr Derek A. Bosman
Consultant Otolaryngologist
The James Cook University Hospital
Marton Road
Middlesbrough TS4 3PW, UK

Professor Mike G. Bramble
Department of Gastrointestinal Unit
The James Cook University Hospital
Marton Road
Middlesbrough TS4 3BW, UK

Mr David Chadwick
Consultant Urologist
The James Cook University Hospital
Marton Road
Middlesbrough TS4 3BW, UK

Dr Stephen Chay
Staff Grade Doctor
Intensive Care Unit
The James Cook University Hospital
Marton Road
Middlesbrough TS4 3BW, UK

Dr Basant Chaudhury
Consultant Physician
University Hospital of Hartlepool
Holdforth Road
Hartlepool TS24 9AH, UK

Dr Fiona Clarke
Consultant Intensivist
The James Cook University Hospital
Marton Road
Middlesbrough TS4 3BW, UK

Mr John R. Clarke
Consultant Ophthalmic Surgeon
The James Cook University Hospital
Marton Road
Middlesbrough TS4 3BW, UK

Dr Ian Conacher
Consultant Anaesthetist
Freeman General Hospital
Freeman Road
Newcastle upon Tyne NE7 7DN, UK

Dr Philip A. Corbett
Surgical SHO
Mersey Deanery
8 Oakdale Road
Liverpool L18 1EP, UK

Professor William A. Corbett
Consultant Colorectal Surgeon
The James Cook University Hospital
Marton Road
Middlesbrough TS4 3BW, UK

Dr Gaynor Creaby
Specialist Registrar Accident and Emergency
St James's Hospital
15 Hyde Terrace
Leeds LS2 9LT, UK

Dr Gerard Danjoux
Consultant in Anaesthesia
The James Cook University Hospital
Marton Road
Middlesbrough TS4 3BW, UK

Sister Gillian Davies
General Theatre
The James Cook University Hospital
Marton Road
Middlesbrough TS4 3BW, UK

Professor Chris Dodds
Department of Anaesthesia
The James Cook University Hospital
Marton Road
Middlesbrough TS4 3BW, UK

Dr Jason Easby
Specialist Registrar in Anaesthesia
The James Cook University Hospital
Marton Road
Middlesbrough TS4 3BW, UK

Mr Jonathan R. Easterbrook
SpR General Surgery
The James Cook University Hospital
Marton Road
Middlesbrough TS4 3BW, UK

Dr Emilio Garcia
Consultant Anaesthetist
The James Cook University Hospital
Marton Road
Middlesbrough TS4 3BW, UK

Dr Simon Gardner
Specialist Registrar in Anaesthesia and Intensive Care Medicine
The James Cook University Hospital
Marton Road
Middlesbrough TS4 3BW, UK

Dr Jacqui Gedney
Consultant in Anaesthesia and Intensive Care Medicine
The James Cook University Hospital
Marton Road
Middlesbrough TS4 3BW, UK

Dr Ronnie J. Glavin
Consultant Anaesthetist
Educational Co-director
Scottish Clinical Simulation Centre
Stirling Royal Infirmary
Stirling FK8 2AU, UK

Dr Steve Graham
Consultant Anaesthetist
The James Cook University Hospital
Marton Road
Middlesbrough TS4 3BW, UK

Dr J. David Greaves
Consultant Anaesthetist
Royal Victoria Infirmary
Victoria Road
Newcastle upon Tyne NE1 4LP, UK

Dr Harry Gribbin
Consultant in Respiratory Medicine
The James Cook University Hospital
Marton Road
Middlesbrough TS4 3BW, UK

Dr Samir Gupta
Neonatal Fellow
Directorate of Neonatology
The James Cook University Hospital
Marton Road
Middlesbrough TS4 3BW, UK

Mr Kyee H. Han
Consultant in Accident and Emergency Medicine
The James Cook University Hospital
Marton Road
Middlesbrough TS4 3BW, UK

Dr Martin Herrick
Consultant Anaesthetist
Perioperative Care Services
Addenbrooke's Hospital
PO Box 93
Cambridge, UK

Dr John Hughes
Consultant Anaesthetist
The James Cook University Hospital
Marton Road
Middlesbrough TS4 3BW, UK

Dr L. Jeyaraj
Specialist Registrar in Anaesthesia
The James Cook University Hospital
Marton Road
Middlesbrough TS4 3BW, UK

Dr Praveen Kalia
Consultant Anaesthetist
University Hospital of Hartlepool
Holdforth Road
Hartlepool TS24 9AH, UK

Dr Deepak Kejariwal
Department of Medicine
University Hospital of Hartlepool
Holdforth Road
Hartlepool TS24 9AH, UK

Dr Khalid J. Khan
Consultant Cardiothoracic Anaesthetist
The James Cook University Hospital
Marton Road
Middlesbrough TS4 3BW, UK

Professor Chandra M. Kumar
Professor of Anaesthesia
Department of Anaesthesia
The James Cook University Hospital
Marton Road
Middlesbrough, TS4 3BW, UK

Dr Tim Meek
Consultant Anaesthetist
The James Cook University Hospital
Marton Road
Middlesbrough TS4 3BW, UK

Dr Robert J.R. Meikle
Consultant Anaesthetist
The James Cook University Hospital
Marton Road
Middlesbrough TS4 3BW, UK

Dr Samit Mitra
Consultant in Accident and Emergency
The James Cook University Hospital
Marton Road
Middlesbrough TS4 3BW, UK

Dr Diane Monkhouse
Specialist Registrar in Intensive Care Medicine
The James Cook University Hospital
Marton Road
Middlesbrough TS4 3BW, UK

Dr Stephen Murphy
Consultant Respiratory Physician
The James Cook University Hospital
Marton Road
Middlesbrough TS4 3BW, UK

Dr Dave Murray
Consultant Anaesthetist
The James Cook University Hospital
Marton Road
Middlesbrough TS3 4BW, UK

Dr Peter Newman
Consultant Neurologist
The James Cook University Hospital
Marton Road
Middlesbrough TS4 3BW, UK

Dr Barry Nicholls
Consultant Anaesthetist
Tauton and Somerset Hospital
Musgrove Park
Taunton TA1 5DA, UK

Dr James Park
Consultant Anaesthetist
The James Cook University Hospital
Marton Road
Middlesbrough TS4 3BW, UK

Mrs Maureen Pearce
Neurology Clinical Nurse Specialist
The James Cook University Hospital
Marton Road
Middlesbrough TS4 3BW, UK

Dr Kathryn A. Price
Consultant in Anaesthesia and Intensive Care
Newcastle General Hospital
Newcastle upon Tyne NE1 4LP, UK

Dr Nigel Puttick
Consultant Anaesthetist
The James Cook University Hospital
Marton Road
Middlesbrough TS4 3BW, UK

Dr David Reaich
Consultant Nephrologist
The James Cook University Hospital
Marton Road
Middlesbrough TS4 3BW, UK

Dr Chandrika Roysam
Consultant Anaesthetist
Freeman Hospital
Newcastle-upon-Tyne NE7 7DN, UK

Dr David Ryall
Consultant Anaesthetist
The James Cook University Hospital
Marton Road
Middlesbrough TS4 3BW, UK

Miss Helen R. Simpson
Consultant in Fetal Medicine
The James Cook University Hospital
Marton Road
Middlesbrough TS4 3BW, UK

Mrs Christine Sinclaire
Acute Pain Clinical Nurse Specialist
The James Cook University Hospital
Marton Road
Middlesbrough TS4 3BW, UK

Professor Sunil Sinha
Professor of Paediatrics and Neonatal Medicine
The James Cook University Hospital
Marton Road
Middlesbrough TS4 3BW, UK

Dr E. Sowden
Specialist Registrar in Medicine
The James Cook University Hospital
Marton Road
Middlesbrough TS4 3BW, UK

Dr Mike J. Stewart
Consultant Cardiologist
The James Cook University Hospital
Marton Road
Middlesbrough TS4 3BW, UK

Mr Roger Strachan
Consultant Neurosurgeon
The James Cook University Hospital
Marton Road
Middlesbrough TS4 3BW, UK

Miss Carol Tennant
Resuscitation Department Manager
The James Cook University Hospital
Marton Road
Middlesbrough TS4 3BW, UK

Dr Mike Tremlett
Consultant Anaesthetist
The James Cook University Hospital
Marton Road
Middlesbrough TS4 3BW, UK

Dr Christopher J. Vallis
Consultant Paediatric Anaesthetist
Royal Victoria Infirmary
Newcastle upon Tyne NE1 4LP, UK

Dr Mark Weatherhead
SpR Respiratory Medicine
The James Cook University Hospital
Marton Road
Middlesbrough TS4 3BW, UK

Dr Oliver Weldon
Consultant Anaesthetist
Freeman Hospital
Freeman Road
Newcastle upon Tyne NE7 7DN, UK

Professor Robert Wilson
Professor of Surgery
The James Cook University Hospital
Marton Road
Middlesbrough TS4 3BW, UK

Dr Judith C. Wright
Consultant Anaesthetist
The James Cook University Hospital
Marton Road
Middlesbrough TS4 3BW, UK

Preface

Many practical procedures are performed in the management of patients in the operating department, intensive care, high dependency and immediate postoperative care units. Most of the practical procedures are described in major textbooks of anaesthesia and intensive care but these books may be heavy and immediate access may be difficult when the procedure is carried out on patients.

The purpose of this thin and light book is to include everyday practical that are performed in the management of patients. Each chapter is organised by introduction, relevant anatomy, physiology, how to do the procedure, indications, contraindication and complications. The 'how to do' sections will contain practical tips with photographic and other illustrative materials so that readers can easily understand the procedures.

The book is intended for those involved in the conduct of anaesthesia and the management of patients in the intensive care, high dependency and postoperative care units. Practicing anaesthetists, trainee anaesthetists, examinees, intensive care nurses, anaesthetic nurses, recovery nurses, operating department assistants and medical students will find this book of immense value. The book should also be of interest to others in surgical and other medical specialities.

Professor Chandra M. Kumar
Professor Chris Dodds

Section 1

Basic Skills

1

Setting up an intravenous infusion

Gerry Appleton

Most patients in hospital environments receive medication, fluids and electrolytes by intravenous (IV) infusion. Volumetric pumps and syringe drivers are used to deliver these medications and to control the flow and rate at which they are infused.

In some clinical areas such as the Intensive Care Unit it is not uncommon to have multiple infusions in progress with ten or more pumps controlling patient medication and fluid delivery.

IV infusions are the avenue for delivery of many high risk drugs such as morphine, heparin, potassium and insulin and therefore safety is paramount in all aspects of the preparation and management of intravenous infusion therapy.

Preparation of infusions

Practitioners are required to adhere to and apply their local drug administration policy to their practice, what we suggest in this section is good practice and technique that should underpin and compliment the requirements of that policy.

Any infusions should be drawn up and prepared in a clean environment. Sterile needles and syringes should be used and practitioners should thoroughly wash their hands prior to beginning of the procedure. The use of filter needles is the optimum method of avoiding contaminants in the prepared infusions such as glass splinters. Evidence suggests that the use of an in-line-filter can help in reducing the incidence of infection from fungi and bacteria. It is good and safe practice that two practitioners make certain safety checks before even preparing the drugs for administration.

- The patient's details should be checked on the prescription chart and identification band. Name, date of birth, hospital identification number and any patient allergies should also be checked.
- The drug should clearly be prescribed using its generic name.
- The amount and type of diluents should be checked along with any further IV fluid that may be required to administer the drug.
- Any special instructions should also be clearly documented on the prescription chart and checked e.g. rate of administration.

Labelling of infusion syringes and bags

Infusions should be labelled in accordance with hospital drug policy but again good practice is suggested here that can compliment local procedure. The patient's name, the generic name of the drug or drugs and doses within the infusion, the type and amount of diluents used should be clearly printed on the infusion label.

The time that the infusion was prepared and when it will expire should also be documented on the drug added label along with the initials of the practitioner that prepared the infusion and the one who checked it. It is essential that the strength/concentration of the infusion is also clearly identified on the label; this enables more accuracy in ensuring the patient receives correct dosage over the correct time (e.g. 1 mL = 1 mg or 1 mL = 80 mcg).

Sometimes higher concentrations are required to be infused if a patient is being fluid restricted. In these circumstances especially if standard regimens for infusions are used, there is a potential risk of drug errors occurring. If a higher strength infusion is prepared this should be clear on the label—writing the strength in red ink and starring it to ensure that it is immediately noticeable to practitioners checking the infusion prior to starting it off.

The infusion line should also be labelled at the point where it connects to the patient's intravenous access. This is done using a 'flag'—the name of what is infusing through that line and again the concentration per mL should be clearly seen on the label. This tells practitioners immediately what is being infused on each line/lumen of the available access. It is particularly useful when multiple infusions are in progress and essential if inotropic drugs are being infused.

Inotrope infusions

Some infusions can have a profound effect on a patient's haemodynamic status and they can become very sensitive to changes in rate or breaks in the infusion of the drug. Accidental bolus can cause episodes of extreme hypertension and tachycardia and breaks in infusion can cause severe hypotension and cardiac instability.

There are several safety aspects in the management of inotropic infusions that must be followed:

- All inotropes should be managed on a labelled dedicated inotrope lumen on a central or long line.
- Three way taps should be closed to infusions that are not running.
- Inotropes should not be managed on a peripheral line.
- Never give a bolus of inotrope infusion.
- An infusion should be checked by **two practitioners** prior to being inserted into the infusion pump and if not started **immediately** by **two practitioners** again prior to starting the infusion.
- Always follow the guidelines for safe 'piggy backing' of inotrope infusions.

Piggy backing of inotrope infusions

Because of the potential haemodynamic compromise and instability associated with inotrope infusions it is essential that they are not allowed to run out and then be changed as other infusions are. To prevent problems occurring piggy backing of infusions is required. This simply means establishing the next infusion before the expiring infusion has run out with minimum impact on the patients haemodynamic status.

Guidelines

Ensure that the infusion is checked by two practitioners prior to starting it even if it is already in the pump and was checked earlier. Check not only the drug but also the concentration.

Start the new infusion at the same rate as the existing infusion.

Slowly reduce the rate of the expiring infusion intermittently, observing the patients clinical haemodynamic status. A transient increase in the new infusion may be required if the patients blood pressure does become compromised by the changeover.

Once the expiring infusion is stopped switch off the infusion pump and turn off its respective three way tap on the central line.

2

Intravenous drugs

Gerry Appleton

Intravenous (IV) drug therapy is now seen as an everyday procedure used in all areas and aspects of the clinical environment. The skill is now so widely used across the spectrum of the multidisciplinary team there can sometimes be a tendency to assume that that the procedure is routine and without associated clinical problems.

Although relatively infrequent complications can and do occur, in this chapter we will examine the safe and correct methods for preparing and administering IV drug therapy therefore minimising the risks of potential complications occurring.

Benefits of intravenous administration

There are many benefits for administering prescribed medication intravenously, first and foremost that it enables far greater control over both dosage of the required drug but also over the rate of administration and bioavailability. The venous circulation facilitates an equal distribution of the drug administered throughout the blood stream enabling a quicker onset of the required effect. This makes IV administration the method of choice in emergency situations such as cardiac arrests.

Intravenous administration ensures an effective absorption into the body and is also used where patients have gut absorption problems or who may be nil by mouth.

Safety

Safety is paramount in all aspects of this procedure; it is essential that practitioners know fully their Trust's drug administration policy.

The skill is performed within the individual boundaries of their own scope of professional practice and ultimately they are accountable.

> Always ensure that you know the drug you are giving, its effect and its possible side effects
>
> If not... do not give it!

Trust drug administration policies differ from area to area but safety aspects of the technique are emphasised throughout. It is good and safe practice that two practitioners make certain safety checks before even preparing the drugs for administration.

- The patient's details should be checked on the prescription chart and identification band. (Name, date of birth, hospital identification number and any patient allergy.)
- The drug should be clearly prescribed using its generic name.
- The amount and type of dilutant should be checked along with any further IV fluid that may be required to administer the drug.
- Any special instructions should also be clearly documented on the prescription chart and checked, i.e. the rate of administration.

Preparation and administration

Infection control

Along with safety, measures to ensure prevention of infection should be utilised at all times through each stage of the procedure. The following good practice tips can ensure this:

- Always wear an apron and gloves.
- Aseptic technique throughout is the key preventative measure in reducing the likelihood of infection associated with IV therapy.
- All cannula, ports and taps should be occluded with an obturating cap when not in use.
- Evidence suggests that the use of in line filters can reduce the incidence of infection from fungi and bacteria.
- Always draw up drugs using sterile needles and syringes, this can minimise contaminants such as glass splinters. The use of filter needles can eradicate contaminants.
- Keep dressings clean and dry to cannulae and lines and observe the site for signs of infection.

Procedure

- It is important to select the most appropriate port for administration, there may just be a single, peripheral cannula or there may be a multi lumen central line with several ports to choose from. Therapies in progress on various lines obviously will affect which administration port is selected.
- If using an in line filter check that it is patent and within its useable date, if there is debris present or visible blockages the filter should be renewed.
- Check the line site to ensure the cannula or line is in place and that there is no sign of infection or inflammation.
- All drugs to be administered should be drawn up separately in individual syringes; they should never be mixed together.
- Documentation with each drug recommends the appropriate volume of dilutant to use and which ones are compatible when mixing. Some trusts have local standardised regimes for diluting drugs such as antibiotics.
- Ensure that drugs are completely dissolved in the dilutant before drawing up, do not give the drug if a cloudy precipitate is seen or an unexpected change in colour occurs.
- Use an alcohol swab to clean the port prior to giving the drugs.
- The line/cannula should be flushed prior to administration to ensure patency.
- Drugs should be infused slowly one at a time with the patient's condition observed/monitored continually throughout the administration process.
- To avoid any chemical interaction between drugs being given (this is rare) it is recommended that the line is flushed with saline between each administration.

> Stop administration immediately if:
>
> - There is any sudden change in the patients visible condition.
> - There is any sudden change in the patient's vital signs.
>
> Draw back on the line to remove as much of the infused drug as possible and get medical assistance immediately

- Once all the drugs have been administered the filter and line should be flushed with saline to infuse any remaining medication

and maintain line patency. Check that all connections on taps, lines and filters are secure and that ports are capped off.
- If the line or cannulae is not in permanent use it is recommended that it is flushed with a heparin saline solution in order to maintain patency.

Allergy and anaphylaxis

Allergic and anaphylactic reactions can occur extremely quickly because substances are being infused directly into the circulation. It is important to be able to recognise an evolving reaction and know what to do about it.

In an allergic reaction the patient may develop a rash with generalised itching, their breathing may become wheezy and in severe allergic reactions they may also develop acute dyspnoea.

An anaphylactic reaction is life threatening, it will have a sudden onset with the patient complaining of feeling faint, short of breath and developing bronchospasm. Acute hypotension can present very quickly along with classic signs such as facial swelling, rash and itching.

If a suspected reaction occurs you need to act quickly. Stop the drug administration and get senior help immediately. IM adrenaline is usually the first line treatment.

Drug errors

You may make a drug error… you may find a drug error.

Don't panic!

Check the patient is OK, then inform the senior medical and nursing staff.

Psychological aspects

Don't forget to think about your patients. They may be anxious and worried about what you are doing or giving them. A few words from you can make a big difference.

- Always inform the patient of what you are doing and why.
- Remember some drugs can be painful when administered through peripheral lines e.g. Propofol.
- Warn the patient of any effects that a drug may have on them.

Summary

- **Always adhere to your Trusts drug administration policy.**
- **Ensure you are confident and competent in this area before using this technique in practice. You are accountable.**
- **Never give a drug that you don't know.**
- **Safety is paramount at all times.**
- **Measures must be taken to prevent cross infection.**
- **Act quickly and get help in the event of an adverse reaction.**
- **Keep patients informed.**

3

How to perform a venous cannulation

Chris Dodds

Introduction

Venous access is one of the most fundamental skills in clinical practice. It is essential for resuscitation of ill patients, for many types of drug administration and for the maintenance of fluid balance in fasted patients.

The anatomy of the venous system is an important element on the road to success and should be remembered prior to trying to cannulate a vein. The veins are low pressure vessels with a series of valves within the lumen to encourage venous return to the heart. The vessel wall is muscular and has an autonomic supply as has the arterial vasculature. The veins in the limbs are arranged in arcades for the counter-current temperature control, and their flow is regulated as one of the bodies' mechanisms to maintain core temperature. This implies that cold will lead to venous constriction (harder to cannulate) whilst warmth will lead to vasodilatation (easier to cannulate).

Access to the vein is through a series of barriers of variable resistance and with discrete functions. The first is obvious, but its function is often ignored. The skin acts as a very effective barrier to infection and this is enhanced by the keratin layer remaining desiccated. It also acts to warn of dangerous environments by nocioception, and whilst the degree varies with the site, all procedures on the skin cause pain. Below the skin is the vascular sub-cutaneous fat layer. It is of low resistance but may be large enough to hide the veins!

Direct puncture of the skin breaks this protective barrier and increases the risk of infection, whilst occlusive dressings will hydrate the keratin layer and reduce its effectiveness in this area.

The pain of cannulation is related to the site chosen and the size of the cannula. Movement of the cannula once inserted remains painful for the entire duration of the cannulation—fix it securely.

Equipment

Non-slip gloves—they do not need to be sterile
2 mL syringe with 1% lidocaine and a 25G needle
5–10 mL syringe with normal saline
Tourniquet—capable of one-handed use
A range of venous cannulae
A fixation dressing—non-occlusive
Good light

Technique

- Wear gloves.
- Clean the skin if it is dirty.
- Keep the limb dependent at all time.
- Apply the tourniquet—it does not need to be very tight!

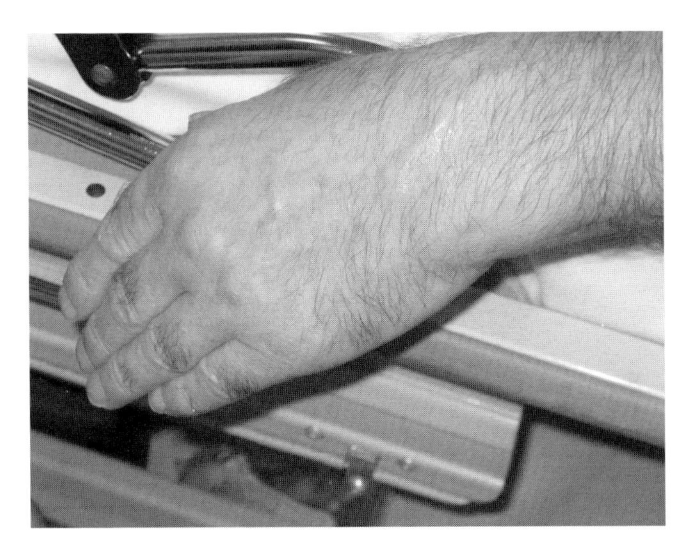

Figure 1. Position of hand to help gravity fill the vein.

- Identify a junction of the veins.
- Raise a dermal wheal with the local anaesthetic (instant anaesthesia) or a subcutaneous bleb (this takes over a minute to work—wait for it).
- Keep traction in the line of cannulation—to prevent folding of the skin.
- Approach the vein parallel to the surface of the skin (the veins usually stand out).
- Smoothly insert to needle through the skin, though the subcutaneous fat and into the vein.
- A sensation of a 'pop' may be felt, there may be a flashback of blood into the cannula, and visualisation of the cannula in the vein are all key end-points.
- Lift the tip of the cannula to prevent it going straight through the back of the vein, and whilst lifting, glide the cannula further into the vein. The larger the gauge of the cannula, the longer the distance between the needle tip and the plastic cannula.
- Once in the vein, release the tourniquet.
- Lift the limb above the heart—this limits the need to press over the cannula tip, an action which can perforate the vein in frail, elderly patients.

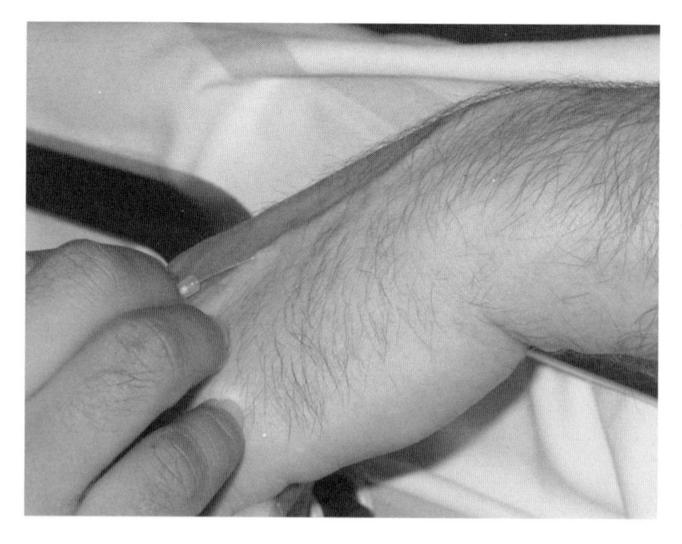

Figure 2. Venepuncture.

- Remove the needle and either cap or connect the IV infusion to the cannula.
- Secure the cannula with the dressing.
- Safely dispose of the sharps yourself!

Key points

- Skin barrier
- Vascular damage
- Neuronal damage
- Embolic problems
- Errors of administration

- Use gravity to fill the vein
- Warm the limb
- Avoid multiple stabs—venous constriction will occur!
- Choose the correct size cannula for the task—the bigger ones are easier to insert!
- Use local anaesthesia
- Transilluminate
- Use saline not water to test the vein.
- Fast and smooth entry
- Always flush the cannula with saline after every drug administration

Factors to consider

Cannula size

The use of the cannula will determine the size you use. If drug therapy is the priority then placing the smallest cannula into the largest vein will limit the potential vasculitis that commonly occurs and means the system will last longer. The relatively high blood flow through the vein will dilute the drug. If rapid fluid therapy is necessary then the largest gauge cannula should be used. There is little indication for using a medium gauge cannula—'just in case'.

Smaller cannulae are harder to insert because they can flex at the skin boundary and enter the vein at an acute angle, and go straight through.

Local anaesthesia

This should always be used for any cannula above a 22G cannula (Blue) because the pain caused by inserting cannulae of greater gauge is increasingly worse than that of injecting the local anaesthesia. 1% lidocaine should be used because 2% is painful. Topical gels and creams are useful in children and some adults, but they take a minimum of 30 minutes to work, and because of the occlusive dressings used to keep them in place, the skin become hydrated and thickened.

4

Cannulation of peripheral arteries

Fiona L. Clarke

The most commonly used site is the radial artery at the wrist. The ulnar artery is used infrequently, and should be avoided if the ipselateral radial artery has already been cannulated. The dorsalis pedis artery is usually used in the foot. The tibialis anterior artery can be used, but is again best avoided if the dorsalis pedis on that side has already been used, because of the risk to peripheral perfusion from thrombosis. More proximal arteries can be used if peripheral cannulation fails e.g. brachial or femoral arteries. Femoral arterial lines are the most likely to become infected. Cannulation of central arteries assumes that collateral arterial supply will perfuse the distal limb if thrombosis occurs.

Modified Allen test

This should be used to check that ulnar artery flow is sufficient to perfuse the hand before attempting to cannulate the radial artery. It is not a completely reliable test and false positive and false negative results can be obtained. Ask the patient to clench their fist tightly, and then apply sufficient digital pressure to the radial and ulnar artery to occlude both of them. In an unconscious patient, elevate the arm to reduce blood flow, and then occlude the arteries. Extend the fingers. After the hand is open, release the pressure over the ulnar artery, and look for a blush of blood returning to the hand and fingers through the palmer arch arteries. If the hand remains pale, release the pressure over the radial artery and look for changes in perfusion. Make sure that the fingers and hand are not hyperextended as this can give misleading results. The original Allen test was performed on both hands simultaneously with one artery occluded in each hand.

Complications of cannulation

Major complications occur in less than 1% of cases.

Early
Technical failure
Haematoma and bleeding
Radial artery spasm and peripheral ischaemia
Intimal dissection and peripheral ischaemia
Embolic phenomena and peripheral ischaemia
Infection

Late
Infection
Peripheral gangrene from prolonged ischaemia or emboli
Pseudoaneurysm formation
Arteriovenous malformation

Choice of cannula

A 20G cannula should be used in adults, 22G or 24G in children. These can be inserted as a cannula over needle or using a Seldinger technique. The cannula should have no injection port and may or may not have wings depending on personal preference. Cannulae are available with devices to prevent the spillage of arterial blood e.g. Flo-switch®.

Technique

Palpate the radial artery at the wrist to identify a point where the pulse is strongest. It is helpful to extend the hand slightly by placing a bag of intravenous fluid under the wrist, or a rolled up towel. Hanging a bag of fluid from several fingers with the hand extended at the side of the bed or trolley has also been recommended. Overextension should be avoided as this may make pulsations more difficult to feel.

Wash your hands and wear sterile gloves.

Disinfect the skin, and use a sterile drape, especially if using a Seldinger technique.

Infiltrate the skin and subcutaneous tissues on either side of the artery with 2–5 mL of plain lidocaine. Lidocaine will anaesthetise the skin and also cause a sympathetic block of the nerves around the artery, reducing the chance of arterial spasm, so should also be used in the unconscious sedated patient. If time permits (e.g. a planned change of cannula in an awake ICU patient) amethocaine gel (Amitop) or EMLA cream may to placed over the site and covered with an occlusive dressing for 30–60 min before cannulation. Insert the cannula at a 30–45° angle to the skin. The artery is a peripheral structure, and if you miss it and go deeply into the wrist, you will hit the periosteum of the radius and cause pain. When a flashback of blood is obtained, advance the cannula over the needle before withdrawing the needle. The walls of arteries are thicker than vein walls, and it is possible to get an initial flashback of blood before the whole bevel of the needle is within the lumen of the artery. If you feel resistance, try gently rotating the cannula on the needle, or altering the angle of the needle relative to the skin and then try to advance the cannula. The cannula should slide in as easily as a venous cannula.

If you have decided to use a Seldinger technique, you will be able to see if pulsatile blood spurts out of your needle. This helps show if you are in the correct position in the correct vessel, but is messy. Advance the guide wire up the needle, making sure to insert the softer, more flexible end first. The guide wire should slide smoothly into the artery. You may feel the change in resistance as it leaves the tip of the needle, but nothing further. Remove the needle over the guidewire, and then insert the cannula over the guidewire, making sure that a small part of the guidewire sticks out of the end of the cannula. You should hold this part of the guidewire, and then slide the cannula over the guidewire into the artery. Remove the guidewire, and connect to a pressurised flush system or a syringe of saline with three-way tap and short extension set. Check that you can aspirate blood, and then flush the line. The cannulae should be secured in place by stiches or thin tape, and then covered by transparent sterile dressings. The line should be clearly identified as an arterial line, and colour coded three-way taps used, to try to minimise the risk of inadvertent intra-arterial injection of drugs.

- Use peripheral arteries first.
- Do not use both co-lateral arteries on the same limb.
- Arteries are rarely deep structures.
- Always use local anaesthesia.
- Avoid hyperextension if using the radial artery.
- There should be no resistance once the cannula is intraluminal.

- Always check the entire pressure system for air bubbles.
- Use a sterile technique especially if using a Seldinger technique.
- Colour code the lines and connections.
- Secure the cannula.
- Cover with occlusive dressings.

Further reading

1 Furhman TM, Pippin WD, Talmage LA, Reilley TE. Evaluation of the collateral circulation of the hand. *J Clin Monit.* 1992; 8:28–32.

2 Scheer BV, Perel A, Pferffer UJ. Clinical Review: Complications and risk factors of peripheral arterial catheters used for haemodynamic monitoring in anaesthesia and intensive care medicine. *Crit Care*. 2002;6:199–204.

5

Maintaining an airway

Tim Meek

Introduction

Maintaining an airway in a patient is a core skill useful to anyone working in a clinical environment. Patients may need airway maintenance as a result of an unexpected event such as cardiac or respiratory arrest, or as a part of the anaesthetic sequence, at any time from induction to recovery. Airway maintenance is needed if a patient is not breathing, or if a patient is breathing, but has an obstructed airway. Generally, you will perform this manoeuvre either in a highly supervised environment (e.g. anaesthetic room, recovery room), or whilst 'holding the fort' waiting for help to arrive (e.g. cardiac arrest). Depending upon the location, the equipment to hand will vary slightly, but the principles are the same. Whatever the situation, a patent airway is a basic physiological requirement. Without it, oxygenation, and therefore life, is impossible. Manikin-based training is useful, but there is no substitute for demonstration in the calm environment of the anaesthetic room and recovery room.

Airway maintenance can be divided into four parts:
Providing oxygen
Optimising position
Opening the airway
Supporting ventilation (if required)

Providing oxygen

Initiating oxygen administration should be a reflex action. This will be delivered either via an oxygen mask, or via a breathing circuit, depending upon the location and the patient's condition.

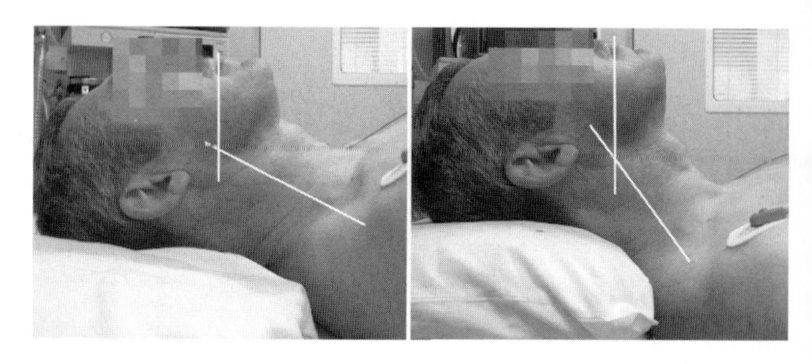

Figure 1. By changing a flat pillow (left) for a larger one (right) the head becomes more extended on the neck and the neck becomes more flexed on the thorax. The oral and pharyngeal axes (superimposed) are brought more nearly into line.

Optimising position

In order to make ventilation easier, the patient should have the neck flexed on the thorax, and the head extended on the neck. This position is often likened to 'sniffing the morning air', or 'sipping a pint of beer'. It requires proper positioning of the patient's head on the pillow. In this position, the axes of the mouth and pharynx are brought more into line than when the patient is lying flat (Figure 1).

Opening the airway

This step aims to create an unobstructed airway for breathing/ventilation. If appropriate, remove any obstructing matter from the mouth and pharynx under direct vision. Use suction apparatus if necessary. Perform a chin lift and/or a jaw thrust; this lifts the tongue from the soft palate. It is best performed by hooking fingers of one, or both hands behind the angles of the jaw (Figure 2).

If needed, an oropharyngeal airway can be inserted: The appropriate size airway is the same length as the distance from the angle of the mouth to the tragus of the ear (or alternatively from the centre of the mouth to the angle of the jaw).

Insertion should be performed gently. Sometimes it is necessary to insert the airway upside down and rotate it, being careful not to damage or dislodge the front teeth (Figure 3).

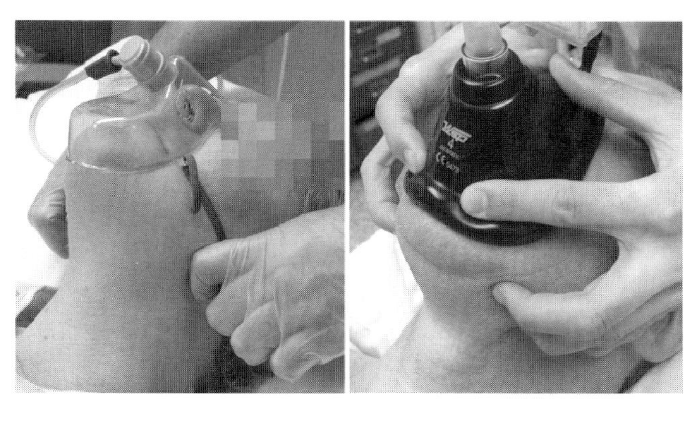

Figure 2. Opening the airway. The fingers are hooked behind the angle of the jaw, and the jaw is lifted forward as gently as possible. It is possible to hold a facemask and perform a jaw thrust at the same time (right).

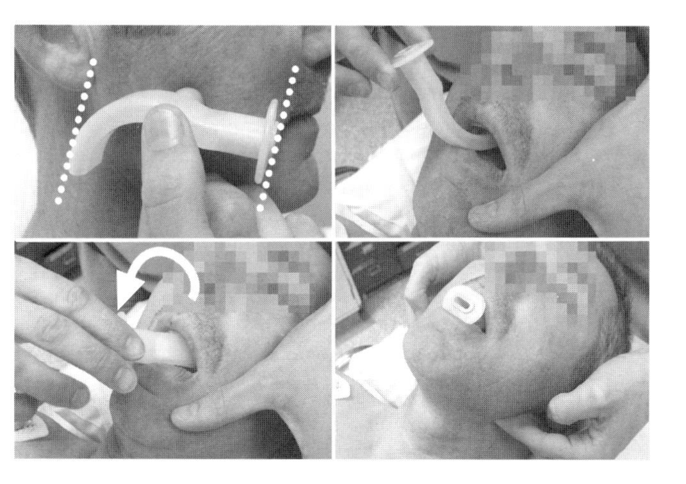

Figure 3. Inserting an oro-pharyngeal airway. The appropriate size of airway is as long as the distance from the angle of the mouth to the tragus of the ear (top left). The airway is inserted upside down (top right) and is rotated through 180° (bottom left), whilst being gently advanced into its resting position (bottom right).

These measures should provide a clear airway. If the patient is breathing, this should be evident—look, feel and listen:

You should see the chest rise and fall.

You may feel breath if you place your face close to the patient's. At the same time, you may also hear breathing.

You may hear breath sounds on auscultation with a stethoscope.

If there is no evidence of breathing, either the airway is still obstructed, or the patient is not making respiratory efforts. If the airway is still obstructed, repeat the above steps.

Obstruction of the airway is suggested by:

Noisy, stirtorous breathing (snoring).

'Tracheal tug' (watch the front of the neck—the trachea can be seen to move down on inspiration).

Paradoxical movement of the chest and abdomen (normally the chest and abdomen move out during inspiration; if obstruction is present, the abdomen moves out, but the chest moves in—also called 'see-sawing').

If the patient has a patent airway and is not making respiratory efforts, you will need to consider how to support ventilation.

Supporting ventilation

Slightly different equipment will be available for bag and mask ventilation, depending upon the location. Generally, the choice will be:

Anaesthetic circuit (anaesthetic room or operating theatre).

'C-circuit' (recovery room).

Self-inflating bag and mask (resuscitation trolley).

Whichever is used, the principles are the same.

Bag and mask ventilation should be considered a two-person manoeuvre until you are experienced:

One person maintains the airway and holds the mask, as above.

A second person squeezes the bag to ventilate the lungs (Figure 4).

A ventilatory rate of 12/min, with a tidal volume of 10 mL/kg is appropriate.

As part of cardiopulmonary resuscitation, there should be two breaths to fifteen chest compressions but with no pause between the compressions for the breaths. Look for evidence of ventilation—the

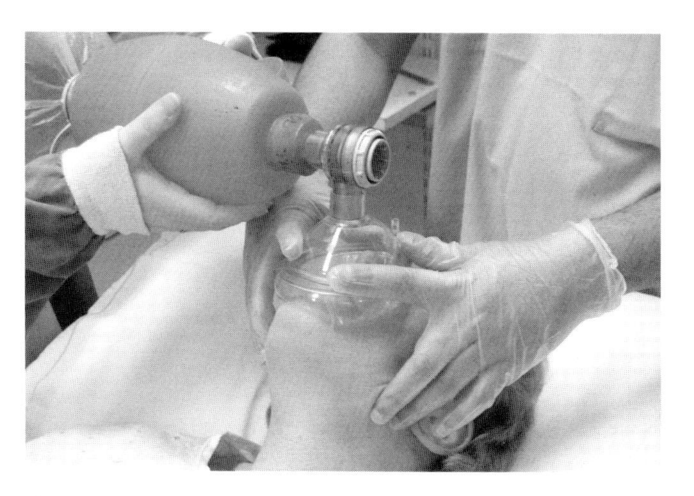

Figure 4. Supporting ventilation. This photo shows two person bag and mask ventilation, using a self-inflating bag.

chest should rise with each breath. Beware of inflating the stomach, which increases the risk of regurgitation. Inflation of the stomach is usually due to:

Failure to position the patient's head correctly or open the airway adequately (see above), or:

Over-enthusiastic squeezing of the bag.

The Laryngeal Mask Airway™ (LMA)

The LMA (Figure 5) is an airway device with an inflatable cuff, which sits in the hypopharynx, above the laryngeal inlet.

It may provide easier airway control in situations where facemask ventilation is difficult or impossible. It has the additional benefit of freeing the operator's hands. It can be used for spontaneous respiration or for controlled ventilation. It is important to recognise however that it does not protect the airway from aspiration of regurgitated stomach contents. Insertion of the LMA is often quite straightforward (Figure 6), but just like other airway maintenance techniques, requires supervised practice.

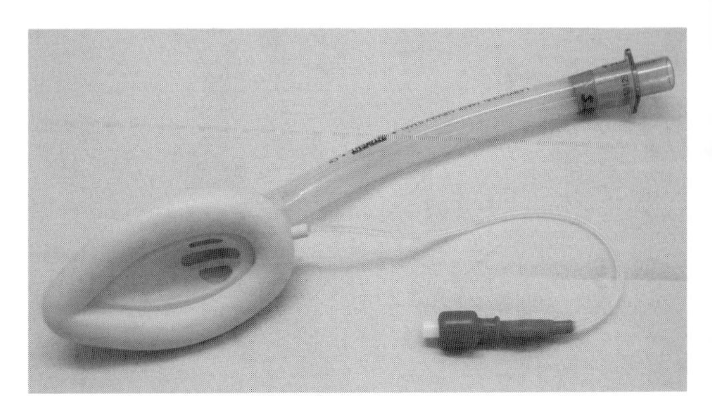

Figure 5. The Laryngeal Mask Airway ™ (LMA).

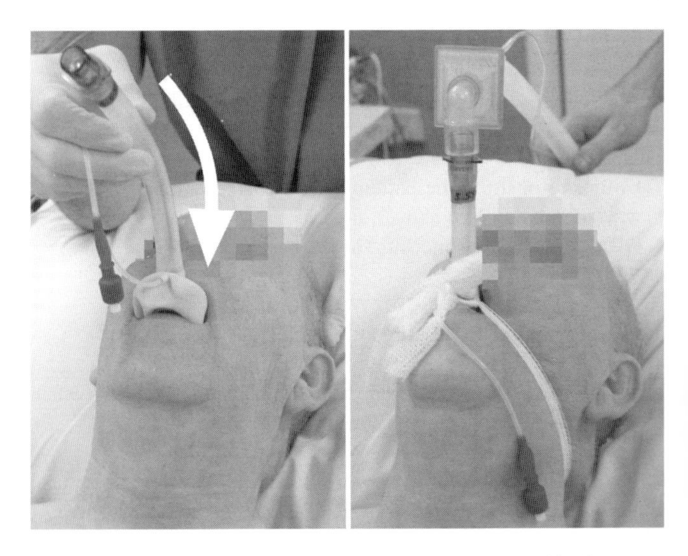

Figure 6. Insertion of an LMA. Left: the head is supported in the 'sniffing the morning air' position. The lubricated and deflated LMA is inserted into the open mouth and advanced gently until resistance is felt. Right: once a satisfactory position is achieved, the cuff is inflated and the LMA secured.

Its use may appear in future Advanced Life Support guidelines, and therefore it may become commonplace on resuscitation trolleys.

- Proper patient positioning is a key requisite.
- An oro-pharyngeal airway can transform an impossible airway into an easy one—have a low threshold for trying one.
- Consider bag and mask ventilation to be a two person manoeuvre—even experienced anaesthetists get help sometimes.
- Beware of inflating the stomach—this is exceptionally common when inexperienced.
- Maintaining an airway is a deceptively complex skill—make opportunities to practice.
- Aim to spend time in the recovery room—it is often overlooked, but is an excellent place to observe and practice basic airway skills.
- At cardiac arrests, the patient's pillows are commonly removed as a reflex action—replace them before attempting ventilation.

Further reading

1 Stone DJ, Gal TJ. Airway management. In: Miller RD, editor. *Anesthesia.* 5th ed. Philadelphia: Churchill Livingstone, 2000;1414–1451.

2 International Liaison Committee on Resuscitation. Adult basic life support. *Resuscitation*. 2000;46:29–71.

6

Intubation skills

Tim Meek

Introduction

Intubation of the trachea is clearly a vital skill for anaesthetists. It can also be useful to clinicians in other areas in an emergency. However, it is important to recognise that it is not a skill which is acquired quickly and if there are any doubts, it is always safer to rely on simple airway maintenance skills (see Chapter 5). It cannot be overstated that the consequences of getting tracheal intubation wrong can be disastrous. The basic skills of intubation can be learned on manikins, but are most realistically demonstrated by an anaesthetist in the anaesthetic room.

Whether as part of an anaesthetic, or in an emergency, the principles of tracheal intubation can be divided into four stages:

- Preparation
- Laryngoscopy and intubation
- Confirmation of tube placement
- Ventilation

Preparation

- Prior to an anaesthetic, it is usual to make an assessment of the airway, in order to predict difficult intubation:
  - The range of movement of the neck is assessed—can the patient achieve the ideal intubating position?
  - The Mallampati test assesses mouth opening, whilst Patil's test assesses thyromental distance (see Chapter 30 for detailed explanation).
- Basic equipment for safe and successful intubation (whatever the situation) are: a laryngoscope (and spare), a variety of tracheal tubes, means of ventilation (including oxygen supply), a means

of confirming tube placement, suction equipment and possibly some form of intubation aid.

- In theatre, there will be more specialised intubation aids and laryngoscopes, and special theatre trolleys and tables.

Laryngoscopy and intubation

- To facilitate laryngoscopy, the patient must be in the 'sniffing the morning air' position, as described in Chapter 5. This helps to create a more direct line of vision to the larynx.
- If possible, the patient is allowed to breathe 100% oxygen for 2–5 minutes. This 'pre-oxygenation' means that the patient's functional residual capacity contains 100% oxygen, providing a reservoir, should intubation and/or ventilation prove difficult.
- Drugs are administered to attenuate the haemodynamic response to intubation, to induce sleep, and to cause neuromuscular blockade (paralysis).
- In emergency situations, one or more of the above drugs may be omitted.
- Once adequate depth of sleep and paralysis are achieved, laryngoscopy is performed.
- A variety of laryngoscopes exist; until experienced, it is best to start with a basic curved blade scope (Figure 1).

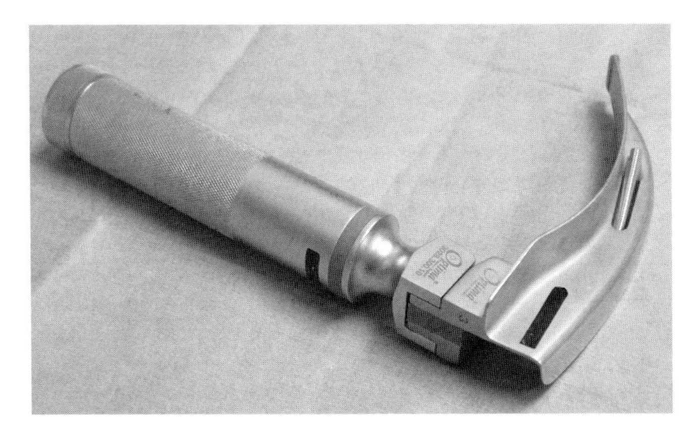

Figure 1. A typical adult curved-blade laryngoscope.

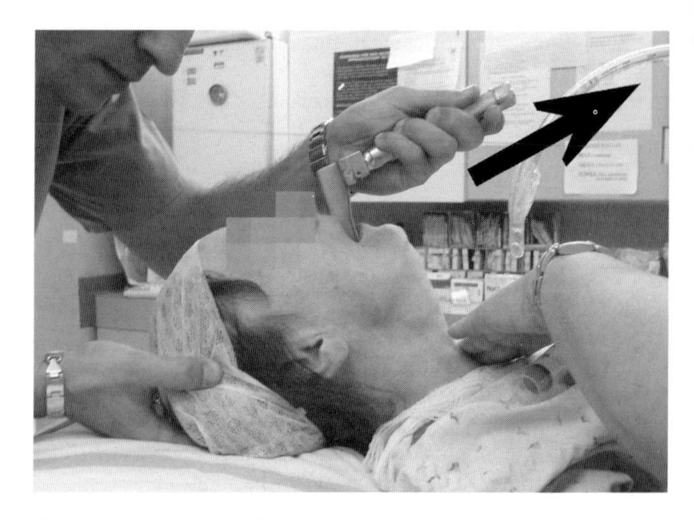

Figure 2. Laryngoscopy. The operator's right hand is supporting the head, whilst his left hand pulls the laryngoscope straight along the handle's axis. There is no rotation or leverage of the handle.

- The laryngoscope is held in the left hand, and is used to sweep the tongue over to the left, and lift it into the floor of the mouth.
- The laryngoscope is pulled along the axis of its handle, and is never used as a lever (Figure 2).
- Great care must be taken not to catch the lips, or damage the teeth. Both of these are commonly done by inexperienced operators.
- The basic elements of laryngoscopy can be practiced on a manikin, although they are not particularly lifelike. Unfortunately, there is no substitute for demonstration by an anaesthetist in the anaesthetic room.
- Once laryngoscopy is performed, the resulting view is graded from 1 (best) to 4 (worst).
- A grade one view is shown (Figure 3).
- The tube is passed with the right hand.
- If intubation is not achieved within two attempts, do not persist. Return to bag and mask ventilation and reassess the patient's position and your laryngoscopy technique. Wait for expert help if possible.
- The typical tube size is 9 for a man, 8 for a woman, but a smaller tube may be necessary (the size refers to the tube's internal diameter in millimetres).

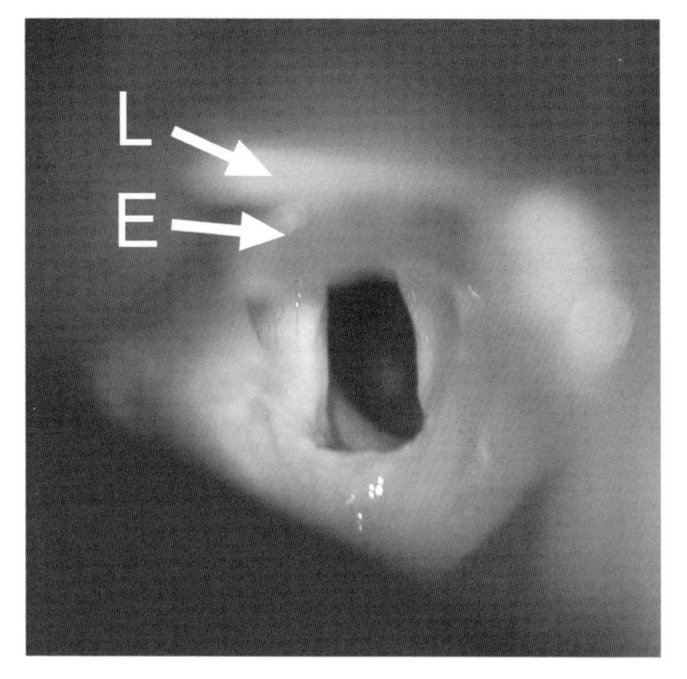

Figure 3. A 'grade 1' (best view) laryngoscopy. The laryngoscope blade (L) and epiglottis (E) are in front of the plane of focus and are indicated for clarity. The tracheal aperture can be clearly seen. The vocal cords are the pale, parallel structures which sit either side of the aperture. (Part of a tracheal ring can also be seen, at the lower left corner of the aperture.)

- The typical distance to insert the tube is 21 cm for men, 19 cm for women (distances measured at the teeth—the tubes have centimetre gradations marked on the side).
- The cuff is inflated just sufficiently to obliterate any air leak.
- The tube is secured.

Confirmation of tube placement

The following are all used to confirm tube placement within the trachea:

- Tracheal tube seen to pass between the cords.
- Air leak disappears when cuff inflated.
- Chest rises upon squeezing bag.

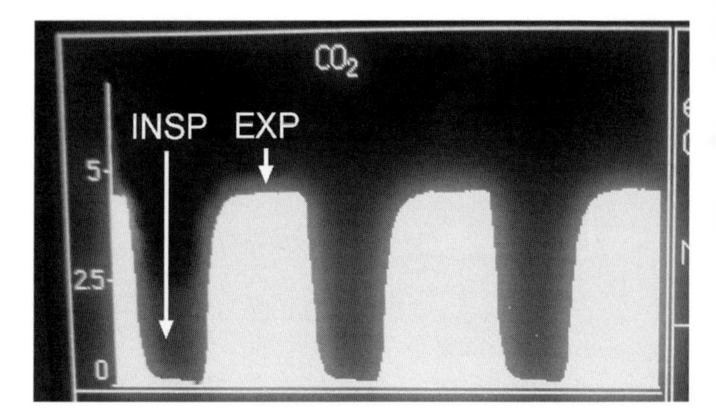

Figure 4. A capnograph tracing in a healthy individual under anaesthesia. The end expiratory (or 'end tidal') CO_2 is about 4.5%, whilst the inspired CO_2 is zero.

- Air entry heard bilaterally (apices and bases).
- No sounds heard upon auscultating stomach.
- CO_2 detected in expired gas.

Of all the above, the last is the most reliable. A typical CO_2 trace from a theatre capnograph is shown in Figure 4 (simpler CO_2 detection devices are available for resuscitation trolleys).

Remember though, for CO_2 to reach the lungs, there must be a cardiac output. If cardiac output is markedly reduced, there will be less CO_2 exhaled from the lungs. If there is no cardiac output (cardiac arrest), no CO_2 will be exhaled.

Unrecognised oesophageal intubation may result in hypoxia, with consequential neurological damage. If you are uncertain of correct tracheal placement of the tube, it is safest to take out the tube and revert to bag and mask ventilation. Remember the aphorism: ***'If in doubt, take it out.'***

Ventilation

- Typical young adult ventilatory parameters are: tidal volume 10 mL/kg, frequency 12/min.

- An adequate tidal volume corresponds with a rise in the chest of 2–3 cm.
- The gas mixture used to ventilate the lungs depends upon the clinical situation:
  - Anaesthesia: oxygen in either air or nitrous oxide, with an anaesthetic agent;
  - Cardiac arrest: 100% O_2.
- During CPR, the ratio of chest compressions to breaths is 15:2 without stopping compressions.

> - Proper patient positioning is a key requisite.
> - Laryngoscopy is a complex skill—do not expect to be proficient immediately.
> - Manikins do not resemble real patients—make opportunities to accompany an anaesthetist and see the real thing.
> - Do not persist if you cannot intubate—after two failed attempts, revert to bag and mask ventilation and re-assess the situation.
> - Capnography is the best method of confirming tracheal tube placement.
> - Unrecognised intubation of the oesophagus can be catastrophic—always have a high index of suspicion.
> - Remember: ***'If in doubt, take it out.'***

Further reading

1 Stone DJ, Gal TJ. Airway management. In: Miller RD, editor. *Anesthesia*, 5th ed. Philadelphia: Churchill Livingstone, 2000;1414–1451.

2 International Liaison Committee on Resuscitation. Adult basic life support. *Resuscitation*. 2000;46:29–71.

7

Assessment of consciousness

Roger Strachan

Introduction

Consciousness is a state of awareness of yourself and your environment. Loss of this awareness occurs with impaired consciousness, and at the extreme, coma is when the awareness is lost entirely. The assessment of conscious level is very important in all branches of medicine. Every doctor and nurse, and many other health professionals, will be faced with assessing and treating patients who have an impaired conscious level, because the causes of impaired consciousness are so varied and extensive. In considering these causes, a useful mnemonic to remember is TVMEDIC:

- T = Trauma
  - Head injury
- V = Vascular
  - Cerebrovascular disease (e.g. stroke, subarachnoid haemorrhage)
  - Cardiovascular disease (cardiac failure, dysrrhythmias)
- M = Metabolic
  - Hypoxia, diabetes, hyponatraemia, myxoedema, renal failure, liver failure
- E = Epilepsy
- D = Drugs
  - Depressant drugs, overdose, CO poisoning
- I = Infection
  - Meningitis, encephalitis, brain abscess, empyaema
- C = Cerebral
  - Any cause of raised intracranial pressure (e.g. tumour, hydrocephalus)

Even these causes are only a few examples. Consciousness depends on the ability of complex parts of the brain to be structurally and functionally intact. Structural damage will always lead to functional impairment of that part of the brain, but functional impairment without structural damage may occur, for instance with drugs or biochemical disturbance. In the latter circumstances, patients may demonstrate differing or variable states of arousal, with impairment of conscious level being reversible.

Anatomy and physiology

Consciousness has two major components: the level of *arousal* which depends on the function of the reticular activating system (RAS) in the upper brain stem (midbrain), and *cognitive function*, dependent on higher cortical function. This latter function is especially well-developed in humans. The reticular activating system lies at the centre of the brain stem, from the medulla to the midbrain. It receives input from every major sensory pathway. The cerebral cortex is activated by the reticular activating system, but also inputs to it, so there are several complex feedback pathways. The number of components that contribute to the RAS is so large that it is not a specific anatomical structure, more a functional unit. There are however three major projections to the cerebral cortex: via the thalamic nuclei, via the hypothalamus to the limbic system, and more diffuse pathways to the cerebral hemispheres via the midbrain raphe and locus ceruleus. It is the interaction between the RAS and the cerebral cortex that controls the level of activity within the neocortex, influencing the state of awareness. Sleep and coma are similar in many respects, but not the same. Sleep is a physiological active and coordinated process. Patients 'awaking' from a coma show many sleep-like qualities, but there are nevertheless differences in the expression of awareness and higher cortical activity. The physiological overlap between sleep and coma is still not well understood.

Assessment of conscious level

Almost 30 years ago, Teasdale and Jennett introduced the Glasgow Coma Scale, or GCS.[1] Prior to this, describing conscious level in patients was open to linguistic interpretation, often based on terms such as confused, drowsy, obtunded, stuperose, unconscious, and so on. There was a need to more accurately describe conscious level without this being affected too much by observer bias, and therefore a need to develop a scale that could be understood and reproduced by all health professionals. It is based on a 15-point scale (not 14), divided into three categories: Eye opening (E, 4 points), Verbal response (V, 5 points), and Motor response (M, 6 points) (Table 1).

The maximum score, in a fully conscious patient, is 15 and the minimum score is 3 (not 0!) in a deeply unconscious patient. Knowledge of the GCS is extremely important since it is now the universally and internationally accepted scoring system to measure conscious level.

The GCS can only be applied to older children, teenagers and adults. Simpson and Reilly[2] modified the GCS for use in children

Table 1. The Glasgow Coma Scale.[1]

Eye opening	4	Spontaneous
	3	To speech
	2	To painful stimuli
	1	None
Best motor response *[Upper limbs]*	6	Obeys commands
	5	Localizes
	4	Withdraws (normal flexion)
	3	Abnormal flexion
	2	Extends
	1	None
Verbal response	5	Orientated
	4	Confused
	3	Inappropriate words
	2	Incomprehensible sounds
	1	None

Table 2. Modified GCS for children.[2]

Eye opening		As adult scale	
*Best motor response** *[Upper limbs]*	6	Obeys commands	>2 years
	5	Localizes	6 months–2 years
	4	Normal flexion	>6 months
	3	Abnormal flexion	<6 months
	2	Extends	
	1	None	
*Verbal response**	5	Orientated to place	>5 years
	4	Words	>12 years
	3	Vocal sounds	>6 months
	2	Cries	<6 months
	1	None	

* Score highest appropriate for age.

and infants, sometimes known as the Adelaide modification (Table 2). The highest score appropriate for the child's age is used. For example, a child of nine months who opens his or her eyes spontaneously (E = 4), localizes to pain (M = 5), and is vocalising (V = 3) will score a maximum of 12.

How to assess patients with impaired consciousness

Eye opening

Eye opening is perhaps the easiest category to score. It will be obvious observing the patient if the eyes opening spontaneously (E = 4). Ask the patient a simple question, or to 'open their eyes' (to speech, E = 3). Induce a painful stimulus, such as squeezing an earlobe, pressing on the supra-orbital nerve above the eye, or pressure on a nail bed (to pain, E = 2). Clearly, despite maximal stimulation, if there is no eye opening, the patient scores E = 1.

Verbal response

In patients who are able to respond to verbal questioning, asking them who they are, where they are, what has happened, why they are in hospital, etc, will establish if the patient is orientated in time, place and person (V = 5). It will also establish if they are confused (V = 4). If the patient makes entirely inappropriate verbal responses, often just swearing or shouting, they score V = 3. Grunting, moaning, or otherwise incomprehensible sounds scores V = 2. No verbal response at all, to verbal questioning or any stimulus (e.g. pain) scores V = 1.

Motor response

This is often the most difficult category to accurately score and does depend more on eliciting appropriate clinical signs and understanding the reasons behind different motor responses. It is the best motor response that is recorded. On questioning, and asking the patient to perform basic tasks like 'squeeze my fingers,' will establish if they are obeying commands (M = 6). If you induce an irritating or painful stimulus, and the patient makes a purposeful movement to remove the stimulus, they are localising and score M = 5. If inducing a painful stimulus on the head or face provokes only a random non-directional flexion response of the upper limbs, but a response which is nevertheless normal in the way the limb moves, this is a simple flexion withdrawal response and scores M = 4. If a similar stimulus causes an *abnormal flexion* response—flexion of elbows, pronation of forearms, and flexion of wrists—M = 3. If the response is to extend the limb at elbow and wrist with supination of the forearm, this is an *extensor* response, M = 2. No response at all, despite maximal stimulation, M = 1.

The difference between a normal motor and abnormal response is crucial, because this demonstrates the difference between general depression of conscious level at a cortical level and brain stem dysfunction more commonly due to structural damage or compression of the brain stem. The difference between abnormal flexion and extension to pain is also important, because it indicates at what level the brain stem is damaged or dysfunctional. Abnormal flexion is a *decorticate* response, where there is physiological disconnection of the cerebral hemispheres from the brain stem at the level of the diencephalon (basal ganglia e.g. thalamus, caudate nucleus, upper midbrain). If the physiological disconnection is anatomically lower at the level of the lower midbrain and brain stem, then the patient is *decerebrate*, and demonstrates extensor posturing. Often these responses are mixed, if the cause of coma is due to damage at different levels within the brain stem and diencephalon.

Investigation of patients with impaired consciousness

Clearly in some patients the cause of an impaired conscious level is obvious e.g. after injury, drug overdose, or near-drowning. In others, the cause may be more obscure, and remembering the mnemonic TVMEDIC helps to systematically identify the likely aetiology of the impaired consciousness. If a patient has been found unconscious, and there is no evidence of injury, consider the following:

- As full a history as possible must be obtained from any professionals that are available to provide information, including paramedics or the patient's GP (if known) or other individuals such as friends or relatives.
- A full clinical examination should be performed looking for evidence of injury and neurological abnormalities.
- Basic cardiorespiratory measurements are taken—pulse, blood pressure, respiration rate. Arterial blood gases and an ECG will help to exclude respiratory causes of coma (hypoxia, hypercarbia) or a cardiac dysrhythmia.
- Patients who have been lying for some time, especially in cold conditions, may be hypothermic. Core temperature should be

measured. Cerebral metabolic rate can fall by 5% for each 1° C fall in body temperature, and below 30° C patients can be in coma. A high temperature, particularly in children, can cause drowsiness and is an indication of infection.

- A biochemical profile is essential, including urea and electrolytes, blood sugar and liver function tests (e.g. renal failure, hyponatraemia, hypoglycaemia, liver failure).
- Consider a drugs overdose. Serum drug levels can be taken. It is helpful to know the patients drug history, but this information is seldom immediately available. Searching for patient medical cards (e.g. diabetic, steroid) might prove useful. An alcohol level is important in patients smelling of alcohol. Extreme intoxication can easily mimic deep coma.
- A CT brain scan is essential in cases of trauma or if no obvious cause for impaired consciousness is found, particularly if a cerebral event is considered. This is essential if lumbar puncture is required.
- Children will usually have a responsible adult with them, if there is a legitimate cause for their impaired consciousness. This may not be true in cases of trauma or illicit drug abuse.

Always

- Remember the mnemonic TV MEDIC.
- Learn the Glasgow Coma Scale thoroughly and know how to apply it.
- Have a systematic approach to the assessment of patients with an impaired conscious level.

Never

- Assume the cause of impaired consciousness. It is always unclear until the patient has been fully examined and appropriately investigated.

Further reading

1 Teasdale G, Jennett B. Assessment of coma and impaired consciousness. A practical scale. *Lancet*. 1974;2(7872):81–84.
2 Simpson D, Reilly P. Paediatric coma scale. *Lancet*. 1982;21:450.
3 Plum F, Posner JB. *The Diagnosis of Stupor and Coma*, 3rd ed. Philaedelphia, F. A. Davis Company, 1982. ISBN 0-8036-6993-3.

Roger Strachan

8

Taking consent

Barry Nicholls

Definition of consent

"Consent is a patient's agreement for a health professional to provide care."

It is a general legal and ethical principle that the valid consent must be obtained before starting treatment or physical investigation or providing personal care for a patient. Consent may be verbal, non-verbal (presenting an arm for the pulse to be taken) or in writing. All are valid in law as long as they are given freely, without coercion by a competent person and with full understanding of the implications and outcomes.

A competent adult has the fundamental right to give or withhold consent to any medical examination, investigation or treatment. This right is founded on the moral principle of respect for autonomy or 'self-rule'—personal freedom in thought, action and decision-making.

While there is no English statute setting out the general principles of consent, case law ('common law'), has established that touching a patient without valid consent amounts to an assault against the person and may constitute a civil or criminal offence of battery.

Consent must not be obtained under duress or coercion and the patient must be fully 'informed.' This means that a suitable knowledgeable doctor has to explain to the patient the nature, purpose and material risks of the proposed procedure. Failure to provide sufficient information to the patient to make an informed choice about whether to accept the treatment recommended may constitute a breach of the doctors 'duty of care.' If as a result the patient suffers harm then they may pursue their claim in negligence against the health professional involved. Poor handling of the consent process may also result in complaints from patients through the NHS complaints procedure and professional bodies (General Medical Council) resulting in disciplinary action or even dismissal.

Consent is not just a signature it is a process and part of the patient's journey, commencing with the first contact. The patient needs to be informed throughout care, both verbally and by supporting written information. The validity of the consent doesn't depend on the signature, but on the adequacy of the explanation given to the patient before he or she makes their decision. (Patient centred approach.)

For many physical contacts between a doctor and patient (e.g. simple clinical examination), consent is implied and does not need to be sought, formally or informally. But for a procedure with a more material risk, the patient's specific agreement should be obtained, either verbally or in writing.

Written consent is usual for all major procedures, particularly those involving general anaesthesia. Written consent isn't absolutely necessary to defend an action for negligence or assault, but it provides important documentary evidence that consent has been obtained (though the 'informed' nature of that consent may still need to be amplified in the clinical notes).

The purpose of consent in law

- **Legal purpose**: to provide those concerned in the treatment with a defence to a criminal charge of assault or battery or a civil claim for damages for trespass to the person. Consent transforms an otherwise illegitimate procedure into a legitimate one. Consent does not provide them with a defence to a claim that they negligently advised a particular treatment or negligently carried out.
- **Ethical purpose**: of recognising and respecting a patient's right to self-determination.

  Prima facie, every adult has the right and capacity to decide whether or not he/she will accept medical treatment, even if refusal may risk permanent injury to his/her health or even lead to a premature death.
- **Clinical purpose**: of enlisting the patient's faith and confidence in the efficacy of treatment.

Case law on consent has evolved significantly over the last decade. Further legal developments are occurring all the time and it is advised that legal advice should always be sought if there is any doubt about the legal validity of a proposed intervention. Whilst much of the case law refers specifically to doctors, the same principles will apply to other health professionals involved in treating or caring for patients.

The Human Rights Act 1998 (UK statute October 2000), further impacts on UK law, bringing it into line with Europe and the rights enshrined in the European Convention on Human Rights. In future the courts will be expected to take into account the case law of the European Court of Human Rights in Strasbourg, as well as the English case law. It is too early to predict the influence this will have in the future but the articles that are relevant in medical law are:

Article 2	Protection of the right to life
Article 3	Prohibition of torture, inhumane or degrading treatment or punishment
Article 5	Right to liberty and security
Article 8	Right to respect for private and family life
Article 9	Freedom of thought, conscience and religion
Article 12	Right to marry and found a family
Article 14	Prohibition in enjoyment of Convention rights

Who can give consent?

1. Adults >18 years
2. Children/young persons 16 years and over (consent)
   Family reform act 1968, s8
   'The consent of a minor who has attained the age of 16 years to any surgical, medical or dental treatment which, in the absence of consent would constitute a trespass to his person, shall be as effective as it would be if he were of full age; and where a minor has by virtue of this section given a valid consent to any treatment it shall not be necessary to obtain any consent for it from his parent and guardian.'
3. Minors-children less than 16 years of age
   Children below 16 years have the right to self-determination as long as they can show that they have sufficient understanding and intelligence to make the decision.
   The 'Gillick competence' or 'mature minor' test
   '... as a matter of law the parental right to determine whether or not their minor child below the age of 16 will have medical treatment

terminates if and when the child achieves a sufficient understanding and intelligence to enable him or her to understand fully what is proposed.'

However as the understanding required for different interventions will vary considerably, a child under 16 may therefore have the capacity to consent to some interventions but not others. It is good practice to involve the young person's family in the decision making process, unless the young person specifically wishes to exclude them.

Who can refuse consent?

1. Adult >18 years
2. Child or young person with capacity <16 years or 16–17 years

Where a young person of 16 or 17 who could consent to treatment in accordance with Section 8 of the *Family Law Reform Act*, or a child under 16 but Gillick competent, refuses treatment, this refusal can be overruled by either a person with parental responsibility for the child or the court.

- In accordance with the 'welfare principle': that the child's 'welfare' or 'best interests' must be paramount.
- Restricted to occasions where the chid is at risk of suffering 'grave and irreversible mental or physical harm.'
- All parental/persons with parental responsibility decisions can be overruled by the court if the welfare of the child so requires.

In accordance with The Children Act 1989 persons who have parental responsibility and can give consent include:

- A child's parents if married to each other at the time of conception or birth.
- The child's mother, not the father if they were not married unless the father has acquired parental responsibility via court order or a parental responsibility agreement or the couple subsequently marry.
- The child's legally appointed guardian.
- A person in whose favour the court has made a residence order concerning the child.
- A Local Authority designated in the care order in respect of the child.

- A Local Authority or other authorised person who holds an emergency protection order in respect of the child.

Elements of consent

For consent to be valid it must be given voluntarily by an appropriately informed person (the patient or where relevant a person with parental responsibility if patient is <18 years of age) who has the capacity to consent to the proposed treatment/care in question.

Capacity

"The ability or power to do, experience or understand something."

In order to have capacity in the context of consent a patient needs to be able to:

- Comprehend information presented to them clearly
- Believe it
- Retain it long enough to consider it, and make a decision

Patients may have capacity to consent for some intervention and not others depending on the nature of the procedure. Adults are presumed to have capacity, but where doubt exists the health professionals should assess the capacity of the patient for the decision in question. If help in assessing a patient's capacity is needed, you should consult guidance issued by professional bodies (BMA—Assessment of Mental capacity—guidance for doctors and lawyers).

A person lacks capacity if some impairment or disturbance of mental functioning renders the person unable to make a decision whether to consent to or refuse treatment. That inability to make a decision will occur when:

a. The person is unable to comprehend and retain the information which is material to the decision, especially as to the likely consequences of having or not having the treatment in question; [and]
b. The patient is unable to use the information and weigh it in the balance as part of the process of arriving at a decision.

Capacity may affected by

- Age*
- Mental Health (confusion)*

- Physical health (pain, medication, infection, shock)
- Fear
- Language, culture and religion
- Competence and skills of the health professional(s)

* (age, mental health illness and learning disabilities do not automatically impair capacity).

Lack of capacity can be

- Temporary
- Permanent
- Fluctuating

Capacity should not be confused with a health professional's assessment of the reasonableness of the patient's decision. A patient is entitled to make whatever decision they wish based on their own religious beliefs or value system, even if it is perceived irrational by others, as long as they understand what is entailed and the consequences of their decision.

An irrational decision has been defined as 'one which is so obviously outrageous in its defiance of logic or of accepted moral standards that no sensible person who had applied his or her mind to the question could have been arrived at.'

Note: When a patient lacks capacity (an 'incapable' adult) under English law, no one is able to give consent to the examination or treatment of this adult. Parents, relatives or members of the health care team cannot consent on behalf of such an adult.

In such cases the treatment offered to this patient should be that which is in the patients 'best interest.' Best interest is not confined to medical best interest; it should take into account the patients values and principles when competent. In deciding what options may be reasonably considered as being in the best interests of the patient, you should take into account:

- Options for treatment or investigation which are clinically indicated;
- Any evidence of the patient's previously expressed preferences, including and advanced statement;
- Your own health care teams knowledge of the patient's background, such as cultural, religious, or employment considerations;

- Views about patient's preferences given by a third party who may have other knowledge of the patient, for example the patient's partner, family, carer, tutor-dative (Scotland) or person with parental responsibility;
- Which option least restricts the patient's future choices, where more than one option (including non-treatment) seems reasonable in the patient's best interest.

Voluntariness

To be valid consent, consent must be given voluntarily and freely without coercion, subtle pressure or fraud to accept or refuse treatment.

Pressure may be exerted by:

- Partners
- Family
- Health professionals
- Authorities (involuntary detention–prison, mental health institutes)

Information

To give valid consent the patient needs to understand in broad terms the nature and purpose of the procedure. Any misrepresentation of these elements will invalidate consent. Although informing of the nature and purpose will validate consent as far as any claim in battery is concerned, it is not sufficient to fulfil the legal 'duty of care' with respect to negligence. A legal duty of care has always been applied to diagnosis and treatments with negligence being implied if practice falls below that of a 'responsible body' of medical opinion held by practitioners skilled in the field in question (known as the 'Bolam test'). Recent medical case law *Sidaway 1985* brought the disclosure of information into line with diagnosis and treatment, implying that disclosure of medical information should be subject to the Bolam Test. *Sidaway* whilst accepting the Bolam simpliciter (Bolam test in principle), also states that it would be negligent to withhold or not disclose information about a risk so obviously necessary, even if a 'responsible body' of medical opinion would not have done so.

The law on information disclosure has been firmly rooted in the doctor's duty of care, not the patient's right to know. This has been upheld by the Bolam test, which implies that the duty of care is for the doctor to give the information, which he feels, is appropriate for the patient. Developing negligence case has curbed the Bolam test for diagnosis and treatment.

> '… if, in a rare case, it can be demonstrated that the professional opinion is not capable of withstanding logical analysis, the judge is entitled to hold that that body of opinion is not reasonable or responsible…' (1997) 39 BMLR 1, per Lord Brown-Wilkinson.

Although the *Bolitho* ruling (new Bolam) has not been specifically applied to information disclosure, more recent case law has shown that the courts are prepared to challenge the 'responsible body' of medical opinion. It is now clear that the courts will be the final arbiters of what constitutes responsible practice, although most health professions set their own standards, which are not law but will often exceed the legal requirements.

As a result of *Sidaway* and more recent case law it is advisable to inform patients of any risks material or general that would fall into the categories below:

- *'Obviously necessary'*—the judge might in certain circumstances come to the conclusion that disclosure of a risk was so obviously necessary to an informed choice on the part of the patient that no reasonably prudent medical man would fail to disclose it.
- *'Special risks'*—there is no doubt that the doctor ought to draw attention of a patient to a danger which may be special in kind or magnitude or special to the patient.
- *'Significant risk'*—significant risk which would affect the judgement of a reasonable patient must be disclosed.

Note: The law does not set a quantitative value of risk to be disclosed e.g. greater than 10%, it relates to the above recommendations.

When supplying information

- Patients must be given sufficient information, in a way that they can understand, in order to enable them to exercise their right to make informed decisions about their care.
- Use up-to-date written material, visual and other aids to explain complex aspects of the investigation, diagnosis or treatment.
- Allow patients sufficient time to reflect before and after making a decision.

The information supplied to the patient should include

- Explanation of the problem
- Treatment options (alternatives)
- What the surgery involves (diagrams)
- Risks and complications
- Benefits/post operative expectations
- Evidence-based
- Regularly updated/customisable

Who should obtain consent?

It is the responsibility of the doctor or person providing treatment or undertaking the investigation to discuss and obtain the patients consent. This person will have comprehensive understanding of the procedure and treatment, how it is carried out and the risks attached. Where this is not practicable this task may be delegated to a person as long as they:

- Are suitable trained and qualified;
- Have sufficient knowledge of the proposed investigation or treatment, and understanding of risks involved.

Key points on consent: The law in England, see Appendix 6.

9

Taking an ECG

Chandrika Roysam

Introduction

The electrocardiograph (ECG) is a recording of the cardiac electrical activity. The electrical signal is far smaller than that generated by the myocardium, but is attenuated by the resistance of the contents of the thorax, chest wall and finally the keratin layer of the skin. Amplification and filtering of the signal is used to retain fidelity of the electrical activity, but muscle artefact and mains interference may still distort the signal.

The ECG is used to diagnose or assist in the diagnosis of many cardiac and pulmonary diseases. The ECG must be regarded like any other laboratory test with proper consideration of both uses and limitations. As with any other test, a good recording will facilitate interpretation whilst a poor one may lead to misdiagnosis and incorrect treatment.

Technique

The standard ECG is taken from twelve leads. These leads actually show the difference in voltage between electrodes placed on the surface of the body. The leads can be divided into two groups.

- The six extremity leads
  - Bipolar: I, II and III;
  - Unipolar: avR, avL and avF.
- The six chest leads
  - V1 to V6

All the leads reflect the electrical cardiac cycle with each lead viewing it from a different angle.

The positions of the leads are shown in Figures 1 to 3.

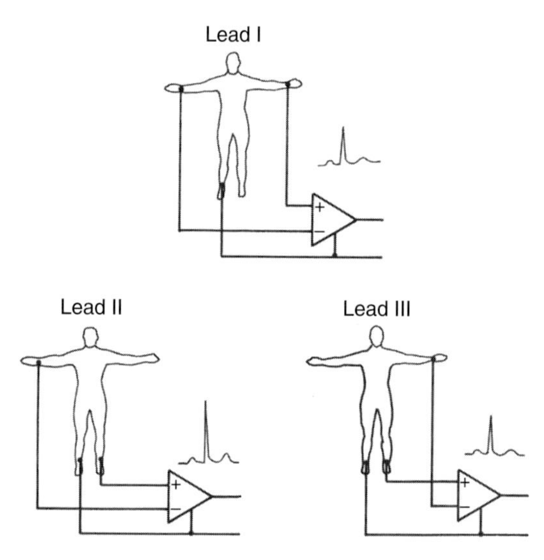

Figure 1. Electrical recording from the bipolar leads I, II and III.

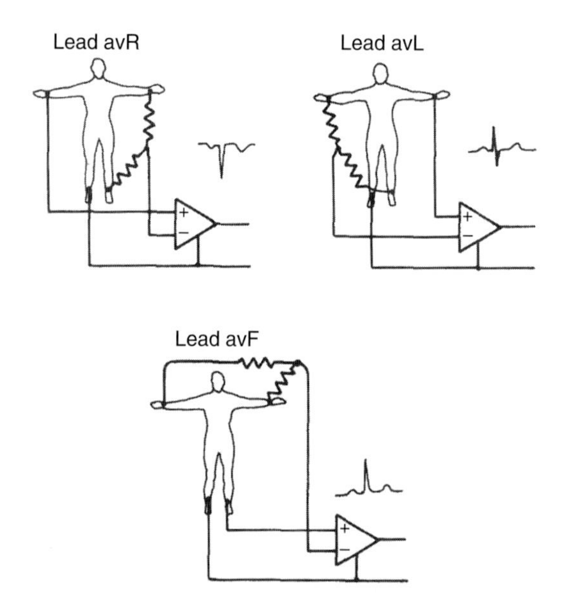

Figure 2. Electrical recording from the augmented (Unipolar) leads avR, avL and avF.

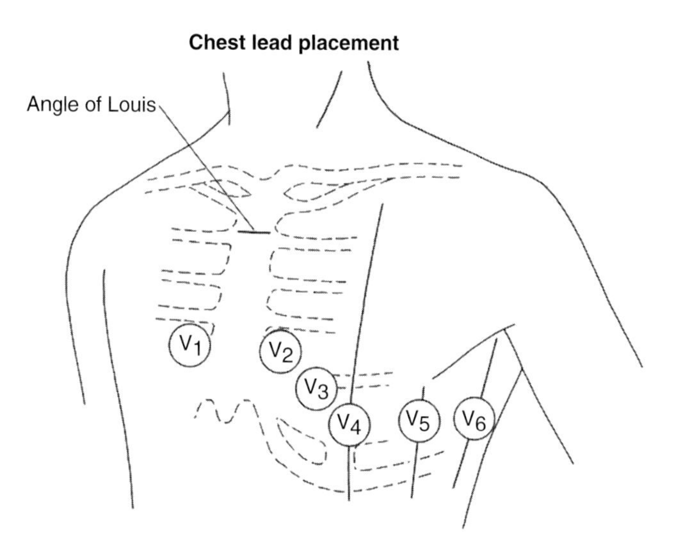

Figure 3. Positioning of the anterior chest leads.

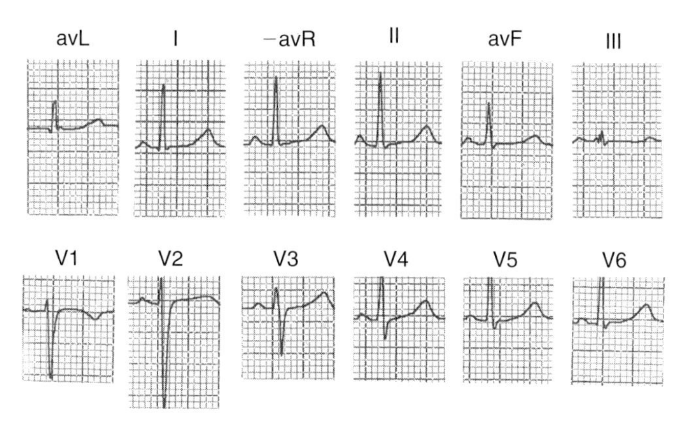

Figure 4. Standard (normal) electrical waveforms from the 12 standard leads.

Practical points

- Always record the patient's name date and time on the ECG strip which will enable future comparisons.

- The machines are usually calibrated with 1 mv = 10 mm. If this is changed for any reason for example a large QRS amplitude, it should be noted.
- ECG paper speed is standardized to record at 25 mm per second. Any variation from this should also be noted.
- The patient should be supine for the recording because any other position will alter the position of the heart within the chest, affecting orientation to the surface leads.
- Electrodes should be selected for maximum adhesiveness and minimum impedance.
- The sites for the placement of electrodes are shown in figures above.
- There should be good contact between the skin and electrodes. Avoid the skin sites with irritation. Surface hair should be shaved and skin cleaned with alcohol wipes.
- The patient should be well relaxed and warm as shivering will produce artifacts on the recording.
- Electrical artifacts should be minimized by disconnecting other nearby devices.

> - Place the patient in a warm and relaxing environment.
> - Ensure that the machine is correctly calibrated and the patient details have been added.
> - Identify the correct lead placements.
> - Clean the skin and securely attach the electrodes.
> - Check for artifacts immediately, it is much safer to repeat the ECG where there is doubt.
> - Remove the electrodes once a good recording has been achieved and allow the patient to get re-dressed.

Further reading

1 Wagner GS, Marriott HJL. *Marriott's Practical Electrocardiography.*
2 Otto CM, Pearlman AS. *Textbook of Clinical Echocardiography.*
3 Conover MB, Bond RJ. *Understanding Electrocardiography.*

10

Interpreting the ECG

Chandrika Roysam

Introduction

The ECG is a recording of the electrical activity of the heart including the conducting nervous system and the myocardial muscle cells.

It records two basic physiological processes.

- Depolarisation (the spread of stimulus through the heart muscle) produces the P wave from the atria and the QRS complex from the ventricle.
- Re-polarisation (the return of stimulated muscle to the resting state) produces the atrial ST segment and T wave (not usually seen on the standard 12 lead) and the ventricular ST segment and T and U waves.

Remember:

- The ECG does not directly measure the mechanical function of the heart.
- The ECG does not directly depict abnormalities in cardiac structure; however, some structural abnormalities do have characteristic ECG patterns, for example mitral stenosis and pulmonary embolism.
- The ECG does not record all the electrical activity of the heart, only those currents that are transmitted to the area of electrode placement. Whilst the 12 leads in the Standard ECG are designed to collect as much electrical information as is possible from the surface, there are some 'electrically silent' areas of the heart.

Reading the ECG

Much of the information provided by the ECG is contained in three parts.

- The timing of the ECG record:
  - The four basic intervals on the ECG are
    - The heart rate;
    - The PR interval;
    - The QRS interval;
    - The QT interval.
- The morphologies of the principal wave forms
- The electrical axis of the heart

Calculation of heart rate

When the heart rate is regular count the number of large boxes between two successive QRS complexes and divide this into 300.

If the heart rate is irregular count the number of cardiac cycles every six seconds and multiply by 10.

The PR interval

The PR interval is measured from the beginning of the P wave to the beginning of the QRS complex. This represents the time it takes for the stimulus to spread through the atria and pass through the AV junction. Normal PR interval is 0.12–0.2 s.

The QRS interval

This represents the time required for a stimulus to spread through the ventricles. Normal QRS interval is 0.07–0.10 s.

The QRS interval is prolonged in bundle branch blocks, hyperkalaemia, following treatment with some drugs (quinidine, flecainide, and tricyclic antidepressants) and ventricular ectopic beats.

The QT interval

This is measured from the beginning of the QRS complex to the end of the T wave. The normal values for the QT interval depend on the heart rate and hence another index the QTc interval has been devised.

$$QTc = QT/\sqrt{\text{RR interval}}$$

Normal QTc is <0.44 s

This is prolonged in a number of conditions for example myocardial infarction, subarachnoid haemorrhage, hypothermia, drug therapy (for example sotalol, procainamide, or disopyramide), hypocalcaemia and hypokalaemia. QT prolongation may predispose patients to potentially lethal ventricular arrhythmias.

The principal waveforms

P wave

The P wave, which represents atrial depolarisation, is a small deflection before the QRS complex that can be either positive or negative. The P wave duration is normally less than 0.12 s. The P wave amplitude is normally less than 0.25 mV in all leads.

The P wave contour is normally smooth. Tall peaked P waves are seen in right atrial abnormalities and wide, sometimes notched P waves are seen in left atrial abnormalities.

QRS complex

Ventricular depolarisation consists of two sequential phases.

- The first phase is stimulation of the ventricular septum from left to right. This produces a small 'r' wave in the right chest leads and a small 'q' wave in the left chest leads.
- During the second phase of ventricular depolarisation, the stimulus spreads simultaneously outward through the left and the right ventricles. Because the left ventricle has more mass than the right, it produces a tall R wave in the left chest leads. The polarity of the wave changes as the sensing electrodes progress across the chest until there is a deep S wave in the final V5/V6 position.

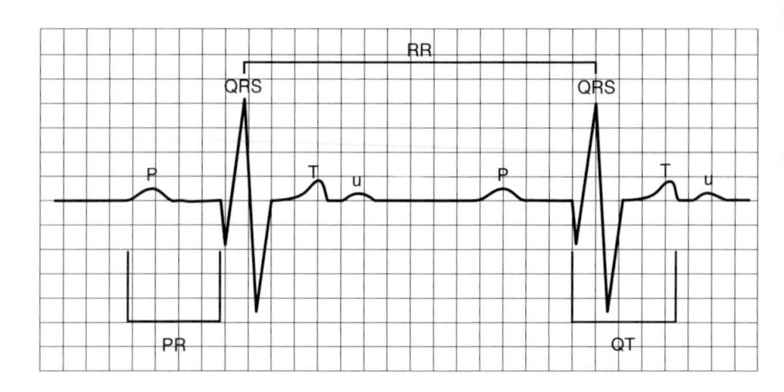

Figure 1. The normal ECG with the key waveforms and intervals identified.

- Loss of normal R wave progression from V1 to V5 may indicate loss of myocardium after an infarction.
- On the other hand reversal of this sequence with larger R waves in the right chest leads may indicate right ventricular hypertrophy.
- In the limb leads the shape of the QRS complex varies with the electrical axis of the heart.

ST segment

The ST segment is that portion of the ECG from the end of the QRS complex to the beginning of the T wave. It represents the start of ventricular repolarization. The normal ST segment is **isoelectric** but it may be slightly elevated or depressed normally by less than 1 mm. Pathological conditions like myocardial infarction produce characteristic deviations of the ST segment. The junction between the end of the QRS and the beginning of the ST segment is called the J point. Characteristic J point elevation is seen in hypothermia.

T wave

The T wave represents part of ventricular repolarisation. It normally has a peak closer to the end than the beginning. The normal T wave follows the direction of the main QRS complex in any lead. The T wave may be normally negative in V1 and V2 but always becomes positive by V3. T waves can be inverted in myocardial ischaemia, bundle branch blocks and ventricular overload.

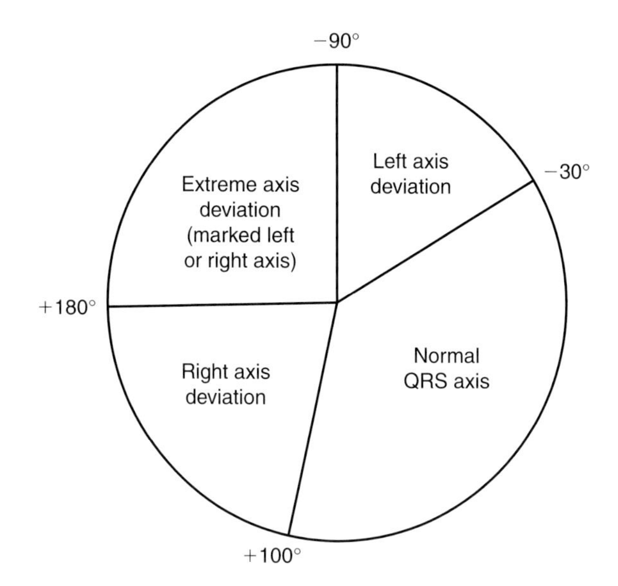

Figure 2. The calculation of the electrical axis grid.

Tall T waves are seen in hyperkalaemia, hyperacute phase of myocardial infarction, left ventricular hypertrophy and occasionally in acute pericarditis.

U wave

The U wave is a small rounded deflection sometimes seen after the T wave. Its exact significance is not known. It is thought to represent the last phase of ventricular repolarization. and prominent U waves are characteristic of hypokalemia.

The electrical axis of the heart

The depolarisation stimulus spreads through the ventricles in different directions at any given time. The mean QRS axis describes the general direction in the frontal plane toward which the QRS complex is predominantly directed.

To calculate the QRS axis, all the extremity leads are arranged in the form of a hexaxial diagram.

- The axis will be directed midway between the positive poles of any two leads that show R waves of equal height.

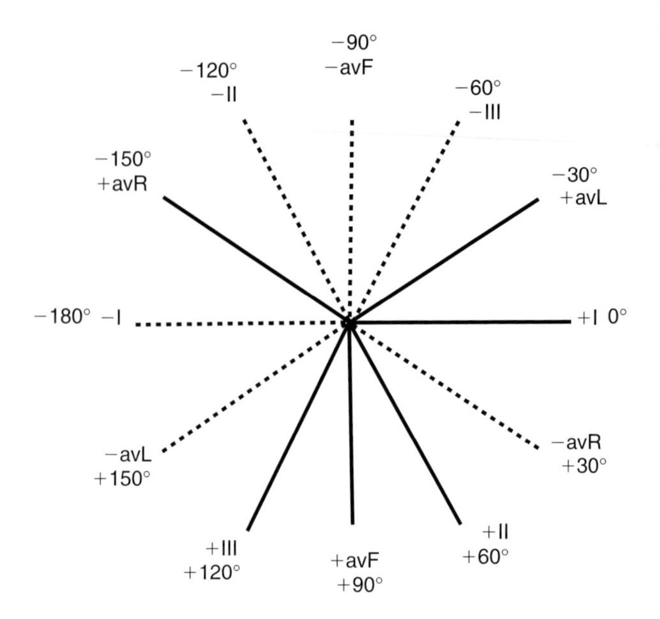

Figure 3. Axis deviations.

- The axis will be at right angles to any lead that shows a bi-phasic complex.
- The normal QRS axis lies between −30 and +100.
- An axis more negative than −30 is left axis deviation (LAD). This is seen in patients with left anterior hemiblock and left ventricular hypertrophy.
- An axis more positive than +100 is right axis deviation (RAD). This is seen in right ventricular hypertrophy, chronic lung disease and left posterior hemiblock. It is occasionally seen in normal people.

> - Check for the correct patient.
> - Check the calibration and correct paper speed.
> - Rate?
> - Rhythm?
> - Morphology?
> - Axis?
> - Finally define the differential diagnosis.

Summary

Accurate interpretation of an ECG warrants a systematic approach.

- Identification: check patient details.
- Standardisation: make sure that the ECG is properly calibrated (1 mv = 10 mm, paper speed 25 mm/s).
- Rhythm: normal sinus rhythm or otherwise.
- PR interval: short PR interval with wide QRS indicates Wolf Parkinson White syndrome. Prolonged PR interval signifies first degree heart block.
- P wave size: tall P wave may be a sign of R atrial hypertrophy (p – pulmonale).
- QRS width: wide QRS indicates conduction defect or an ectopic beat.
- QT interval: may be a hidden clue to electrolyte disturbances.
- QRS voltage: low voltage may result from pericardial effusion, emphysema or hypothyroidism.
- Mean QRS axis: check to see if any axis deviation is present.
- R wave progression may be poor in myocardial infarction.
- Abnormal Q waves : prominent Q waves in II, III and avF may indicate an inferior wall infarction.
- ST segments: look for abnormal ST elevations or depression.
- T waves: look for polarity and size. Tall T waves may indicate hyperkalaemia.
- U waves: may be a sign of hypokalaemia.

The final ECG reading will have a list of findings and a possible explanation of these findings; for example a prolonged QT interval and prominent U waves consistent with hypokalaemia or drug effect.

Further reading

1 Wagner GS, Marriott HJL. *Marriott's Practical Electrocardiography*.
2 Otto CM, Pearlman AS. *Textbook of Clinical Echocardiography*.
3 Conover MB, Bond RJ. *Understanding Electrocardiography*.

11

Simple local anaesthetic techniques

Dave Murray

Introduction

Simple local anaesthetic techniques refer to infiltration anaesthesia, field blocks and minor nerve blocks. They allow the practitioner to perform a variety of minor procedures with little discomfort to the patient. It may allow an operation to be performed in a patient who is not fit for a general anaesthetic.

Anaesthesia occurs due to the action of the local anaesthetic on sensory nerve endings or minor peripheral nerves. Local anaesthetic diffuses into the nerve and prevents transmission of impulses along that nerve. Relatively large volumes of anaesthetic are required to produce anaesthesia compared with, for example, performing a major nerve block. This is not a problem with minor surgery. However with more major surgery, this increases the likelihood of systemic toxic reactions.

Indications include

- Minor superficial surgery e.g. removal of skin lesions, wound suturing and toilet;
- Wound infiltration for post-operative analgesia;
- Invasive procedures e.g. insertion of chest drains, central lines, large intravenous cannulae.

Cautions

Due to the increased risk of toxicity, a reduction in dose is required with the following:

- Extremes of age
- Low cardiac output states, e.g. cardiac failure
- Hepatic impairment

Contraindications

- Patient refusal
- Allergy to local anaesthetic
- Infection at injection site
- Significant bleeding diathesis

Drugs

The two agents most commonly used are lidocaine and bupivacaine.

Lidocaine

Lidocaine is available in 0.5%, 1% and 2% dilutions, with or without epinephrine. It is short acting and causes some degree of vasodilatation. The maximum dose of plain lidocaine is 4 mg/kg (Table 1). Onset of action is usually 2–3 minutes for infiltration anaesthesia, and the duration of action may be up to 45 minutes if epinephrine (adrenaline) is added.

Adding epinephrine to lidocaine causes localised vasoconstriction. This reduces washout of drug from the tissues and both prolongs the duration of action and allows an increase in the maximum dose because of reduced systemic absorption. It also reduces bleeding at the site of surgery. It is unnecessary to use concentrations greater than 1:200,000 (2 μg/mL). The maximum dose of epinephrine is 500 μg for an adult. It must never be used in areas supplied

Table 1. Maximum doses and volumes of local anaesthetics for a given weight of patient.

Drug	Maximum dose	Drug concentration (%)	Maximum volume (mL) Patient weight 30 kg	50 kg	70 kg
Lidocaine	4 mg/kg	0.5	24	40	56
		1	12	20	28
		2	6	10	14
Lidocaine with adrenaline	7 mg/kg	0.5	42	70	98
		1	21	35	49
		2	10	17	24
Bupivicaine/ levobupivicaine	2 mg/kg	0.25	24	40	56
		0.5	12	20	28

by end arteries such as digits, earlobes, nose and penis. It also needs to be used with caution in patients with hypertension and thyrotoxicosis. The addition of epinephrine to lidocaine increases the safe maximum dose to 7 mg/kg (Table 1).

Bupivacaine

Bupivacaine is available in 0.25% and 0.5% solutions. It is longer acting than lidocaine, but takes longer to work. It is not available with epinephrine as there is little advantage to be gained by its addition. Bupivacaine consists of two optical isomers (the D- and L- form) in equal proportions. Levobupivacaine is a relatively recent development and is the L-isomer of bupivacaine. It has the same anaesthetic qualities as bupivacaine, but a wider therapeutic profile. It is therefore safer and should ideally be chosen in preference to bupivacaine when larger doses are used. It is also available as 0.25% and 0.5%. The maximum dose of bupivacaine and levobupivacaine is 2 mg/kg (Table 1).

Dose calculation

Confusion may arise due to the fact that maximum dose of local anaesthetic is expressed as milligrams per kilogram (mg/kg), whereas the drug is labelled as % concentration. However calculation of the maximum volume of anaesthetic is relatively straightforward. To calculate milligrams of local anaesthetic in each mL, multiply the % concentration by 10. This then allows the maximum volume of a particular local anaesthetic to be calculated (Table 2).

Procedure

Obtain the patient's history including any allergies and their weight.

Explain the procedure to the patient and gain consent. Explain that the initial injection will usually sting. Also explain that once the block is established, they may feel pressure around the site but not pain. Maintain verbal contact with the patient during the procedure.

Calculate maximum dose of local anaesthetic and decide on appropriate concentration and volume. If a large volume of anaesthetic is required due to the size of the surgical site, then the concentration

Table 2. Examples of dose calculation for local anaesthetics.

E.g. 1
(i) Maximum dose of bupivicaine = 2 mg/mL
(ii) For a 70 kg adult, maximum dose is:
70 kg × 2 mg/kg = 140 mg
(iii) 0.5% bupivicaine contains 10 × 0.5% = 5 mg per mL of bupivicaine
(iv) Therefore maximum volume is:
140 mg ÷ 5 mg/mL = 28 mL of 0.5% bupivicaine

E.g. 2
(i) Maximum dose of lidocaine with adrenaline = 7 mg/kg
(ii) For a 70 kg adult, maximum dose is:
70 kg × 7 mg/kg = 490 mg
(iii) 1% lidocaine contains 10 × 1% = 10 mg/mL
(iv) Therefore maximum volume is:
490 mg ÷ 10 mg/mL = 49 mL of 1% lidocaine
(v) 2% lidocaine contains 20 × 2% = 20 mg per mL
(vi) Therefore maximum volume is:
490 mg ÷ 20 mg/mL = 24.5 mL of 2% lidocaine

will need to be reduced (twice the volume of 0.5% lidocaine can be used compared with 1%). Avoid giving the maximum dose of local anaesthetic at the outset, as this means that it will not be possible to supplement the block if required.

Consider whether intravenous access is required. It should be obtained in all cases where there is an increased likelihood of toxicity occurring; such as when using large doses of local anaesthetic or in patients in whom a dose reduction is necessary. However, toxicity may occur even with a small amount of inadvertent intravascular injection.

Prepare equipment: skin preparation, syringe, needle, and local anaesthetic. Pay particular care to whether epinephrine free local anaesthetic is being used.

Identify landmarks, taking particular note of any veins.

Clean skin in a manner appropriate to the procedure being performed. Introduce needle, aspirate (to exclude intravascular injection) then inject slowly. Small veins may collapse under negative pressure so the inability to aspirate does not guarantee that the injection is not intravascular. If blood is aspirated, withdraw or advance the needle and aspirate again.

Use a small needle for the first injection. It will cause less pain and allow subsequent injections to be made using a larger needle with less discomfort.

If further injections are required, endeavour to insert the needle through a previously anaesthetised area.

Subcutaneous injections that raise a skin wheal are painful regardless of needle size used. The injection should be made intradermally.

Wait for the block to work. This will be longer with more dilute concentrations of local anaesthetic.

Test for adequacy of anaesthesia before proceeding. Believe the patient if he complains of pain.

Give any additional oral analgesia before the block wears off.

Document technique in patient notes.

Local infiltration

This is suitable for

- Insertion of chest drains, central lines, etc.;
- Suturing of clean lacerations. Infiltrating around the wound by inserting the needle from within the wound, rather than through the surrounding skin, will reduce pain due the lack of nerve endings within the wound itself;
- Post-operative analgesia.

Equipment

Lidocaine with or without epinephrine, bupivacaine, levobupivacaine.
5, 10 or 20 mL syringe.
25G (orange) needle for initial injection, then 23G (blue) or 21G (green) needle for subsequent injections.

Field block

This is a technique in which a wall of local anaesthetic agent is placed around the area to be operated on (Figure 1). It is suitable for:

- Minor surgery on areas where infection exists, e.g. incision and drainage of abscess. If local anaesthetic were to be injected into

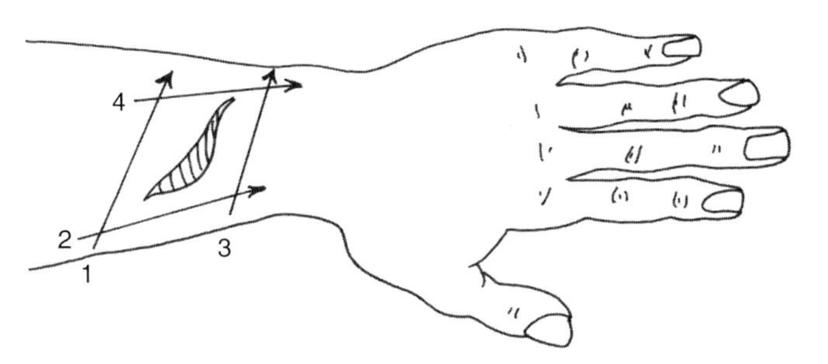

Figure 1. Field block. The order in which injections are performed is shown. Note that subsequent injections are made through previously anaesthetised skin.

an area where infection is present, the block is very likely to be ineffective. The acid environment due to infection prevents the action of local anaesthetic agents. A field block must therefore be used instead.

- Wound toilet. Injecting local anaesthetic at the wound site would risk introducing infection from the wound into surrounding areas. A field block reduces this risk as the anaesthetic is placed a distance from the wound.
- Removal of skin lesions.

Equipment

Lidocaine with or without epinephrine, bupivacaine, levobupivacaine.
5, 10 or 20 mL syringe.
25G (orange) needle for initial injection, then 23G (blue) or 21G (green) needle for subsequent injections.

Digital nerve block

This is a minor peripheral nerve block, and allows surgery on the distal two-thirds of the fingers and toes. The digit is supplied by a dorsal and palmar nerve on each side of the digit (Figure 2). Onset of block is usually within 2–3 minutes, and lasts for 45–60 minutes.

Equipment

2–5 mL of plain lidocaine. Epinephrine must not be used.
5 mL syringe.
23G (blue) or 25G (orange) needle.

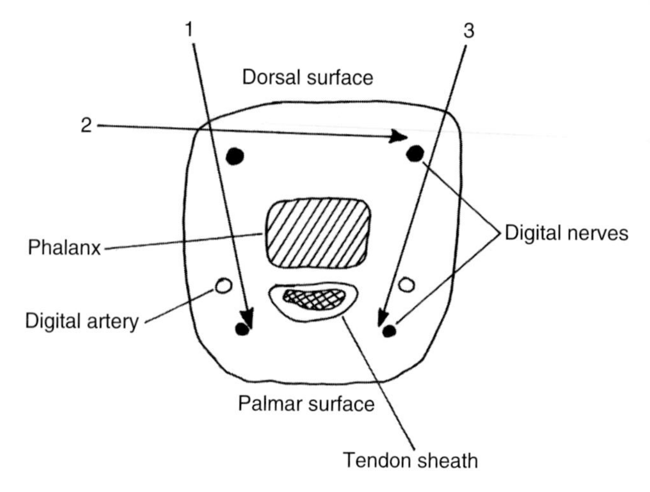

Figure 2. Digital nerve block. The order in which injections are performed is shown.

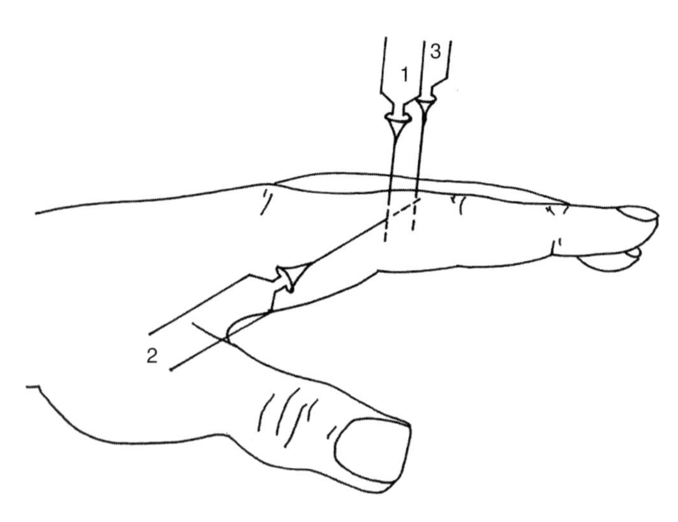

Figure 3. Section through a finger at the proximal phalanx showing the site of the dorsal and palmar digital nerves. The order in which injections are performed is shown.

Technique

Introduce the needle close to the web space at the proximal phalanx on the dorsal side of the digit, and advance until it is felt tenting the palmar surface (Figure 3).

Aspirate and inject 0.5–1.5 mL of local anaesthetic while withdrawing the needle.

Repeat along the dorsal surface and on other side of the digit.

Do not use epinephrine

Although sometimes called a ring block, local anaesthetic should not be injected circumferentially around the digit. Ischaemia may occur due to vaso-occlusion caused by the volume of local anaesthetic.

Complications

Failure of block
If the block wears off before the procedure is complete, further local anaesthetic may be given, provided that the total amount given does not exceed the maximum dose. It may be necessary to perform a peripheral nerve block more proximally (less local anaesthetic will be required), or a general anaesthetic may ultimately be required.

Paraesthesia
If injecting near a site of a peripheral nerve, paraesthesia will be caused if the nerve is touched. If so, withdraw the needle and continue to inject. Injection into a nerve will cause damage.

Toxicity
Toxicity affects the central nervous and cardiovascular systems. It may occur due to direct intravascular injection or due to systemic absorption of local anaesthetic. Symptoms will occur immediately with direct intravascular injection. If due to systemic absorption, they usually develop within 10–25 minutes, as this is when peak plasma concentrations occur.

Early neurological symptoms are usually mild, such as circumoral paraesthesia, tinnitus, light-headedness, visual disturbances, and garrulousness. Maintaining verbal contact with the patient may allow detection of such symptoms before they become more severe. With more severe reactions convulsions, loss of consciousness and apnoea may occur.

Initial signs of cardiac toxicity are hypertension and tachycardia due to blockade of central nervous inhibitory centres. These may progress to hypotension, bradycardia, arrhythmias, and cardiac arrest.

Treatment of toxicity

- Stop injection
- Call for help
- Maintain airway
- Ensure adequate ventilation
- Administer oxygen
- Obtain intravenous access if not already available.

Always

- Assemble all equipment prior to starting the procedure.
- Calculate the maximum dose of local anaesthetic prior to starting the procedure.
- Obtain intravenous access if there is risk of toxicity.
- Ensure you have paid particular attention to whether you are using epinephrine free lidocaine.
- Use a small needle first.
- Aspirate before injecting.
- Try to make subsequent injections through previously anaesthetised skin.
- Give the block time to work before starting the procedure.
- Maintain verbal contact with the patient throughout the procedure.
- Believe the patient if he complains of pain.
- Observe the patient for 30 minutes after infiltrating local anaesthetic.

Never

- Exceed the maximum dose of local anaesthetic.
- Use epinephrine in appendages.
- Raise a skin wheal, as subcutaneous injection is painful.

- Hypotension—give 500 mL of intravenous fluid and raise the patient's legs
- Convulsions—give diazemuls 5–10 mg i.v. slowly
- Arrhythmias—usually resolve spontaneously. Treat if they are causing cardiovascular compromise. If cardiac arrest occurs, there may be resistance to DC shock for up to 30 minutes. Ensure normokalaemia and correct acidosis.

Further reading

1 Covino BG. Pharmacology of local anaesthetic agents. *Br J Anaesth.* 1986;58:701–716.
2 Reynolds F. Adverse effects of local anaesthetics. *Br J Anaesth.* 1987;59:78–95.

12

Basic suturing techniques

Philip A. Corbett and William A. Corbett

Introduction

Manual surgical skills have been learnt throughout the ages by observation, supervision and practice. Reading a chapter in a book is no substitute for practical training but it is possible to explore some of the principles and practices that are used by reading. The principles behind direct closure of wounds depend on understanding how they heal, and why close apposition of the tissues is so important.

The majority of cases that need suturing involve apposing the skin after minor surgery or trauma (Figures 1–3).

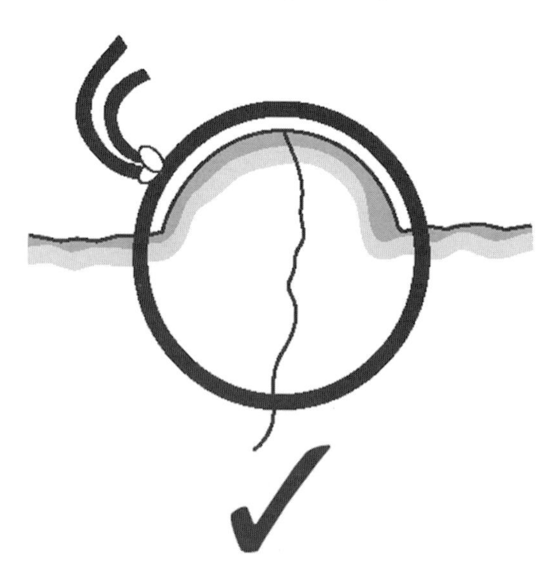

Figure 1. Simple suture closing the deep layers.

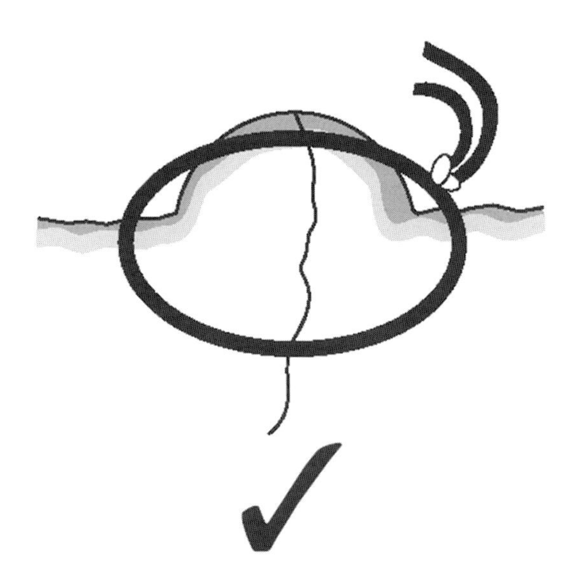

Figure 2. Vertical mattress suture where the top of the wound is closed as well as the deeper layers. Note the slight eversion of the skin.

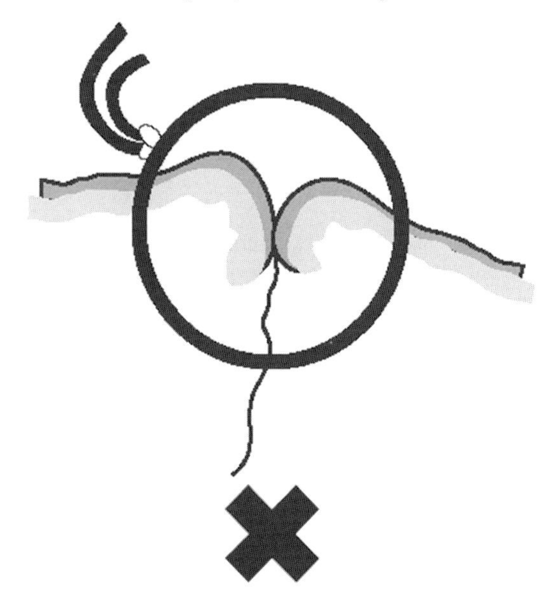

Figure 3. Everting, over-tightened suture.

Table 1. Removal time for sutures.

Region	Removal time
Head and neck	5 to 7 days
Trunk and upper limbs	7 to 10 days
Lower limbs	10 to 14 days

Wound healing

Wound healing has three phases. An inflammatory phase lasting 48 hours is followed by a proliferative phase, which produces an extracellular matrix that fills the defect in the tissue. Angiogenesis and epithelialisation occur simultaneously in this phase. A final maturation phase produces the final appearance and strength of the scar. This process varies with the area of skin and this determines how long the sutures need to remain in place.

Prompt wound healing is dependent upon the presence of viable tissues with an adequate blood supply. It is retarded by the presence of infection, foreign bodies and dead tissue, poor blood supply, steroid therapy, anaemia, jaundice, persistent hyperglycaemia and malnutrition.

Ways of healing

Primary intention

Apposition of the cut edges, e.g. by suturing, promotes direct healing of the tissues and reduces the inflammatory and proliferative responses. Healing times are shorter, scars are smaller and stronger. However, contaminated wounds have an increased risk of infection, which may present as an abscess or as cellulitis. Abscesses can be drained but in the pre-antibiotic era (or in parts of the world where their use is limited) a spreading cellulitis not halted by wound drainage could be fatal even for the fit and young.

Secondary intention

The wound is left untouched to heal by a process of granulation tissue formation and contraction of the wound size with the spread of epithelium from the edges to cover the defect. This is a slow but relatively safe means of wound healing as colonisation of the wound surface by commensal organisms is inevitable but invasive infection is unlikely. However, the final scars are bigger and weaker. Healing times are prolonged during which the exposed surface is prone to further damage.

Sutures

Suture materials are classified as either absorbable or non-absorbable. The majority in use today are synthetic and may be braided or monofilament. The suture material is presented according to its size or gauge. The typical range of suture gauges in general use are from 1 (heaviest), through O, 2O, 3O, 4O, 5O, to 6O (lightest).

Needles

These may be straight or curved, the former used largely for skin closure, and they have differing point shapes. Round bodied points are used in gut closure for instance, whilst cutting points are necessary for skin, fascia and other tough tissues.

Knots

General principles

- The knot must be secure.
- The knot must be as small as possible to minimise its potential as a locus for infection and reduce tissue reaction.
- The knot should be tied so that it lies 'flat,' to avoid the formation of a slip knot.
- The knot should be tied at a tension appropriate to the tissue. The degree of tension should be just sufficient to approximate and immobilise tissues, as greater constriction of the tissues will impair blood supply, resulting in ischaemic necrosis and wound breakdown.
- The suture should never be grasped by artery forceps or needle holders, as this damages and weakens the material. The exception is the free end of the suture, when performing a tie using instruments, which is cut off and discarded.

There are many different types of knot but the commonest are the Reef, Granny and Surgeon's knots (Figures 4 and 5).

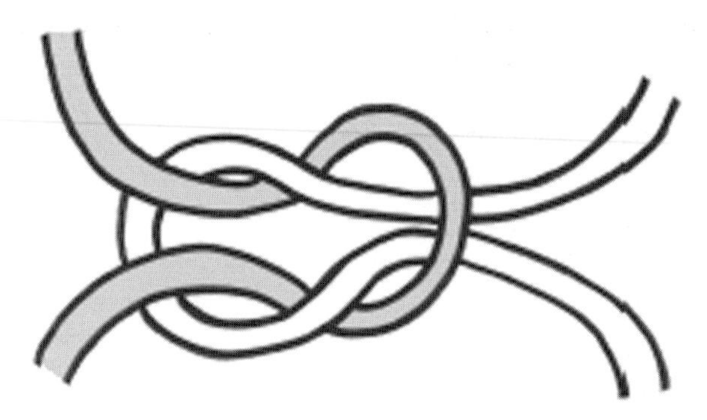

Figure 4. A Reef knot—this can also be tied as a sliding knot.

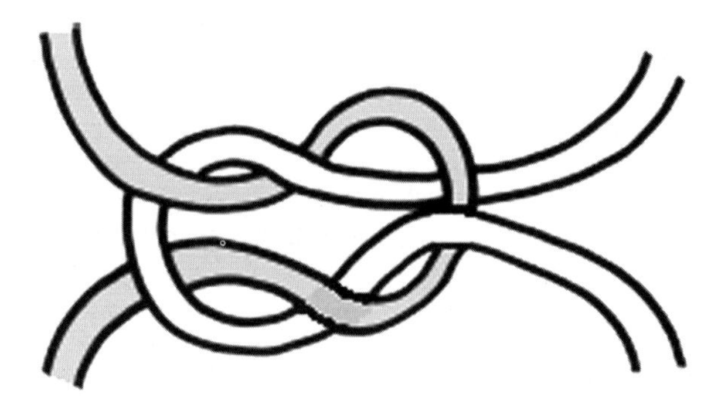

Figure 5. A Granny knot—this can also be used as a sliding knot.

Suturing

There are two basic techniques—interrupted and continuous suturing. The former is the most commonly used after trauma whilst the latter, if used subcuticularly, gives a much better cosmetic result.

Basic technique: interrupted sutures

The wound or incision should be clean and composed only of viable tissue. Burnt areas from diathermy heal badly. After scrubbing up and wearing gloves and either gown or apron the patient needs to be prepared. The skin should be cleaned with an antiseptic solution and the wound draped with sterile sheets.

The equipment necessary includes:

- Gauze swabs
- Local anaesthetic
- Syringes and fine needles
- A range of sutures
- Suture holding forceps
- Toothed tissues forceps
- A blade/scalpel
- Dressing pad
- Disposal system for the sharps

After cleaning the wound edges (and injecting local anaesthesia if necessary—see Chapter 11) hold the edges of the wound together and check that they will appose without distortion. Place the first suture in the centre of the wound and work from either side of that halving the distance between the sutures each time.

Hold the needle about 1/3 of its length from the centre of the needle and rotate it through the skin and out of the deeper part of the wound. Re-enter the opposite side at 90° to the cut surface and exit through the skin directly across from the initial entry point. Tie a single throw and tighten until the two edges are just apposed and slightly everted. Avoid over-tightening as this will impair healing and make the scarring worse. Tie at least one more throw to create a reef knot and to secure the suture. Hold the suture up and cut it so that it is no longer half the length of the distance to the next suture. This makes it easier to remove and stops it being included in the next stitch.

For a simple continuous suture the next bite is taken without tying the previous stitch leading to a series of mattress sutures as the wound is closed (Figure 6). The same can be done just below the skin (subcuticular) with better cosmetic results.

Common problems

- 'Dog-ears': If larger stitch intervals have been taken on one side than the other, the left over skin on one side forms a 'dog-ear'. Such loose skin heals poorly and is unsightly. If one is

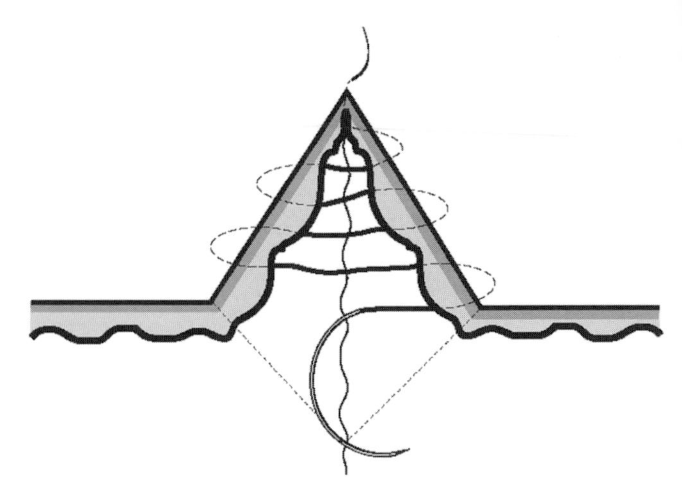

Figure 6. Continuous subcuticular suture.

formed, the wound must either be re-stitched or the excess skin excised and the defect closed.

- Peri-oral wounds: Get an expert to assess and repair these!

Further things to do

There is no substitute for practical training. The skills of knot tying and suturing cannot be learnt from a book and there are many more techniques of knot tying and suturing that require observation, experience and practice. A good way to start is to attend a **Basic Surgical Skills** course. Courses are run by the Royal Colleges of Surgeons and at other venues throughout the country.

Contacts

Royal College of Surgeons of England
35–43 Lincoln's Inn Fields
London WC2A 3PE
UK
website: www.rcseng.ac.uk

Royal College of Surgeons of Edinburgh
3 Hill Place
Edinburgh EH8 9DS
UK
website: www.rcesd.ac.uk

Royal College of Surgeons and Physicians of Glasgow
232–242 St. Vincent Street
Glasgow G2 5RJ
UK
website: www.rcpsglasg.ac.uk

13

Scrub/sterile techniques

Gillian Davies

Hand washing has become a major issue in hospitals in recent years due to the increase in Hospital Acquired Infection (HAI) and more so in the peri-operative environment.

The peri-operative environment has an even more active role in hand washing and that is the procedure for Surgical Scrubbing. Techniques employed by peri-operative personnel when preparing themselves to take part in a sterile procedure can be varied. Standardised practice of aseptic technique should be used throughout the peri-operative environment. All health care professionals undertaking surgical scrubbing should implement guidelines using evidence-based practice. Each hospital will have a set of Guidelines and Policies for a Scrubbing up Protocol to be adhered to by health care professionals.

The aim of surgical scrubbing is to effectively reduce the number of micro-organisms on the skin by mechanical washing (NATN, 1998). Infection control precautions are vital when undergoing any surgical technique procedures. Cross infection occurs when an individual has direct physical contact with the source of the infected organism. Dirty hands are the most significant method of cross infection; effective hand washing prior to any clinical procedure being carried out can largely eliminate the spread of cross infection. Universal precautions for infection control apply in the peri-operative environment.

The procedure for scrubbing up has been based on a technique of surgical scrubbing for five minutes for many years; however until recently this was not research based. There are a variety of antiseptic agents in use at present such as povidone iodine, chlorhexidine and aquasept. A standardised technique of practice is recommended (ICNA, 1996; NATN, 1998) and (AORN, 1999).

Guidelines for surgical scrubbing

- Good standards of personal hygiene are recommended in the peri-operative environment.
- All staff should be dressed in the appropriate theatre attire before beginning a surgical scrub.
- Clean mask, protective eye wear/face shields, should be worn during the procedure when aerosolization or splashing of blood or body fluids is possible.
- Protective eye wear, spectacles or splash visors should be positioned and secured. All hair should be covered with a surgical hat.
- Clean hands and nails. Nails should be short and free from nail polish and artificial nails. Artificial nails can harbour fungal organisms.
- No jewellery should be worn.
- There should be no breaks/abrasions on hands or arms.
- Protective clothing (lead/plastic aprons) should be donned and comfortable. Sterile gown, disposable scrubbing brush with nail cleaner, two hand towels and appropriate sized sterile gloves are available and opened according to manufacturer instructions.
- Taps and antiseptic dispensers should have elbow adjustments provided.
- Staff should also ensure the water is of a comfortable temperature and should provide a steady flow. Warm water removes less of the protective oil of the skin.
- The hands must be above the level of the elbows. Water should flow from the least contaminated to the most contaminated.
- Washing in a circular action helps remove micro-organisms.
- Interlacing the fingers and thumbs cleans the interdigital spaces.
- Rinsing is performed from fingertips to elbows, do not vigorously shake hand and arms to dispel water.
- Movements are steady.
- Care should be taken not to splash theatre clothing.

Procedure for surgical scrub

- The hands and arms are rinsed under running water, 5 mL of antiseptic solution are dispensed into the palm of the hand and the hands and arms are washed to the elbows. The lather is then rinsed off under the running water, allowing the water to run downwards towards the elbows.

- Reapply the antiseptic solution to the hands and mid forearms, dispense antiseptic solution onto a sterile nailbrush and scrub nails thoroughly (a sterile nailbrush must be used for the first scrub of the day). Any dirt under the nails should be removed using the nail cleaner provided with the disposable nailbrush.
- Reapply antiseptic solution to the hands and wrists ensuring the digital spaces between fingers are cleaned thoroughly. Rinse hands and arms allowing the water to run downwards towards the elbows ensuring the hands and arms are elevated away from the body. Taps should be turned off using the elbows.
- The hands and arms are dried using a sterile towel for each hand and arm (two towels are recommended).
- Drying should start at the fingertips, using a corkscrew motion work towards the elbows. The towel should cover the drying hand to prevent contact with the arms. The skin should be blotted dry rather than rubbed.
- The towel should be discarded immediately after use, do not transfer towel to drying hand for disposal.

Donning of surgical gown

- Gown and gloves must be donned using an aseptic technique following the scrubbing up procedure.
- Gowns are single use and come in sterile packets of differing sizes, made of a non-permeable material in a wrap around style, covering the wearer from neck to calf.
- Gowns provide a barrier against micro-organisms. Worn over the correct theatre attire.
- Gowns must have cuffed sleeves ensuring the sleeves are kept securely in the surgical gloves at the wrist.
- Gowns must be donned using an aseptic technique following the scrubbing up procedure, ensuring they touch only the inside of the gown. Pick up gown at inside shoulder area, let gown unfold gently, away from any unsterile surfaces, slide arms into armholes, hands and fingers remain inside cuff of gown to allow donning of gloves using closed method.
- The circulating person assists the scrubbed person by tying the gown.

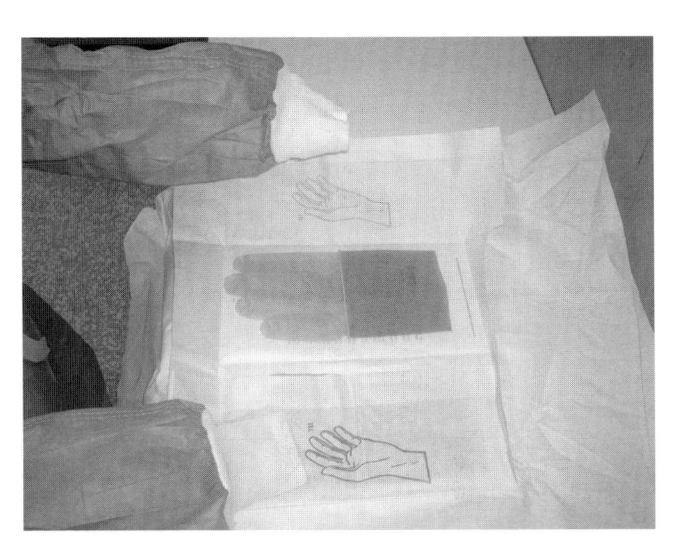

Figure 1. Keeping hands and fingers inside gown sleeves, grasp knitted cuff in palm of hands.

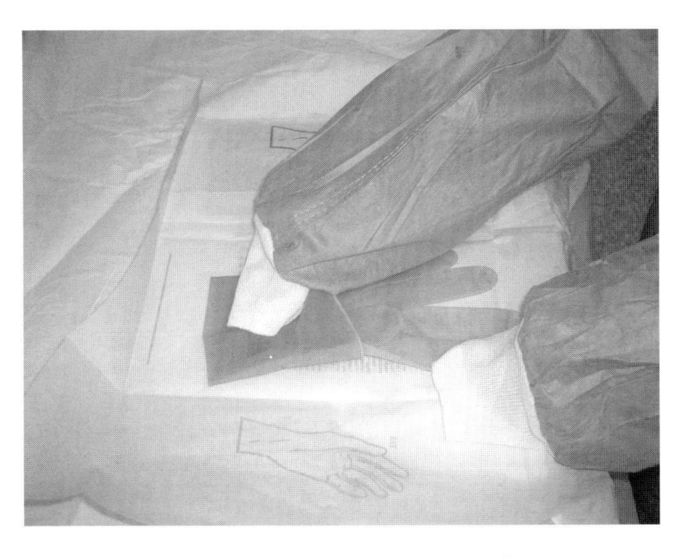

Figure 2. Turn glove packet around and open so that fingers are pointing towards you.

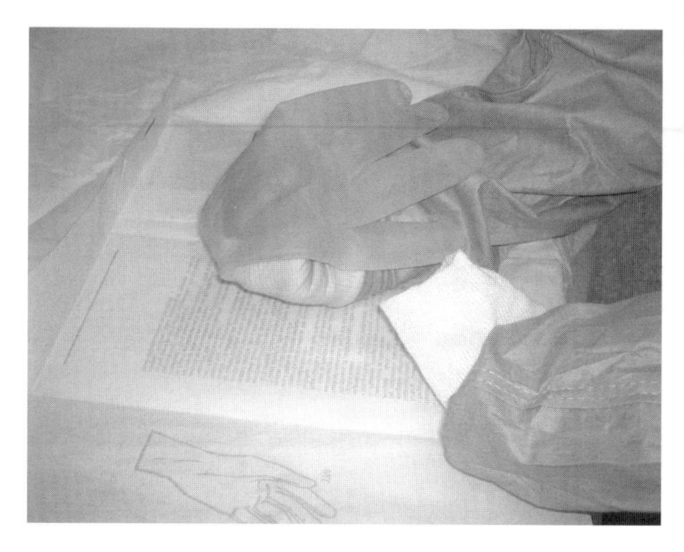

Figure 3. Using right hand thumb and forefinger, take hold of right glove cuff, lining up glove thumb with your thumb. Pick up glove, turn hand over so that glove rests on forearm.

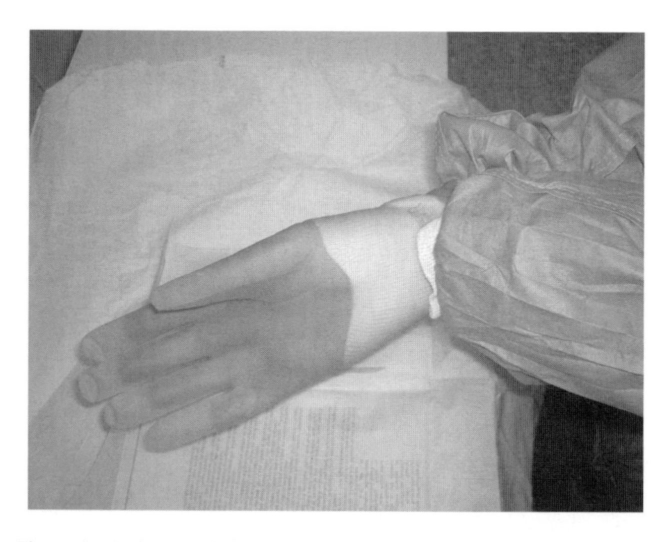

Figure 4. Using your left-hand (still inside gown) pull edge of glove over your right hand. Wriggle fingers and thumb into place as gown and glove slide together up your arm. The glove is now fully on.

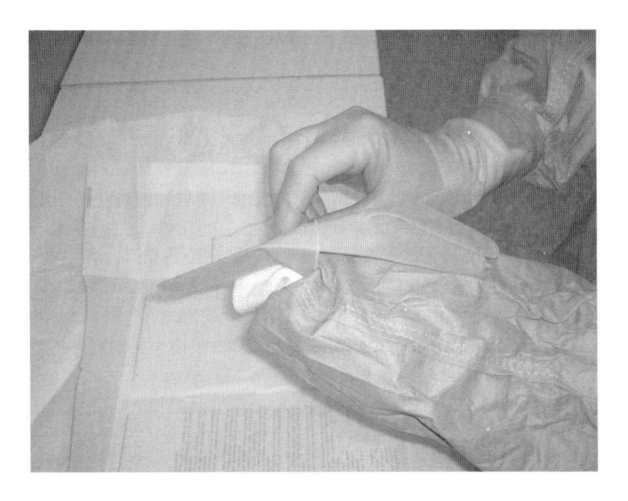

Figure 5. Pick up left glove with left hand and repeat procedure using gloved right hand to pull edge of glove over left hand, pull glove into place.

Gloving procedure

Closed method

The closed method of donning gloves is recommended, however the open method is still in use. Poor technique will compromise sterility whichever method is used.

- Keeping hands and fingers inside gown sleeves, grasp knitted cuff in palm of hands.
- Turn glove packet around and open so that fingers are pointing towards you.
- Using right hand thumb and forefinger, take hold of right glove cuff, lining up glove thumb with your thumb. Pick up glove, turn hand over so that glove rests on forearm.
- Using your left-hand (still inside gown) pull edge of glove over your right hand.
- Wriggle fingers and thumb into place as gown and glove slide together up your arm.
- The glove is now fully on.
- Pick up left glove with left hand and repeat procedure using gloved right hand to pull edge of glove over left hand, pull glove into place.

The arms must be kept at or above waistline level at all times. Only the front of the gown from shoulder to waist is regarded as sterile.

Other important points

The arms are never folded and when not involved in a sterile procedure the palms of the hands should be together. A scrubbed practitioner should never turn his/her back on the sterile trolley and should only pass in a back to back motion ensuring the sterile field is not compromised. If at any time the sterile gloves are compromised they should be discarded and replaced using the same method of gloving technique. At the end of a surgical procedure when discarding the gown and gloves, the gown is removed first then the gloves. They should be disposed of according to the local policy.

Sterile technique

The knowledge and application of aseptic technique used by the perioperative staff influences the patient's surgical outcome. The Health Care Professionals involved in the surgical procedure are responsible for providing a safe environment for the patient.

Measures to prevent surgical wound infection include provision of supplies and equipment, which are free of microbial contamination at the time of use. Sterilisation provides the highest level of assurance that an object is free of viable microbes. Disinfection reduces the risk of microbial contamination but without the same level of assurance.

Maintaining asepsis and limiting the risk of contamination best achieves a safe environment. The basic principles of aseptic technique prevent contamination of the open wound, isolate the operative site from the surrounding unsterile physical environment and create and maintain a sterile field around the patient, so that the surgery can be performed safely.

The sterile field should be constantly monitored and maintained. Personnel participating within the sterile procedure must stay within the sterile boundaries, and a wide margin of safety should be given between scrubbed and non-scrubbed persons.

All staff need to be aware of correct methods for opening sterile packages to avoid contamination of contents. All pre-sterilised articles must be checked for damage and expiry date prior to use. Any packs found to be in an unsatisfactory condition must be discarded.

To reduce the risk of cross infection the following should be kept to a minimum: Talking, movement, number of personnel in the theatre, opening and closing of doors, exposure of wounds, disturbance of clothing and linen. Care must be taken to maintain the sterile field at all times.

Patient preparation

Skin preparation
The area may need to be shaved according to type of surgery, usually pre-operatively to reduce the risk of infection. The skin is prepared with a suitable antiseptic, i.e. aqueous betadine or 0.5% chlorhexidine in alcohol, mucous membrane with normal saline. This will remove dirt and bacteria from the skin and provide an antiseptic cover for the skin surface.

Draping
Sterile drapes are used to provide a safe barrier between sterile field and non-sterile parts of the patient's body, preventing cross infection and contamination of the surgical wound. Disposable drapes are in use in most operating areas and used according to manufacturer recommendations. The drapes are sterile and pre-packed for single use only. Usually it is necessary to have two sterile people to position the sterile drapes to leave only the operative site exposed ready for surgery.

Further reading

1 Recommended Practices for Surgical Scrubs. *AORN J.* 1999; 69(4), 842–850.
2 Infection Control Nurses Association (ICNA). 1996. *Hand Hygiene. ICNA-Sims Portex Teaching Pack for Infection Control.*
3 McLatchie GR. *Oxford Handbook of Clinical Surgery*. Oxford Medical Publications.
4 National Association of Theatre Nurses. *Principles of Safe Practice in the Perioperative Environment*, revised 1998.
5 Kumar B. *Working in the Operating Department*, 2nd ed. Churchill Livingston.

Gillian Davies

14

Simple patient monitoring

Nigel Puttick

Introduction

This section covers the basics of physiological monitoring in the ward or high dependency unit (HDU); monitoring for operative procedures is covered in Chapter 43. It is important to state at the outset that simply monitoring a patient is of little clinical value; the parameters measured are only useful if they are observed, recorded, interpreted, and acted upon. Patient monitoring is not confined to 'monitors'—clinical observations are equally important. The true value of technology in monitoring is that it either extends our ability to observe beyond that which we can measure directly with our senses, or automates the process so that frequent or continuous recording is possible. It is now routine practice to monitor ECG, non-invasive BP and oxygen saturation at the bedside using a small, integrated monitor. Together with simple clinical observations and measurements, and appropriate investigations, it should be possible to identify and manage most early physiological changes before they become problematic. Recognition of a sick patient is a vital skill, identifying deterioration even more so. It is important to seek help early, in order to prevent further deterioration and pre-empt cardiorespiratory arrest. In this short section it is not possible to be comprehensive, but I hope to illustrate some of the ways in which simple monitoring can aid and inform clinical judgment.

Respiratory monitoring

Respiratory rate is best and most easily observed visually, by counting over a minute; while doing so you will also be able to assess other aspects of the patient's respiration. While some ECG monitors measure respiratory rate by impedance change, this method is not always reliable.

Tachypnoea is commonly due to hypoxia or metabolic acidosis and is an important warning sign of deterioration due to many causes. An increasing rate to over 30 is cause for immediate concern. The character of the respiratory pattern is also relevant; rapid shallow breathing is inefficient (dead space forms a greater fraction of tidal volume) and tends to be associated with a rising CO_2. It is very tiring to maintain rapid respiration, and when the respiratory musculature becomes fatigued the rate drops, which is a sign of exhaustion and impending ventilatory failure. This is best assessed by regular, accurate recording of the respiratory rate.

In the postoperative patient, increased respiratory rate can be due to pain, especially in association with a painful abdominal wound. Conversely, central respiratory depression induced by opiate analgesia or respiratory inadequacy due to a high epidural block must be recognized and managed. Postoperative Acute Pain protocols should always include advice on management of respiratory depression.

To assess the pattern of respiration, consider the posture and effort, whether the accessory muscles are being used, whether there is recession of the intercostals, if expansion is symmetrical, and whether the patient is able to converse in unbroken sentences. Abdominal distention will limit diaphragmatic excursion—this is an important cause of rapid, shallow breathing, and is worsened by pain (e.g. peritonitis). An elderly patient with COPD may not tolerate the added respiratory embarrassment of peritonitis or a painful wound. A patient with a critical upper airway obstruction or severe acute asthma may only be able to breathe adequately in the sitting position: being unable to breathe comfortably while lying down is an important sign.

Oxygenation is now easily measured using a pulse oximeter. This is the monitor *par excellence* which extends our senses, as it measures arterial oxygen saturation non-invasively and in real time. Visual assessment of skin or mucous membrane colour is highly unreliable, being dependent on skin type, adequacy of circulation, haemoglobin level, and ambient lighting. Be aware however of the potential problems of pulse oximetry. An adequate oxygen saturation (SpO_2) is not evidence of adequate respiration, as it does not measure CO_2. In a patient receiving supplementary oxygen, the SpO_2 may remain high in the presence of worsening respiratory depression or even critical airway obstruction; when the situation worsens further the SpO_2 drops suddenly. On the other hand, in conditions where gas transfer is compromised the SpO_2 is a good guide both to pulmonary function and effectiveness of therapeutic efforts such as oxygen administration, physiotherapy or bronchoscopy. An adequate SpO_2 on air (>92%) is an important measure of recovering lung function, in both medical and postoperative settings. Conversely, an oxygen saturation less than 90%, or falling, on added oxygen is evidence of serious respiratory impairment.

Expired CO_2 is not easy to measure accurately unless end-tidal gas can be sampled. In practice this is only achievable in an intubated patient. Sampling from within a facemask will not be quantitative owing to a variable degree of dilution with room air or oxygen, giving only a crude indication of respiratory rate; arterial blood gas analysis is required.

Cardiovascular monitoring

Heart rate can be monitored from several sources: ECG, non-invasive BP, and pulse oximeter. The pulse oximeter is often the most reliable source, but does give the peripheral pulse rate. The ECG rate may differ, especially if there are arrhythmias, and the difference can provide useful diagnostic information. Be aware of ECG artefacts such as a high amplitude T wave (possibly due to electrode position or lead selection) leading to a display of double the actual heart rate, or a low amplitude QRS reading intermittently and displaying an apparent bradycardia: look at the trace, and check the pulse manually yourself if in doubt. Tachyarrhythmia is common in acute physiological disturbance, especially hypovolaemia, electrolyte abnormalities, hypoxia, and pain. Remember that myocardial infarction can be silent in the acutely unwell, and may present as a new arrhythmia: consider checking the cardiac enzymes. It can be difficult to assess the fine detail of the ECG on a bedside monitor, particularly arrhythmias or ST changes, and a 12-lead ECG may be necessary for clarification.

Blood pressure is now rarely taken manually, as automated non-invasive BP (NIBP) monitors are common. However there are many potential problems with NIBP monitors. Correct cuff size is important for accuracy, and arrhythmias or shivering may prevent the monitor from making a reading successfully. Most importantly, NIBP monitors do not generally perform well on hypotensive patients. If in doubt, take the BP manually yourself, especially if you are basing your management on the result. Remember these monitors cycle intermittently or manually: so check at what time the reading displayed was actually taken.

Peripheral circulation can be usefully assessed by colour, capillary refill, and peripheral temperature. Pulse oximetry does not work well if the peripheries are shut down by hypovolaemia or arterial disease. An adequate peripheral circulation together with a normal BP and heart rate is a good indication of a normovolaemic patient with a normal cardiac output. On the other hand, cold peripheries with tachycardia and normal BP may suggest compensated hypovolaemia, while warm peripheries with low BP can occur in sepsis.

Central Venous Pressure (CVP) can be monitored on the ward, HDU and ITU. This is now normally measured using a transducer, rather than a fluid column, and recorded in mmHg. As the measured value is small relative to atmospheric pressure, usually in the range 5 to 15 mm Hg, the transducer position is critical to accurate and repeatable readings. You should always aim to position (and zero) the transducer at the level of the right atrium—and to move its relative location depending on the position of the patient. If ignored, this can lead to large errors which can in turn be misunderstood and lead to erroneous treatment. An unexpected change in CVP should always lead you to check the transducer position and zero before giving fluids or drugs. Other errors can arise from catheter position, for example in the right ventricle (high, pulsatile) or in the neck veins (low, damped) so check the position on CXR. You should remember that this is invasive monitoring with potential serious complications such as air embolism, blood loss and sepsis. Accurately measured CVP in a patient with normal cardiac function is a very good guide to fluid replacement, particularly if considered along with other information such as urine output.

Invasive Arterial Blood Pressure (IABP) is normally only monitored on HDU or ITU. This is because it is mostly used in patients receiving active treatment with cardiovascular drugs such as inotropes or vasodilators, or in whom continuous BP monitoring is required. Like CVP, it has serious potential complications including distal arterial occlusion, blood loss and sepsis. Compared to CVP, the measured value is relatively large, usually in the range 50 to 200 mm Hg, and so the transducer position is less critical though you should still aim to level (and zero) it at the height of the heart. There is sometimes poor correlation between IABP and NIBP, as they are based on different physical principles. An arterial line is very useful, but not essential, when serial blood gas measurements are desired.

Temperature

Mercury thermometers are considered unsafe, and have been replaced by ear thermometers. The readings are not necessarily identical, as they use different principles. The trend is of course more important than the absolute value, and so a uniform technique is required. In theatre it is common to measure both core and peripheral temperature, as the difference gives a useful indication of filling of the vascular compartment, but this is not often done on the ward or HDU. Peri-operative normothermia is now recognized as being of great importance. As a cold patient rewarms, vasodilatation may unmask hypovolaemia previously compensated by vasoconstriction. Methods of measuring temperature continuously in the ward or HDU include adhesive skin sensors and a urinary catheter with temperature sensor to measure intravesical (core) temperature.

Fluid balance

In any unwell patient, fluid balance should be measured as accurately as possible, to monitor and preserve renal function and to prevent fluid overload or dehydration. With IV fluids and a urinary catheter (preferably with a volumetric bag) this is straightforward, but charting should be hourly, accurate and meticulous. Remember to account for other fluid losses, in particular from the GI tract, drains, and fistulae. Consider whether clinical signs such as thirst, tongue appearance, and skin turgor are in accord with your measurements, and consider outflow obstruction in the event of anuria. Urine output is often a reflection of cardiovascular performance and may switch on or off dependent on blood pressure, CVP or cardiac output, so is an important indicator of deterioration or recovery. In adults the minimal acceptable urine output is 0.5 mL/kg/hr.

Neurological assessment

The Glasgow Coma Score (see Chapter 7) is not a subtle measure of conscious level, and is mainly useful in the management of severe impairment. A falling GCS is an ominous finding, and below 8 the patient will not be able to maintain a safe airway and should be intubated. However, the GCS does not differentiate minor to moderate degrees of confusion. Confusion can be a very sensitive indicator of physiological derangement, especially in the previously neurologically intact patient. It may result from a variety of causes including hypoxia, hypercapnia, and electrolyte disturbance and should be considered an important sign of deterioration.

Abdominal assessment

An intra-abdominal emergency is a common cause of deterioration in the elderly and unwell. Ileus, perforation, peritonitis and sepsis must be recognized promptly and changes monitored and recorded. Measure girth to assess progressive distension, listen for bowel sounds, elicit tenderness, and seek surgical advice promptly if necessary. Acute abdominal distension represents a compartment syndrome in which the increased intra-abdominal pressure shuts off ureteric flow, reduces venous return, and splints the diaphragm. Ultrasound scanning at the bedside is now arguably the most useful and the least invasive or disruptive method of assessing the acute abdomen in a sick patient.

Investigations

Much can now be achieved with hand held analyzers, for example blood glucose and haemoglobin. Arterial blood gas analysis provides much valuable information about a patient's respiratory, cardiovascular and metabolic state, and most analyzers now measure a variety of electrolytes. Using these near-patient techniques saves much time taking samples to the laboratory and waiting for results, and if properly quality-controlled are suitable for making diagnostic and treatment decisions. However daily laboratory measurements of routine biochemistry and haematology should also be ordered. It is helpful to chart all the 'numbers' at least daily on a cumulative chart so that trends can be easily picked out.

Putting it all together

The aim is to identify deterioration and prevent progression to cardiorespiratory arrest. Two complementary approaches are evolving:

Early Warning Scoring (EWS) systems for detection and Outreach services for intervention. Neither is yet fully clinically validated but they are increasingly employed worldwide. An EWS system requires careful monitoring and rule-based decision making, triggering a request for assistance once a threshold is reached. Outreach teams can be nursing or medical based: what is most important is the ability to intervene effectively, appropriate action being taken either within the ward setting or by transfer to HDU or ITU. Most EWS systems track five physiological parameters: systolic blood pressure, heart rate, respiratory rate, temperature and higher neurological function. Specificity is improved by incorporation of urine output and oxygenation. If a formal EWS is in use in your institution, familiarize yourself with its use and find out who to call for assistance. Even without a scoring system, careful consideration of consecutive recordings of monitored variables should enable you to detect the deteriorating or at-risk patient and to initiate early appropriate action. At hand-over, run through the physiological systems and the results you have observed, identify significant changes, and have target ranges either to be achieved or if breached, will prompt further action by your colleagues.

- The aim is to recognize the sick patient, and to prevent or reverse physiological deterioration.
- Monitored parameters must be observed, recorded, interpreted and acted upon.
- Understand the operating principles and limitations of monitors.
- Cumulative charts are useful to allow trends to be seen.
- Understand and use an Early Warning Score if implemented locally.
- Know who to call for assistance, and do so before a crisis develops.
- At hand-over, identify key observations and give targets.

Further reading

1 Goldhill DR. The critically ill: following your MEWS. *QJM.* 2001;94:507–510.

2 Subbe CP, Kruger M, Rutherford P, Gemmel L. Validation of a modified Early Warning Score in medical admissions. *QJM.* 2001;94:521–526.

3 Whitehead MA, Puthucheary Z, Rhodes A. The recognition of a sick patient. *Clin Med JRCPL*. 2002;2:95–98
4 Baudouin S, Evans T. *Improving outcomes for severely ill medical patients*. URL: http://www.rcplondon.ac.uk/pubs/ClinicalMedicine/0202_mar_ed3.htm

15

Urinary catheterisation

David Chadwick

Introduction

Catheterisation of the urinary bladder is a commonly performed clinical procedure. The usual indications for catheterisation are as follows: acute or chronic retention of urine, incontinence, immobility, or to allow the accurate measurement of urine output. Other indications include severe haematuria (which may necessitate washouts and irrigation of the bladder), and following surgery to the lower urinary tract. The usual method of accessing the bladder is via the urethra but in some situations the suprapubic route is chosen.

Anatomy

The adult male urethra is approximately 20 cm in length. It begins at the bladder neck and then passes through the prostate and external sphincter before bending anteriorly through 90 degrees to pass through the length of the penis to exit on the glans at the external meatus. The female urethra is 2 cm in length and passes from the bladder neck to the external meatus which is located at the introitus immediately anterior to the vagina.

The bladder is located anteriorly within the pelvis. It is covered with peritoneum on its superior, lateral and posterior aspects. When the bladder is full it can be detected by percussion and palpation of the lower abdomen and by ultrasound examination ('bladderscan').

Technique

Male urethral catheterisation

- The procedure is explained to the patient and consent is obtained.
- The patient lies in the supine position.

- Sterile gloves are worn.
- The external genitalia are washed using a topical antibacterial solution (e.g. cetrimide, aqueous chlorhexidine). The prepuce (if present) is retracted and the glans penis thoroughly cleansed.
- Sterile drapes are positioned. A ‘catheterisation pack’ will contain a sterile drape containing a small circular hole through which the penis can be delivered.
- Lignocaine gel is introduced into the urethra using either a tube and nozzle or alternatively a preloaded syringe. The gel is then held in the urethra by compressing the distal urethra with the index finger and thumb of the left hand whilst the right hand is used to massage the gel proximally towards the base of the penis. It is advisable to wait for a minute or two prior to the passage of the catheter. This allows the patient to relax further and also gives time for the lignocaine to anaesthetise the urethral mucosa.
- The right hand is then used to pass the catheter. To facilitate this, the urethra is straightened as much as possible by gentle pulling on the penis with the left hand and elevating it to an angle of some 60 degrees above the horizontal. The catheter is retained as much as possible within its sterile wrapping to reduce the risk of contamination.

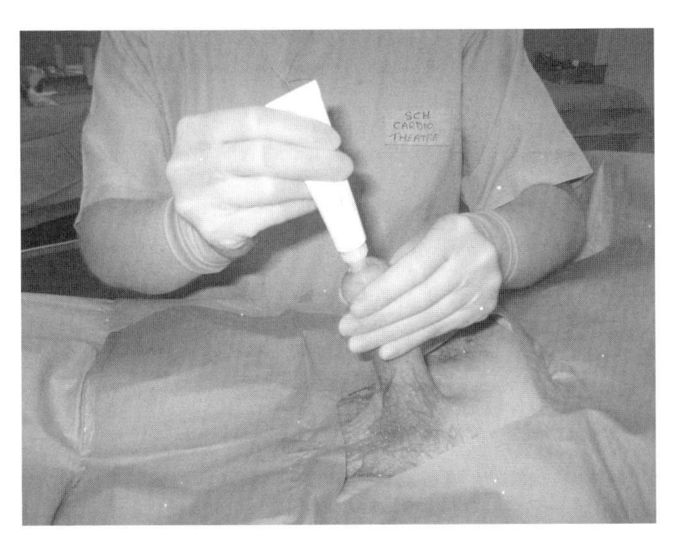

Figure 1. Local anaesthetic gel is introduced into the urethra.

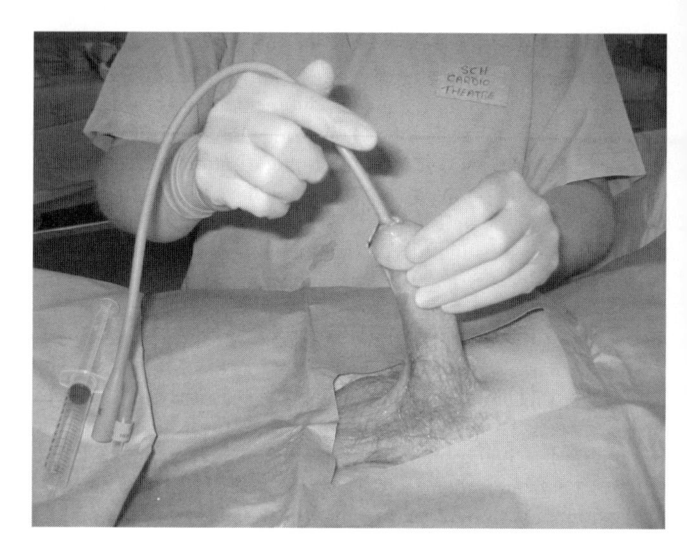

Figure 2. The catheter is passed.

- A minor degree of resistance is often encountered as the tip of the catheter passes through the external sphincter and subsequently the prostatic urethra. This can be the most uncomfortable part of the procedure and it is important to provide words of reassurance and encouragement for the patient.
- If significant resistance is encountered it is important not to try to force the catheter as this can damage the urethra and create a false passage.
- As the catheter enters the bladder urine usually begins to drain. At this point the catheter balloon can be inflated. This is done using a syringe connected to the balloon port of the catheter paying particular attention to the maximum balloon volume as stated on the cuff around the balloon port. Some catheters have inbuilt reservoirs of water which can be released by removing the plastic clip and compressing the reservoir thus allowing the water to be transferred to the balloon.
- If urine does not drain spontaneously this is either because the bladder is empty or a result of the eyes at the tip of the catheter being blocked by lubricating gel. Flushing the catheter with a bladder syringe filled with 50 mL sterile water will usually confirm that the catheter is within the bladder.

- It is important that the catheter balloon is not inflated unless the operator is certain that it is in the bladder. If the patient experiences pain on inflation of the balloon this is a warning that the balloon may still be in the urethra in which case the balloon must be deflated and the catheter repositioned.
- Finally a drainage bag is connected to the catheter and placed in a dependent position on a catheter stand or leg strap or waistband if the patient is to have the appliance concealed under clothing.

Female urethral catheterisation

The principles of female catheterisation are similar to that of the male. The urethra is of course much shorter and it is rare that difficulties are encountered in the passage of the catheter.

- The patient lies supine with the hips abducted and laterally rotated. The knees are flexed to allow the heels to be touching and resting on the examination couch.
- The external genitalia are cleaned (as above) and care is taken to separate the labia and allow inspection and thorough decontamination of the external urethral meatus.
- Following the installation of lignocaine gel into the urethra the catheter is passed and the balloon inflated.

Difficulties with urethral catheterisation

- In the male a tight foreskin (phimosis) may obscure the external urethral meatus. If the foreskin can be opened to allow the passage of the catheter the lubricated tip of the catheter very often finds its own way into the urethra. Alternatively the foreskin can be opened using a pair of artery forceps or can be dilated with dilators.
- A meatal stenosis can prevent passage of the catheter. In this situation dilators (e.g. Lister sounds) can be used to widen the meatus prior to catheterisation. The use of lignocaine gel is essential to minimise discomfort to the patient.
- Obstruction to passage of the catheter more proximally within the urethra may be due to urethral stricture, prostatic enlargement or bladder neck narrowing. Irregular prostatic regrowth or bladder neck stenosis can occur in men who have undergone transurethral resection of the prostate.

- A urethral stricture can be dilated prior to catheterisation but this should only be performed by an experienced practitioner.
- The use of a catheter introducer can facilitate a difficult catheterisation but as with the use of urethral dilators the introducer should be used with care and only in the hands of experienced operators. The curved shape of the catheter introducer allows the operator to keep 'the tip up' in the negotiation of the large prostate or high bladder neck.
- Problems with female catheterisation are rare. Occasionally in the elderly the external meatus can migrate posteriorly as a result of postmenopausal atrophy. Location of the urethra can then be difficult especially when it is located on the anterior vaginal wall. Significant urethral narrowing is rare but in this situation gentle dilatation usually permits easy passage of the catheter.

Suprapubic catheterisation

The usual indication for suprapubic catheterisation is acute retention and a failed attempt at establishing urethral drainage. However, in

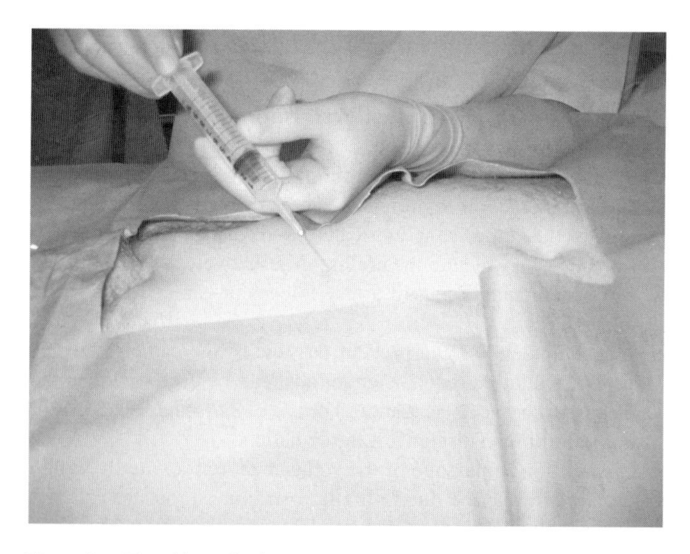

Figure 3. The skin and subcutaneous tissues are infiltrated with local anaesthetic prior to insertion of a suprapubic catheter.

certain situations the suprapubic route is chosen as the method of choice and in many respects it is the easier and safer option.

- It is essential to confirm that the bladder is full or at least of sufficient volume to allow ready access without damage to intraperitoneal structures. This is confirmed by clinical examination (palpation and percussion) or if necessary ultrasound imaging.
- With the patient in the supine position the suprapubic area is exposed and prepared with antiseptic solution and sterile drapes. An area of skin midway between the pubic symphysis and umbilicus is marked. This area together with the subcutaneous tissues, linea alba, and anterior bladder wall is infiltrated with 10 mL of lignocaine 1%.
- A 19G needle connected to a 10 mL syringe is then inserted at 90 degrees to the skin until urine can be aspirated from the bladder. The needle often has to be inserted to the hilt to access the bladder and in the obese patient firm pressure may be required. If urine cannot be aspirated using this technique it is dangerous to proceed with suprapubic catheterisation without the aid of ultrasound guidance.

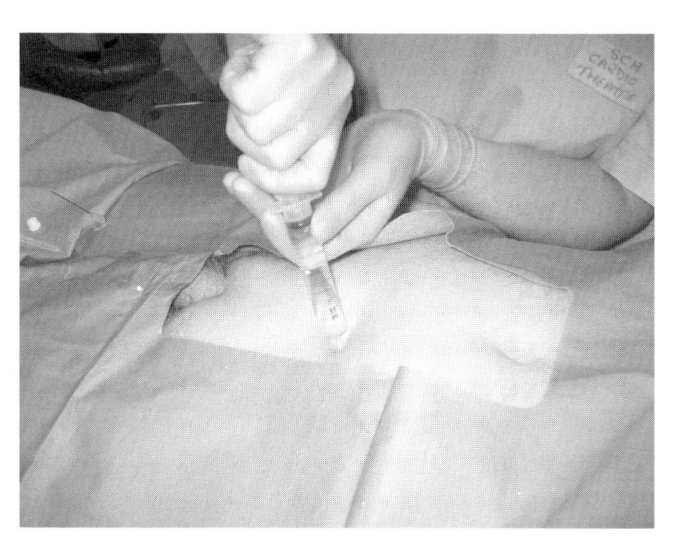

Figure 4. Urine is aspirated via a needle and syringe to confirm the presence of a full bladder.

- A stab incision is made in the skin using a small, pointed scalpel blade.
- The trocar and cannula device (e.g. Adacath®) is then passed firmly through the anaesthetised tissues into the bladder. This requires the use of controlled pressure especially in the elderly male where the bladder is likely to be thick-walled. Removal of the trocar is accompanied by the ejection of urine under pressure and the lubricated catheter is passed quickly through the cannula into the lumen of the bladder. The balloon is inflated prior to removal of the cannula using the tear-off strip of plastic which runs along its length.
- The catheter can be further secured using a silk suture. This can be removed after 10 days by which time the suprapubic track will be mature thus allowing the catheter to be replaced in the event of balloon failure.

Complications

Infection

Bacteraemia and septicaemia can result from instrumentation of the urinary tract and this can include straightforward catheterisation. It is more likely to occur in the following situations and the use of antibiotic prophylaxis is therefore recommended.

- When there has been an indwelling catheter and the catheter is changed
- Chronic retention
- Renal failure
- Urinary tract stone disease

A patient who becomes unwell soon after catheterisation should be treated promptly with a broad spectrum antibiotic with cover against gram negative organisms, e.g. co-amoxiclav, cephalexin, ciprofloxacin. Endotoxic shock can develop and is a life-threatening condition which requires urgent treatment.

Urethral trauma

This results from traumatic catheterisation as a result of excessive force or lack of care in the passage of the catheter. It is more likely to occur in the presence of urethral stricture or an obstructing prostate or bladder neck. Bleeding around the catheter is usually self-limiting.

Diuresis and electrolyte imbalance

This can occur following drainage of a chronically distended bladder and should be anticipated if the residual volume is in excess of a litre. All patients should undergo urgent measurement of serum electrolytes and renal function. If the renal function is impaired or if the diuresis is excessive (e.g. greater than 3 litres per day) then intravenous fluids may be required. Normal saline is recommended with the rate of infusion being dependent on the urine output. Further checks on serum biochemistry are necessary to monitor electrolyte fluctuations and renal function. The development of hypokalaemia will indicate the need for potassium to be added to the intravenous regime.

Damage to intraperitoneal structures

On rare occasions suprapubic catheterisation can cause intraperitoneal damage. This is more likely to occur if the bladder is insufficiently filled or if needle aspiration fails to demonstrate the presence of urine prior to passage of the trocar. The presence of surgical scars on the lower abdomen raises the possibility of intraperitoneal adhesions from loops of small bowel. Suprapubic puncture should not be made at these sites. If signs of peritonitis develop after suprapubic catheterisation a general surgical opinion should be sought and laparotomy may be considered.

Further reading

1 Walsh, Retik, Vaughan, Wein, editors. *Catheterisation*. In: *Campbell's Urology*, 7th ed. Chapter 5, p. 159.
2 Fillingham, Douglas. *Urological Nursing*, 2nd ed. Chapter 5, Catheterisation, p. 90.
3 Bullock, Sibley, Whitaker. *Essential Urology*, 2nd ed. Chapter 2, Anatomy, p. 17.

16

Using a medical simulator

Ronnie J. Glavin

The material in this chapter aims to help you make the most of a visit to a simulation centre.

What is a medical simulator and what is a medical simulation centre?

Quite simply, it is a device to replicate one or more features of a patient. Many of you will have used part task trainers to practice techniques such as intravenous cannulation or urinary catheterisation. The simulators referred to in this chapter contain sophisticated hardware and software and when located in a clinical area allow the management of a clinical episode, especially one where the patient is acutely unwell and in a very unstable condition, for example a patient with chest pain, breathlessness and a low blood pressure. These devices are expensive and are usually housed in a specifically designed centre which will usually have a control room behind one-way glass, an area for briefing and debriefing and audiovisual equipment to record the performance of participants.

Why use simulation?

Many of the advantages of simulation are self evident and will have become obvious when using part task trainers or working with simulated patients in clinical skill centres.

The great strength of a simulation centre is that it provides learners with an opportunity for managing a case by themselves, without direct supervision. This allows learners to make decisions, to see the consequences of those decisions (whether beneficial or harmful) and their actions without any harm to patients. This is then followed by an immediate review of the performance. In real clinical practice it is often very difficult to spend time reviewing a challenging clinical episode because of other demands on the job.

What can I expect to happen at a simulation centre?

Most teaching is based around clinical scenarios. On some occasions, especially in the earlier stages of training, bedside based teaching is used. In scenario based training the learner, working individually or as part of a team, is given a clinical case to manage, such as a patient with post-operative oliguria. The learner has to act as he or she would in the real clinical environment by finding out information from the patient (the manikin can 'speak' and can generate pulses and breath sounds, etc.) and decide what further monitoring, investigations and treatment are required. These have to be performed in real time. If the learner wants to measure the blood pressure then the cuff has to be applied and operated. If intravenous fluids are requested then a bag with a giving set has to be attached and so on. The software modelling allows the manikin's physiology to respond appropriately to drugs administered by the learner. A member of the centre faculty will perform a supporting role, such as a nursing auxiliary, to help locate equipment, etc. In some scenarios other participants play the roles of other health care professionals. On some occasions the scenarios will have a multi-professional team performing the scenario, each performing their own role. Other participants on the course may observe from behind the one way glass or via a live video link. Scenarios usually last from 15–30 minutes. At the end of the scenario the participants and observers review the performance, usually with the aid of the video camera. In bedside teaching a more senior member of staff takes the learners through a case. The patient is likely to be very unstable and very ill and so this would be used to help develop understanding of concepts of pathophysiology or pharmacology in shock or major trauma etc.

The scenario based teaching not only provides practice it also is used to help learners identify their own strengths and weaknesses. Pass/Fail testing does not take place in this kind of visit.

Preparation for the visit

At the time of writing most visits are organised as a component of an attachment. There may be opportunities for a small group of interested learners to arrange a session but few centres have spare capacity.

Practical issues

Most courses at centres will be designed for small groups to maximise the opportunities to get hands on practice. However, a minimum number of participants is usually required to carry out scenarios. If you are unable to attend because of other commitments it is important to give staff at the centre sufficient warning to avoid last minute cancellations.

It is also important to be sure of the directions. Some centres are located adjacent to clinical skills centres; others are in former operating theatres or other clinical areas. They are all signposted but if you do not know what you are looking for you will not find it.

Briefing and orientation are very important to prepare for the rest of the course. Some courses may only have four or five participants so if you are unavoidably detained it is important to let the staff at the centre know so that appropriate arrangements can be made.

Educational preparation

You will be given very little information about the course beyond a general heading e.g. postoperative emergencies in the surgical ward. This is not an oversight. The very nature of the type of cases means that they often arise unexpectedly and unpredictably. Indeed it is difficult to replicate this fully at a centre because the participants are more alert for the unexpected on a course than would be the case in real practice. However, the challenges in the scenarios go beyond diagnosis; they address management, both in terms of specific treatment and more general aspects such as human factors skills. Therefore knowing that this is the scenario with the asthmatic is of little help. The scenarios are not designed to trick people, they are designed to help learners deal more effectively with very real clinical problems.

Preparatory reading also contributes very little to the preparation. My experience is that many of the learners already possess adequate knowledge but either have had scant opportunity to put that knowledge into practice or find that other aspects of management of the case are more challenging.

What can I do to get the most out of the visit?

The key factor is getting into the right frame of mind. Scenario based teaching gives the opportunity to see yourself in action and to identify your strengths and weaknesses. You only do this if you are being honest with yourself. The staff at the centre will do all that they can to create an environment where learners can admit to mistakes or errors without fear of ridicule.

It is also important to act in the way that you normally do. If you behave in a very abnormal manner compared to how you normally act in a clinical setting then it will be more difficult to make inferences from your behaviour. The easiest way to do this is to suspend disbelief and let yourself go into the flow of the scenario. This will be more difficult if you are trying to 'look behind the scenario' by concentrating on what you think 'they' are going to give you in terms of the content of the scenario.

If you are asked to play a supporting role then pay attention to the briefing instructions you have been given. The active participant (hot seater) is centre stage, not the person playing the part of auxiliary nurse or blood porter. It is also important to stay in role during the scenario. There is a natural tendency to want to find out what is happening but it does not help the scenario if the auxiliary nurse is diagnosing second degree heart block. Remember, by staying in role you will help the active participants find it easier to suspend disbelief and everyone will learn more from the scenario during the debriefing.

The scenarios have been designed and developed to bring about some learning objectives. This is less likely to be realised if participants begin to invent details in the scenario. If a chest X-ray is requested then either an actual X-ray or a phoned report will be given. It is inappropriate to ask for the X-ray and then invent the findings.

If you are observing the scenario then ask yourself some questions—What do I think is happening? What would I do now? What is the treatment for this condition?

Remember, it always looks much easier when watching than it does when performing.

Debriefing

Performing in the clinical area is only one part of the educational experience.

Reviewing that performance is equally if not more important and often debriefing lasts longer than the actual scenario. Everyone is there to learn and this will be most effective when the environment allows learners to be honest with themselves when reviewing their own strengths and weaknesses. Negative criticism or ridicule will serve the opposite. In these circumstances people take a defensive position and attempt to justify their actions rather than acknowledge that aspects of their performance could be improved. In courses where everyone takes part in at least one scenario negative criticism is less likely because the ridiculer knows that he or she may in turn be ridiculed. Staff at the centre will do all that they can to create the appropriate environment but it cannot happen without cooperation from the learners. Being honest does not mean denying that events have not gone well. It means acknowledging your limitations. As an observer you can support the active participants by saying if you would have found the clinical challenge difficult or not. As adults you will bring different experiences to debriefing and the facilitator will draw upon these. If you have managed a case similar to that portrayed in the scenario then it is relevant to add this to the discussion.

By the end of the debriefing session everyone, active participants, support cast and observers should have identified some areas of their own practice that could be improved. These can then be used to form a set of learning objectives for the future.

Many people find the experience of watching themselves in action quite daunting, even when managed well. It is important to replay the events in your own mind a few days after the event and go through the list of learning objectives. Staff at the centre are not out to trick you or expose your shortcomings, they are giving you an opportunity to prepare for some real challenges. It is much more daunting to find yourself struggling to manage a real patient.

- The most important thing you can bring on a visit to a simulation centre is an appropriate frame of mind: be honest with yourself, be prepared to participate and be prepared to be supportive of your fellow participants.
- Use the opportunity of managing simulated clinical cases to identify your own strengths and weaknesses.
- Think about what you have learned about yourself and decided what you need to do to improve subsequent performance (all of us can improve our performance).

- Use these areas to form learning objectives for the future and think about where you get the resources you need to help you learn.
- Reinforce what you have learned at the simulator session by using the knowledge and skills in subsequent clinical practice.

What should I do afterwards?

The important points are to work on what you have learned. Use what you have found about your strengths and weaknesses to structure what you need to learn. What resources will you need? Where can you get these?

What you have learned will be best reinforced by gaining further practice. You may not need to do the whole scenario—there may some skills that you can practice with a minimum of equipment and supervision, there may some treatment protocols that are new or updated that may require further study. There may be some aspects of your performance that you can transfer to other situations, especially the human factor skills.

The process of reflection only begins when you have finished the scenario. After a few days think back on your visit, not just your own performance, but the visit as a whole and revise the learning objectives that you have set yourself.

Finally, be reassured. Feedback from participants reveals that the majority find the experience fun as well as being helpful for future clinical practice.

Further reading

1 Greaves DG, Dodds C, Kumar CM, Mets B, eds. *Clinical Teaching: A Guide to Teaching Practical Anaesthesia; Section 3 Using Simulators for Teaching*. Lisse, The Netherlands, Swets & Zeitlinger, 2003.

17

How to prepare to speak at an educational meeting

J. David Greaves

It doesn't matter whether you are talking in your department or to the United Nations; there are some basic rules to observe.

Rule 1: Find out what the person organizing the session expects you to talk about and then stick to that topic

This is a golden rule because by breaking it you risk spoiling someone else's presentation and wrecking the whole meeting. Speakers often make assumptions about why they are being asked to speak. A good organizer will have carefully planned the topics, they will probably coordinate to cover a larger issue and you will have been chosen because they think that your contribution will suit the plan. So, don't make assumptions. Talk to the organizer and find out what they have in mind. Ask them how your topic contributes to the overall scheme. Is the topic absolutely set or can you negotiate a more congenial subject? If there are other speakers with related topics it is as well to contact them if you think that there is any chance of them clashing with your presentation. It doesn't matter how carefully you plan if the preceding speaker gives the talk that you planned to give. I have had the experience of the contributor speaking before me getting up and saying, 'The title I was given was …… but I am not going to talk about that. I am going to talk about ……' He then proceeded to talk on the topic that I had been asked to speak on. I have also been in an audience when four speakers in a session all addressed the same issue! Of course this sort of mix-up is the organizers fault but it would not happen if speakers found out what was expected of them, and liaised with the other speakers. A meeting stands or falls by the quality of a session rather than by individual lectures and as a contributor the quality of co-ordination lies with you.

Rule 2: Each event will need a tailor-made talk

The great and good are often invited to many centres to give a particular talk. They are experts in a field and they can spread their information by talking to large groups. If you are asked to talk you must ask yourself whether you fall into that category. The chances are that you don't, and that you are being expected to tailor your talk to the day's audience. It is quite common for speakers to present a previously prepared talk that was clearly intended for another audience. The more famous the speaker the more likely this is to happen. Even if you are being asked to give a talk that you have given previously you should take the trouble to adjust it to the day's audience.

Rule 3: Know how long you have got and—stick to it

Find out how long you are being given and stick to it. This is another golden rule because again you can wreck the day and spoil other people's presentations. I was once scheduled to speak last before lunch and the preceding speaker spoke for twice his allotted time. Facing a bored, restless, hungry audience, as I mounted the podium the chairman said, 'Please can you cut to ten minutes—Lunch is waiting!' Predictably my presentation was about the worst I have ever done. It is essential to keep to time. Every speaker must cooperate and every chairperson for a session must cut off a speaker at the agreed time; irrespective of whether they have finished. If this happens to you, your presentation will be a disaster. So, know how long you have got, prepare for that time and practise the talk to see how long it takes. Practice run-throughs are faster than real presentations. If you have been asked to speak for fifteen minutes your practice should take ten. If thirty minutes has been allotted, practice for twenty. When you become an experienced speaker you may know more than the meeting organiser and they may give you longer than you need. If you are speaking to an audience of over fifty people you have to be very good or very entertaining to need longer than twenty minutes. Try to persuade the organiser to give you an appropriate time to talk and find out whether the time includes audience questions or whether these are timed separately.

Rule 4: Find out about the facilities

Find out how big the audience will be, and who they are. Talking to an audience of 300 makes different demands to talking to 20 and your planning will need to reflect this. Your visual aids, if you use them, will need to be tailored to the available equipment and to the size of the room. If you plan to use video and sound, then the technical facilities must be available, intact and there must be a technician who knows how to use them. It is no use trying to use felt tip written overheads in a big lecture theatre—they will be too dim.

Rule 5: Plan your talk carefully

When you come to plan your presentation you must give it an overall plan. Don't fire up PowerPoint to make your first slide. You will need an introduction, a summing up and a number of points will be discussed in between. If you have eight points in a twenty-minute talk you will have two minutes for each topic. More sensible is four points for twenty and six for thirty minutes. A lecture will have two or three important messages in it. Plan your talk so that these do not get lost in a gabble of detail that is unimportant. Remember that if your audience really needs to learn all that detail, attending a lecture is a bad way to set about it. Among other things the lecture may set the scene for the hard work of learning, it may describe the importance of different aspects of the learning and set emphasis and it can select a small number of difficult issues and try to clarify them. There is no point in standing up to play the part of a talking textbook. Use examples and stories to make your talk seem relevant and vivid.

Rule 6: Take account of what the audience knows about your topic

Unless you are giving a particular, uncommon type of talk where the whole of a topic must be dealt with, you must select your material to suit the audience. The more mixed the audience, the more difficult this is. If most of your audience are fully conversant with the foundation of what you are going to say, they will loose interest if you repeat it. Doctors often start right at the beginning and try to cover the whole ground, as though they were organising an examination answer. This is a mistake. Find out what the audience knows already, before you start to plan. If you are concerned about this, ring the organiser and ask what the audience will know about specific topics. I advise against asking whether to include a topic, the organiser will usually say yes—they are not planning and delivering the lecture. When the audience has very different levels of information you have to decide where to pitch. This will depend on the purpose of the whole meeting. Organise your presentation to meet the objectives of the whole day. It may be necessary to accept that your talk will be beyond the understanding of some of the audience and this can be helped by careful introduction and summary for each topic. Similarly there may be some experts present for whom your talk is pitched too low. If you are a real expert in your field you may also want to incorporate a couple of advanced points, specifically for these people—but they should be very brief.

Rule 7: Practice your talk

There's no way to become comfortable as a lecturer except through experience. Some events are very scary and no amount of practice will stop you being frightened. Proper preparation can help though. Next time you hear a really good lecturer be reassured that, even though they may have had some natural talent, much of their excellence has been achieved by hard work and practice. Inexperienced presenters should always write out their talk in full rather than using headings. They should then practice. If it's a really high stakes event for you, it is best to practice until you practically know it by heart. Get someone to listen and criticise your performance. Finally do the whole thing, at a lectern, with someone watching. This helps you to get all your timings right, it lets you find phrases that you have written that you can't get your tongue round and it will probably show up if you have any annoying habits. It's not possible to offer coaching advice on paper but there are a number of things to watch out for. Stand still—don't sway and don't pace. If you are able to leave the lectern it's a good idea to move about but not too much. Use your arms for emphasis but practice it in the mirror. You don't want to look like a wind farm. Talk slowly and allow deliberate pauses. Most inexperienced presenters talk much too fast and this makes their tone tedious. Vary the loudness and pitch of your voice. Deliver some sections quietly and then raise your voice for emphasis. Again, enough is enough, you don't want your voice to be coming and going as though you were talking into a gusty wind. Look at the audience and vary where you look. Look to the back as well as the front. Speak to specific individuals in the audience. This makes your delivery look more natural. But, if you get their eye contact, don't hold it, it's very disconcerting for them!

Good, experienced speakers develop an individual style. This includes their delivery, the way they construct their talks and the way they use visual aids. The best way to develop a platform style is to practice and to take note of the way other speakers behave. As regards style, most speakers develop a number of formats that suit them—for instance, shaping a talk around a number of clinical cases with interesting circumstantial detail.

Rule 8: Check the facilities—on the day

Arrive early. You will need to check that you can work the presentation equipment or whether everything will be done for you. Can you operate the auditorium lights? Do you understand how to use the microphone? Many speakers don't use the microphone even though they can't be heard. If there's a microphone—use it. Remember, your mouth is quite near to your ears! Most speakers benefit from amplification—it allows them to talk, rather than shout. Speakers don't use it because they have not taken two minutes to try it out.

Do your audio-visuals project? Run right through your presentation to check that all your slides look right. Sometimes, for a variety of reasons, one or two slides may need to be adjusted.

Make sure that you have a drink of water available.

Rule 9: Listen to the other speakers

Whenever possible a speaker should attend the whole part of the meeting that is relevant to their participation. A good educational event builds the information, insight and understanding of the participants and they will often ask for opinions and advice from presenters throughout the meeting. It is therefore best to set aside the time to attend the whole meeting. There are exceptions. Some meetings have a sequence of presentations that are unrelated, and where each presenter has little expertise in the other fields. More often the speakers are expected to interact as a faculty. If this is the case it is rude to talk and then leave. If you can't afford the time; don't agree to speak. They will find someone else.

Sometimes listening to the other speakers allows you to adjust your talk. If a speaker covers one of your points, or raises an issue that you think you should comment on, then you can take this into account. If a presenter shows a slide that you have also used, then you can delete it. But, beware of fiddling with a PowerPoint presentation at the last moment in case you mess it up.

Rule 10: Avoid jokes

Never tell religious, off colour, racist or sexist jokes. Never stigmatise identifiable groups—such as orthopaedic surgeons! Recently, I spoke at a meeting where an experienced co-presenter told blue and Irish jokes and showed a semi-obscene slide. A number of members of the audience were affronted and even more were made uncomfortable by knowing that their friends were upset. Jokes in general are always risky. Anyone who has told jokes to friends knows that they can go flat. You don't want that to happen in front of a large audience. Cartoons can lighten the mood and get a laugh but they should be relevant and suitable. I have a cartoon that I think is very funny and I have used it in several presentations. Sometimes the audience laughs uproariously but sometimes there is scarcely a titter. If you are worried about the presentation, why take the risk? Humour is however another matter. Most really good presenters use humour. It is usually low key and they often turn it against themselves. Relevant anecdotes are a very good way of introducing a light-hearted element. Doctors love to hear clinical stories and real situations can almost invariably be used to frame the lessons.

- Always talk on what you know.
- Always arrive early.
- Check with the other speakers for overlapping topics.
- Don't use 35 mm slides or overheads.
- Check every PowerPoint slide on the presentation hall computer.
- Time matters—it is far better to finish early than be late.
- Prepare a clear handout well in advance of your lecture.

And lastly—always have a handout. It should not just be a print out of your slides. It should summarise your talk and provide a list of further reading and websites. Your feedback will be much better if you provide a handout!

Good luck!

J. David Greaves

18

Using audio-visual material in presentations

J. David Greaves

Every presenter must both inform and entertain. Entertainment is not just a refinement; it lends a structure to a presentation in a way that can enhance learning. Audio-visual accessories help achieve both the structure and the entertainment. Presentation software has revolutionised the way audio-visual content is used in medical teaching.

Overhead projection

Overheads are useful in small rooms but they are not bright enough for large displays and they are often rather crudely produced using felt tip pens to draw on the transparencies. They are not very versatile with regard to what can be put on the slide. The projector itself is not very expensive, it is uncomplicated and one is usually to be found wherever a presentation is to be made. Overhead transparencies can be printed using a laser printer and this type is relatively durable though it is only black and white. Inkjet printing is always easy to smudge and rub off—even when dry. It is important to use bold large type, as the much-magnified writing will become dim and blurred.

A more recent development of overheads is actually a re-invention of the old epidiascope. The optics of these machines allows the projection of an image of non-transparent material that is placed under it. With these slides can be printed on paper and can be as versatile as the printer allows. The episcope optics are better than those of an overhead projector but the light is still not bright enough to allow large magnification. Episcopes are not widely available.

Slide projectors

For many years slide projectors have been the high quality way of delivering images during lectures. They are now being superseded by computers and video projectors for a number of good reasons. Chief amongst these is the versatility of the image editing facilities of electronic presentation software. Other disadvantages of slides are their bulk, the difficulty of storing them and the difficulty of projecting them without errors. Slides often appeared reversed or inverted, the machine sticks and the slide order often gets mixed up. Another disadvantage of 35 mm slides is the cost of their production.

Until recently it was the PowerPoint devotee who was most likely to encounter projection problems. Now, however, most presenters use the computer and the speaker who arrives with slides may find that the projector in disrepair. A request for 'dual projection', in particular, is beyond the capacity of many lecture theatres.

Electronic presentation software

The new standard for presentations is Microsoft PowerPoint. The technique of making these slideshows can be learned from one of the simple manuals available. These can be used to guide the learner through the stages of making a variety of slides. These will improve with practice. One of the best resources for the novice is a more experienced colleague who is usually very willing to help.

What are its advantages and disadvantages of presentation software?

In my opinion, the biggest snag with PowerPoint stems from its greatest strength—its ease of use. Everyone uses PowerPoint and this has the effect of making presentations monotonous in a number of ways. Most serious of these is the way it imposes uniformity upon lectures. The routine PowerPoint slide designs make very heavy use of a system of headings and bullet points. This dictates a structure. About six bullet points will go on a slide so that is what presenters tend to do. If you want to add extra text or sub-headings on a slide it rapidly becomes cluttered so presenters tend to simplify to a routine of headings and bullets. There is of course nothing intrinsically wrong with this, other than the fact that it stands in the way of a lecturer developing an individual style. Good lecturers have such style in what they say, how they say it and the visuals they use.

Perhaps as serious, is the way that PowerPoint can lead a lecturer to make the text of their presentation into a series of screens that they then read out. Why is the presenter there? If you find yourself dictating from your slides then you could be doing better.

Having said all of which, for the in-department presentation none of these criticisms stand. Compared to other available methods PowerPoint will allow clear, orderly presentations much better than anything else. The bullet point format is OK for the sort of teaching that is usually being done and following the text through the bullet points is less jarring in a small classroom than in a large lecture theatre.

The uses of audio-visual materials—general comments

Your audio-visuals are there to add an extra dimension to the presentation. The audience can now both hear and see what you mean. They show the structure, order and hierarchy of your arguments and highlight the things that you consider important.

They can be used as signboards, 'This is what I am talking about' or as signposts, 'This is the way we are going'. Graphics can show relationships and illustrations of what you are talking about. It is a good idea to start with an introduction slide that shows the arguments you will be developing and end with a conclusions slide. The conclusion slide can often be a repeat of the introduction slide. The slides do not need to stand alone. It does not matter if they do not make sense without your spoken commentary they are intended for a lecture. Many presenters make their display very laborious because they endeavour to make the visuals self-sufficient.

The projection can prompt the presenter. This is not the same as reading out a presentation off the screen. Ideally the prompts to the presenter will not be quite so obvious to the audience. One of the great strengths of PowerPoint is the ease of including pictures. Appropriate pictures can be used as cues. In the previous chapter I emphasised the importance of anecdote and examples in giving relevance to presentations. Pictures of these contexts or objects associated with stories can provide prompts.

The watchword for making any presentation must be 'relevance'. Keep telling them what it means to them. First the presentation must deal with the topic in ways that are useful to the audience. Secondly deal with contexts that your audience understands, use everyday examples that will be familiar to them and tell them stories that they will recognise. All of this will mean that a presentation will need to be modified to specifically fit each audience and on every occasion that it is given.

Ten dos and don'ts for preparing and using visual-aids

Irrespective of the type of presentation system used there are good and bad slides and good and bad ways to use them.

Rule 1: Your material must be legible

It is blindingly obvious that visual aids must be legible and it is perhaps surprising that a warning is necessary. Overhead projectors produce very dim light. The intensity of illumination varies with the square of the distance, so in a large meeting room you can choose between a dim slide projected large or an area of projection that is too small for the audience to read. With this in mind, use dense colours to write and choose a medium point marker. To make really clear overheads print them on a laser printer or copier. If you do this choose fonts that are suitable for the size of your room. The smallest font size that is reasonably legible on an overhead is 20 pt and something over 32 is best. Do not put more than ten lines on an overhead.

Similar caveats apply to 35 mm slides and PowerPoint. Do you want the room to be light or dark when you talk? The background to your slides will provide the level of illumination. Blue backgrounds are common but give a dim light that encourages sleep. Clear or yellow backgrounds make the room lighter. If you use clear screens use very dark type—black is best. If you use dark screens, use a light type—white on blue is suitable. Check that the colour combinations you choose for font and background show up well in the size of room you will be using.

Rule 2: Don't dazzle the audience

Keep your colours simple. Shades of pink, lime green and purple are hard on the eyes. Some projector systems do not show 'designer colours' the same as on the computer screen and unexpected incompatibilities may show up. I recommend sticking to clear primary colours. Limit yourself to a palette of no more than six.

Rule 3: Use appropriate fonts

Use simple fonts that are legible when projected. I restrict myself to three: Times New Roman, Arial and Comic Sans MS. Fancy cursive scripts and novelty items often don't show up well. Also, uncommon fonts may not be resident on the computer you are using for projection, so check before you start. If you think a font may be a problem and it is a 'True Type' font you can use the command 'Embed True Type fonts' from the tools menu, when you save your presentation and the file will incorporate the font information. The most common example of 'font failure' to see is where fancy bullets have been used. The projection computer's best guess at the effect you hoped for can ruin your slide.

Choose fonts that are large enough. I don't use anything smaller than 20 pt. For headings use 36 pt or larger. These large fonts will restrict the number of lines you will be able to get on your screen.

Rule 4: Beware of backgrounds

The PowerPoint system provides many customised backgrounds. These are touted as giving a professional finish to your presentation. A few years ago, when few were adepts, this was the case. Now some backgrounds are so common that they add drab uniformity to a day of presentations. Firstly, be sure that your chosen custom look satisfies the requirements of light, colour and font types that you want. Next, take a look at the layout. Most set-ups restrict your use of the left hand side and top of the slide by having graphics in the background. Do you mind this limitation? Lastly, does the background spoil the clarity of the slide? If you choose to use a custom background remember there is an option that enables you to miss it off individual slides if it is interfering with their clarity.

Rule 5: You don't need a slide for everything

Every point does not need to be on a slide. Your visual aids are to help your audience follow the structure of your talk and to illuminate details. Some presenters, in effect, write the text for their talk on the slides. Whilst there is nothing wrong with this, it means that as well as being visual aids for the talk, the slides constitute the lecturer's notes. This leads to the presenter having far more slides than are necessary and, as each point is an opportunity for digression, there is a big risk of running over time. It also leads to a dull presentation style where the lecturer reads out what is on the screen. It is better to have separate notes and to know your material well enough to know when there is a point to discuss that does not use a slide. If you don't have a slide for everything, however, there is a chance of missing things out. A good way round this is to use pictures and clip art. A graphic can be chosen so as to prompt an anecdote or case history—without actually including any of the text.

Rule 6: Beware of bullets

Bullets lend even more uniformity to presentations. Thirty headings, each with five or six bullet points, may give a clear structure but they lead to a staccato delivery style and none of the slides are interesting or entertaining.

Try breaking lists up and putting each point in a box. The boxes can be any shape, lines and arrows can show connections and the background colour in the box can also be used to demonstrate relationships. Boxes can appear simultaneously, in groups or one at a time providing a further demonstration of relationships.

Check that there is a suitable space between your bullet and the text. It is common to see them cramped together. You can increase the indent after the bullet by viewing the ruler and moving the tabs.

Rule 7: Beware of special effects

PowerPoint allows fancy transitions between slides and the introduction of items separately. These effects can be used to produce 'animations' that appear to make slides build up or perform actions. Some presenters introduce very clear messages in this way and their slide animations are fundamental to the clarity of their message. Others, however, use pointless 'busy' transitions and effects that obscure the message and distract the audience. If you have a slide with five bullets don't introduce them line-by-line unless you have a reason. Let the audience see your five points, give them fifteen seconds to read them and then talk your talk. A similar warning applies to the overhead projector striptease. An overhead is often flashed up and then masked with paper that is then drawn down a line at a time. I think this is very distracting. Again, show your slide and then talk through it. If there are things, results for example, that you don't want the audience to see yet; put them on a new slide with a new heading.

Rule 8: Use 'punctuation' slides

It is well recognised that audiences need a break from concentration. Using an anecdote for instance can do this. The audio-visuals are, however, wonderfully versatile at providing lighter moments. A good picture is worth more than a thousand words. It should be relevant, entertaining or amusing and not offensive. Relevant still photographs taken by the author in the course of work are very useful. I am less sure of pictures of holidays, mountains climbed or the presenter's children (or more often, dog). In my view these fail the task of relevance. Try and incorporate a relevant interesting graphic into every third or fourth slide. There are hundreds of thousands of photographs of every possible situation that can be downloaded from the internet.

Rule 9: Beware of audio and video

Pieces of video are excellent—if relevant. Unfortunately many lecture theatres have underpowered computers that loose the synchrony of sound and vision when projecting, so beware. Video will increase your file size to many megabytes, and can make transporting it into the guest computer a headache. Postgraduate centres are often the final resting ground of tired old machines.

Sound is a particular problem. Many lecture theatres have no audio facility, so if your presentation needs sound you need to check. If you intercalate stray sounds into your presentation the audience may not be expecting them. They are likely to think the sudden sound is something outside the window and you will loose the effect you expected. Sometimes a presentation has been made on a computer with the sound turned off and a slide transition with accompanying audio has been included by mistake. If this happens to you, turn off the sound. I have watched a presenter go through about a dozen slides with a ricocheting bullet effect before someone explained to him how to get rid of it.

Rule 10: Check your presentation on site

When you arrive to give your lecture you must check your presentation. If you are using a projector, load and project all your slides to check they are in order and right way round. It is a wise precaution to write numbers on the mounts of 35 mm slides in case the carousel falls on the floor. It is essential to number overheads. They will fall on the floor. Check that overheads can be read from the auditorium.

Using PowerPoint in a strange environment is a minefield. How are you transporting your presentation? Some institutions will not allow guest laptops to be connected, and you must use a medium with sufficient capacity to transfer your talk. Take two copies. I also make a copy with most of the graphics stripped out so that it will go on a floppy. Some older CD ROMs will not read all formats of read/write discs. Less common media such as Zip discs and USB media may not be available, even if the organiser has told you that they are. If possible email your presentation to be loaded in advance—but do not assume it has been properly loaded. Always test it and have another copy with you.

Incompatibilities of versions of Microsoft Windows and PowerPoint are now less common though it is as well to remember that some lecture theatres may be equipped with versions that are several years out of date. Old software will not project the latest version. Some features of presentations may call for features that are not often used and you may be the first person to reveal that a part of the programme is corrupted. So, test your presentation and project every slide. Failures and unexpected effects and appearances can be mended.

The meeting organiser should know how they want presentations loaded and organised. However they often do not know what they are doing. If this is the case load your presentation onto the host desktop and in so doing give it your name. Sometimes presenters use very similar names such as 'Birmingham Presentation' or 'Lung study', and you may not be sure which is yours. If you are using your own computer turn off any screen-saver and make sure the charger is plugged in and turned on. If the computer is ready and waiting on one of a number of connections to the projector make sure that it is secure and out of the way. If the previous presenter can reach your computer and close the lid, it is common for them to do so. This sabotages all your preparation, as you will have to re-boot.

It is important to avoid all these little pitfalls, not because your audience will notice your amateurish approach but because you will get flustered and this might make you give a bad presentation. Never underestimate how scared you can get in front of an audience.

- Always talk on what you know.
- Always arrive early.
- Check with the other speakers for overlapping topics.
- Don't use 35 mm slides or overheads.
- Check every PowerPoint slide on the presentation hall computer.
- Time matters—it is far better to finish early than be late.
- Prepare a clear handout well in advance of your lecture.

19

Electrical safety

Steve Graham

The use of electricity is one of the major markers of a 'modern' society. This dominates much of medicine's daily activities in one form or another. There are few reasons for deliberately applying electricity to your patients, although when we choose to do so it is often using substantial power. Unfortunately, there may also be many occasions on which you will do so inadvertently, and patients have been injured or even killed on occasions in the past by electrical forces or their consequences. Understanding the effects of electricity is one of the key requirements for using electrical equipment safely.

Terminology

Most materials permit an electrical current to flow through them when they are used to link two points with a potential (voltage) difference. These materials are termed *conductors* of electricity. Conductance occurs by stripping off electrons from the outer shell of atoms and moving them onto the next receiving atom, and so on. In doing this, work is done to move these electrons, and this is described as the material presenting a *resistance* to the flow of current. A material that is resistant to current flow is called a *resistor*, while materials preventing current flow are termed *insulators*. Under extreme conditions even insulators may permit electrical currents to flow. High potential differences can permit currents to flow without direct contact, in the form of electrical sparks. In normal conditions, this will happen when the potential difference between source and target is greater than 600 V per cm of air separation. If normal mains electricity is the source, then such conduction will occur if you place your fingers within 4 mm of the electrical source. If higher voltages are used in the source, then 'safe' distances need to be much greater, or more insulation needs to be present.

Table 1. The effects of passing electricity through a body from one hand to the other.

Current	Effect
>1 mA	Mild tingling noted
>15 mA	Tonic contractions of muscle noted (flexors stronger than extensors); If held in the hand, unable to let go of the current source; Risk of asphyxia from contracture of intercostal muscles
>75 mA	Danger of ventricular fibrillation
>5 A	Tonic contracture of ventricular muscle

Effects of electricity on the normal body

Small amounts of electricity will do little harm to the body. Currents of around 0.5–1.5 mA are normal when using nerve stimulators, and even then effects will only be noted when the needle is close to the nerve. Table 1 lists the effects of higher currents passing through the whole body from one hand to the other. In this it is important to remember that all living creatures are driven by electrical potentials, and that it is possible to disrupt most physiological processes by application of electrical signals. The electrical impulses of heart, nerve and brain are the most obvious, but all cell surface activity is driven by similar potential differences.

Very high currents (with power dissipation of up to 200 W, and potential differences of 9 kV) may be used with cutting diathermy, and this results in local tissue destruction. A large area low resistance return plate is essential if severe burns are to be avoided, and a good insulator (such as rubber gloves) is required to protect the user from an electric shock. The cardiac risks listed in Table 1 result only from that part of the whole current that passes through the heart. If the current is directed through the heart more directly, such as through a wire or catheter directed into the heart, then much smaller currents will produce major cardiac effects. This is termed microshock.

Static electricity

When one material is rubbed up against another electrons may be transferred from one to the other. In this manner a charge may be built up on each material. This is termed *static electricity*. The electrical potential built up this way may be substantial—lightning is an extreme example—but even the static built up on a human being may result in generation of sparks when the carrier is close to an earth point. The effect of such sparks may be treated as any other high potential electrical source. The ability of static sparks to ignite fires in a susceptible environment was the drive to provide operating theatres with a static-free environment. In this context, cotton was the preferred clothing material (silk/nylon discouraged) and all materials were mildly conductive and earthed where possible.

Earth differences

In electrical terminology, an earth is regarded as being at zero potential. In practice, the complex interaction of electrical sources means that the potential at one particular point on the Earth may be slightly different to that of another. If two earth sources with different potentials are connected together then current will flow between them. If a patient is used to link them, then patient injury may occur. Since many pieces of equipment earth the patient as a safety feature, this may represent a significant risk. There are two ways to minimise this problem—most rooms in a building (while they may have many different power supplies) have only one earth source, but at local levels most equipment has metal lugs labelled as *equipotential bonding points*, which may be connected together with good conductors such as copper cables, which will eliminate earth differences.

Capacitative and inductive linkage

Electrical signals can pass between an electrical source and a second conductor without direct electrical current flow. If a positive charge is applied to a surface, then any free electrons in nearby surfaces will tend to be attracted towards it. If this surface was then made negatively charged, then the nearby electrons will be driven away. If a varying charge is applied to that surface (driven by an alternating voltage) then the nearby surfaces will have their electrons repeatedly attracted to and driven away, and behave as if a varying potential had been applied directly to it. This is termed *capacitative linkage*.

When current flows in a conductor, a magnetic field is generated by that current. By a similar process, when a magnetic field moves through a conductor, a current is generated. An alternating current produces a magnetic field that rises and falls with the variation of the current. If this moving magnetic field contacts a second conductor then a varying current will be induced in that second conductor. This is termed *inductive linkage.* Since mains electricity and all electronic equipment use alternating current (AC) sources, this can be a powerful source of induced signals. The risks from these induced currents can be minimised by either keeping potentials low, maximising physical separation (the effects are inversely related to the square of the separation distance), shielding the source of signal (wrapping it in a continuous sheet of metal—often the frame of the device), or directing the currents to flow so as to minimise interactions (this usually means running the source conductors to run pointing directly towards or away from anything where you wish to avoid induced currents).

Pacemakers

A pacemaker is a device that both senses electrical signals and generates a potential that is then conducted directly into the heart via a wire (or two wires, depending on the design). Electrical interference may generate a number of problems.

Powerful electrical signals (such as may be generated by diathermy) can trick the pacemaker into believing that a cardiac impulse has been sensed, and that the demand pacing function may therefore be switched off during the interference. Ideally diathermy should be avoided in patients with pacemakers, with bipolar diathermy being the next best option if unavoidable. If monopolar diathermy must be used, then the earth plate should be used to direct current at right angles to a line joining the operating site to the pacemaker. Cutting diathermy, with its greater power, should be avoided.

The pacemaker provides a direct, highly conductive path for electrical signals into the myocardium. This can then allow relatively small currents to produce substantial cardiac effects (see the effects of MRI).

The presence of a battery and electrical pathways (even more of a problem with implantable defibrillators) means that in the event of someone with a pacemaker having a cardiac arrest, then extreme care should be taken with the high energy of an externally applied defibrillator, as the pacemaker can be damaged or even caused to explode.

Diathermy

Diathermy is a technique where electricity is used to generate heat to coagulate bleeding points or cut tissue. The power utilisation is high (up to 300 W with voltages up to 9 kV at very high frequency—up to 6 kHz), and the risk of electrical damage is high. A clear electrical pathway is essential. Monopolar diathermy uses a point source for effect, with a large neutral electrode for the return pathway. The neutral electrode must be a large area low resistance pathway—modern adhesive gel electrodes are always preferable. The current passed between the two electrodes, and a pathway through the heart MUST be avoided. Particular care is essential if a pacemaker is present (avoiding diathermy is preferable, and if necessary bipolar is better). Bipolar diathermy passes the current between the two points of the diathermy forceps and therefore minimises current dissipation.

Magnetic Resonance Imaging scanners

A Magnetic Resonance Imaging (MRI) scanner is a device that relies on developing zones of high moving magnetic field strengths and high electromagnetic (radiofrequency) signals. Any conductor is linked with these generators through both capacitative and inductive coupling. A conductor in a moving magnetic field functions as one half of a dynamo; in a radio environment it functions as an aerial. As a consequence, powerful signals can be developed in any conductor to either swamp what you are trying to measure, damage the input circuits of the monitor, or even injure your patient. In general, ECG monitoring can be quite dangerous, and pacemakers are absolutely forbidden, while only specially protected electrical equipment can be operated within an MRI environment. The warning signs on the doors should give warning of the level of problems!

Safety standards

Tables 2 and 3 list the safety classifications that will apply to medical devices. If a fault can result in a voltage being applied to the internal framework of the device, and the framework is accessible by the operator, it is necessary for safety that the current be diverted to earth. An earth wire is then mandatory for safety (a Class I device). In Class II devices, it should be impossible to access the interior of the device and an earth connection is not essential. Class III devices are low power, and low voltage, with a low potential for harm. None the less, all electrical devices leak energy to some degree. A separate classification

Table 2. Classification of medical equipment by electrocution risk from contact with the chassis.

Safety category	Properties
Class I	Exposed metal chassis, which must be connected to an earth.
Class II	The internal components are double insulated, and contact with electrical components should be impossible. An earth connection is not required.
Class III	Electricity is supplied at less than 24 Volts.

Table 3. Classification of medical equipment by maximum tolerated leakage currents.

Safety category	Maximum leakage current, normal operating	Maximum leakage current, single fault condition
Class B	0.1 mA	0.5 mA
Class C	0.01 mA	0.05 mA

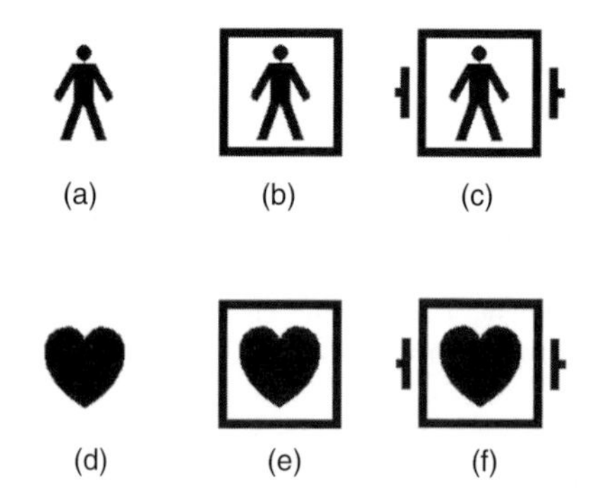

Figure 1. Symbols associated with electrical safety classifications. (a) Class B; (b) class BF; (c) defibrillator-safe class BF; (d) class C; (e) class CF; (f) defibrillator-safe class CF.

system defines the maximum permitted leakage. Class B devices are permitted a higher maximum leakage, and should therefore be used for body surface application only. Class C devices have a lower maximum permitted leakage, and are appropriate for devices such as monitoring systems that introduce a current path closer to the heart. Figure 1 illustrates the symbols that are applied to such devices. Where the term F is added, it indicates that the mains power supply has been isolated from the core of the device (floating power supply).

Defibrillation

A defibrillator is a powerful source of electrical energy, with the higher defibrillator settings generating potential differences of 3–5 kV. As with all powerful tools, you should obtain training in its use before using it on a patient. The energy delivered should be appropriate to the situation and the patient, and as low as possible. There should be good contact with the skin via conductive gel pads to reduce skin resistance. If using electrode gel, be careful that a film of gel does not develop between the two contact points, or the flash from the charge arcing between the two paddles will be impressive and damaging. The current will always take the path of least resistance, so a final check is necessary to ensure that the patient is not in contact with any metal structure (a risk of burns to the patient) or other members of the resuscitation team (a risk of electrocution).

Fire hazards

Hospitals are environments with lots of added oxygen. As a consequence, it becomes easier to burn materials, and any fires burn faster and hotter. In extreme examples, a fire may be so rapid that it presents as an explosion. The closer the fire is to an oxygen source (facemasks, anaesthetic circuits, etc.), the greater the local oxygen concentration, and the greater the risk. With anaesthetic circuits, it is important to note that although the oxygen concentration might be relatively low, the gap is often filled with nitrous oxide, which supports combustion even better than oxygen. Many skin cleaning fluids are based on alcohols, and are therefore flammable, while mixtures containing diethyl ether or acetone are potentially explosive if the vapour is mixed with a spark (such as diathermy, static, etc.) or a heat source in an oxygen-rich environment.

- Electricity is potentially hazardous.
- Always read the manuals before using electrical devices.
- Where possible get specific training in the use of electrical devices.
- Warning symbols are there for a purpose—understand them. They are supposed to be intuitive, but experience suggests otherwise.

20

Writing a discharge letter

Philip A. Corbett and William A. Corbett

Introduction

Producing a discharge letter can be a daunting prospect. What do you include in it and what do you leave out? The answer to these questions lies in the purpose of the letter itself. Discharge letters are an essential means of communication in patient management between primary and secondary care. Relevant clinical information must be shared between health care professionals and so discharge letters should contain information helpful to the process and they should be sent and received in a timely manner. There remains a primary consideration in all these forms of correspondence and that is patient confidentiality.

Interim discharge letter

This should be e-mailed or faxed to the patient's primary care team within 24 hours of the patient leaving hospital. The patient's GP should be informed that the discharge has happened and that the information is being sent. This should be done by a telephone call as all other means of communication have in-built delays. The letter should then be sent.

The discharge letter is a *brief* report that should contain the important information that the patient's GP will need to enable a safe and effective care programme to be achieved. The majority of letters are still hand-written despite the ubiquitous availability of desktop computers. It is a simple task to create a template that can be used for all patients, and then simply completed on discharge. It should always include the following information:

- Full patient details;
- Date and type of admission and discharge;

- Consultant in charge;
- Diagnosis—acute and chronic conditions;
- Key investigations;
- Treatment—surgical, medical and drug;
- Any complications;
- Date and place of follow-up;
- Contact details of the admitting team.

The inclusion of a receipt function on the e-mail or fax will enable the team to confirm in writing that the information has been delivered on time.

Discharge summary

This is usually used as a précis of the whole admission and is used primarily by the hospital medical staff. Long-winded letters, with vast amounts of data, are rarely useful in primary care.

Key information in the summary will include all the major details of the admission and the treatment plan. This encompasses the clinical multidisciplinary team, pathology and other results, expected progress of the patient (for example the need for rehabilitation or palliative care) and of other teams that may need to be involved (Social Services or MacMillan nursing teams for instance). Finally, no discharge summary is complete without the clinical coding being checked for accuracy. This may often be ignored but it is the information upon which all hospital (and specialist) published data is based on.

- Ring the practice to inform them the patient is being discharged.
- Use a template to write the discharge letter to avoid missing out important data.
- Confirm delivery has occurred.
- The summary should be comprehensive and include clinical coding.
- Writing the discharge letter is part of Clinical governance.
- Only write by hand if other people can read it.

Other issues

Patient access

There is good evidence that patients wish to have access to their discharge letters. If this is to be done then their needs must be considered. Plain English terms should be used where possible and abbreviations avoided.

Security

Fax and e-mail systems are not infallible and appropriate protocols must be followed in both primary and hospital settings. Many areas have defined protocols that will ensure that the receiving practice has to confirm their identity before the information if sent. Password protection on computer access is another common solution.

Confidentiality

Every patient has the right to read his or her records. Access to these records by other people has been difficult with written notes but is becoming more likely with electronic data storage. The health services are striving to provide an electronic patient record (EPR) and these security and confidentiality issues will have to be addressed as the EPR is introduced.

Conclusion

The discharge of a patient from hospital to their own home is a dangerous time. Only with the appropriate information provided in a timely manner can the primary care team maintain the process of recovery and ensure that appropriate nursing care, medication, physiotherapy and social care are available for the patient.

Example letter

Dr A Smith
The Surgery
1 The High Street
Anytown
XX1 2YY

Dear Dr Smith

19th February 2003

Re: Brian Jones DOB 13/03/1949
42 Acacia Avenue, Anytown, XY2 3AB

Emergency admission	to ward 8, The James Cook Hospital, on 30 January 2003
Admission Diagnosis:	Large bowel obstruction
Invest. 30/01/2003:	CTscan-obstructing cancer sigmoid colon with liver metastases.
Proc. 30/01/2003:	Radiological insertion of intraluminal colonic stent. IV sedation.
Opn 3/02/2003:	Palliative sigmoid colectomy with primary anastomosis and liver biopsy. GA with epidural analgesia.

Mr Jones postoperative recovery was complicated by acute urinary retention which required replacement of his urinary catheter. The catheter was successfully removed before he was discharged home. There were no other significant complications. The pathology report of the removed specimens confirmed the radiological and operative diagnosis of advanced colonic cancer. His situation was discussed at our regular Colorectal Cancer MultiDisciplinary Team meeting and Mr Jones will see our Oncologist, Dr Black, at The James Cook University Hospital next week. The MacMillan Nurses were present at the meeting and have seen Mr Jones whilst he was on the ward and with his approval they have made arrangements to see him at home within a week of his discharge from hospital.

I saw Mr Jones with his wife on the ward after the operation when all the results were available and explained to them that the blockage in the bowel was caused by a cancer which has been removed. They understand that cancer remains in the liver. I did explain that although his condition was not curable a significant benefit could be obtained from palliative chemotherapy. I recommended that he see Dr Black as arranged in the outpatient clinic to discuss this option.

Discharged home from ward 8 on 19 February 2003

Discharge Diagnosis: Advanced carcinoma of colon with liver metastases

Drugs on discharge:

Coproxamol two tablets 4 hrly as reqd for pain	40 tablets dispensed
Fybogel one sachet twice daily	28 sachets dispensed

Follow-up arrangements:

Surgical outpatient follow-up	11.30 am 13/03/2003.
Oncology outpatient appointment with Dr Black	10.00 am 24/02/2003.

The District Nurse has been asked to visit Mr Jones at home within 24 hours of discharge. The Macmillan Nurse Service will visit within the first week after discharge.

Yours sincerely

A N Other
Consultant Surgeon

Further reading

1 Longstaff JJ, Thick MG, Capper G, Lockyear MA. A model of accountability, confidentiality and override for healthcare and other applications. Fifth ACM Workshop in Role-Based Access Control, Berlin July 2000. ISBN 1-58113-259-X.

Section 2

Higher Skills

21

Sedation

Mike G. Bramble

Introduction

Sedation is widely used by clinicians in hospital medicine, particularly in gastroenterology, gynaecology and radiology but also in chest medicine and cardiology.

The main reason for using sedation as a pre-medication for an endoscopic or minor surgical procedure is patient comfort and to make an investigation, which to many seems unpleasant, into one which can be tolerated and if necessary repeated without the patient experiencing any distress. It is also important in endoscopy to examine the relevant part of the GI tract thoroughly and this may be very difficult if the patient is unable to tolerate the procedure because of discomfort and/or inadequate sedation. Similarly in other branches of medicine patients benefit from the skilled administration of a sedative drug but this must always be delivered in a safe and controlled way.

Physiology

Safe sedation equates to conscious sedation so that verbal contact is maintained at all times. Loss of verbal contact implies that the patient is more deeply sedated than necessary with all the associated risks of a general anaesthetic.

Practicing safe sedation requires a detailed knowledge of how the drugs work and their mode of action. Benzodiazepines in particular have a slow onset of action and carry a risk of respiratory depression in certain susceptible groups of patients.

The definition of conscious sedation is as follows:

> **'a technique in which the use of a drug or drugs produces a state of depression of the central nervous system enabling treatment to be carried out, but during which verbal contact with the patient is maintained throughout the period of sedation … should carry a margin of safety wide enough to render the loss of consciousness unlikely.'**

The effects of sedation are increased in certain situations and it is important for endoscopists to recognise those conditions, which increase the effect of drugs commonly used to achieve conscious sedation. These include:

- **Abnormal lean body mass index**
- **Dehydration**
- **Poor hepatic function**
- **Poor renal function**
- **Cardiac failure**
- **Chronic pulmonary disease**
- **Increasing age**

The UK Academy of Medical Royal Colleges and their Faculties published a working party report in 2001 entitled "*Implementing and ensuring SAFE SEDATION PRACTICES for healthcare procedures in adults*." In this document the recommendation is made that the Royal Colleges define appropriate techniques for each group of specialist procedures and that there is formal instruction on sedation techniques for those practicing in that specialty or training in that specialty. At hospital level trusts are required to appoint a user of sedation and an anaesthetist to lead recommendations covering all users of sedation as part of their practice.

Indications

The indications for sedation relate to the benefits for the patient who might otherwise be distressed by a long or uncomfortable procedure. Sometimes sedation also makes the procedure easier for the clinician carrying out the procedure (particularly in endoscopy where many patients are reluctant to suffer discomfort and have a fear of embarrassing themselves). The main benefits are:

- Patient acceptability;
- Easier for the endoscopist or surgeon;

- Time to perform the procedure;
- Ease of performing the procedure;
- Therapeutic endoscopy.

The risks associated with over-sedation

- Hypoxia;
- Respiratory arrest;
- Cardiorespiratory arrest.

The risks associated with under-sedation

- Invalid consent;
- Withdrawal of consent;
- Injury to the patient, nurse or clinician carrying out the procedure;
- Inadequate examination;
- Complaints;
- Litigation.

The dangers of sedation are minimised by

- Detailed knowledge of the drugs used;
- Inquiry about drug allergy;
- Knowledge of contraindications;
- Knowledge of patient variables.

Important variables

Age
Weight
Previous drug therapy
Alcohol intake
Co-morbidity

How to do the procedure

Basic guidelines

- Irrespective of whether or not the patient is deemed to be 'at risk' all patients should have protected IV access using a plastic cannula.

- Pulse oximetry should be used on all patients and drugs should be available in colour coded syringes.
- Low dose oxygen (2 L/min) via nasal prongs or nasal catheter is safe even for patients with COPD.
- ECG monitoring should to be available if patients are deemed to be at risk of cardiac arrhythmias or critical ischaemia.
- All patients should have a health check questionnaire completed by a competent health care professional such as a nurse or health care assistant suitably trained. This does not absolve the endoscopist or surgeon from the responsibility of making their own assessment of the patient's fitness for the procedure. Special attention should be paid to patients referred from the ward.
- Baseline oxygen saturation measurements are very important in this group, as many are mildly hypoxic before the procedure is commenced.
- DO NOT MEASURE OXYGEN SATURATION ONLY AFTER THE INITIAL INJECTION AS THIS IS TOO LATE!

Which drugs?

The drugs commonly used to achieve conscious sedation are midazolam and diazepam although for colonoscopy and other procedure such as ERCP opiates are often used in small doses to reduce the need for higher doses of benzodiazepines and provide some analgesia during the procedure.

How to make sedation safe

Benzodiazepines

- Be patient (wait 3–4 minutes);
- Use small aliquots (2.5 mg)*;
- Give less, more slowly in the elderly;
- Give minimum sedation required;
- Monitor the effects;
- Have flumazenil available.

*** In older frail patients aliquots of 1 mg are adequate for many patients and even 2.5 mg may induce respiratory depression in a susceptible person.**

Opiates

- Always give the opiate first;
- Avoid in the very elderly;

- Use small aliquots (be prepared to **only** use 25–50 mg of pethidine);
- Do not give more than 50 mg pethidine (or equivalent if fentanyl or alfentanil used);
- Always have naloxone available.

Patient monitoring

It is important to monitor all patients carefully especially during procedures where the lights in the room may be dimmed (radiology or colonoscopy). Pulse oximetry is mandatory and the oxygen saturation should always be >90 %. The nurses and the endoscopist should encourage the patient to relax and breathe normally. Patients should be reassured throughout the procedure and more sedation given only if necessary as determined by any patient distress. This should not include excessive pain.

Remember that there should always be someone whose only task is to monitor the patient. This should not be the endoscopist.

After the procedure

- Check oxygen levels before the patient leaves the endoscopy room.
- If the patient has been heavily sedated oxygen saturations should be measured in the recovery area and oxygen administered if necessary.
- Think about drug reversal with naloxone or flumazenil.

Individuals should review their practice if patients are regularly receiving oxygen post procedure or drug reversal.

- Conscious sedation means maintaining verbal contact.
- Drug distribution may be very slow in elderly patients—take at least a minute between bolus doses.
- Ptosis is one of the cardinal signs of sedation and indicates adequate depth of sedation.
- Recovery may be delayed and clear guidelines for discharge must be followed.
- Practice airway maintenance skills.

Conclusions

- Sedation must be safe.
- Protocols must be in place to ensure patient safety.
- Oversedation is the main danger—be patient!
- Monitoring the patient closely does not substitute for good clinical practice.
- Clinical governance should ensure high standards are maintained.
- Adverse events should be audited on a regular basis.

22

Intravenous regional anaesthesia (Bier's Block)

Chandra M. Kumar

Intravenous Regional Anaesthesia (IVRA) was described originally by a German surgeon, August Bier, in 1908 but became used widely after its re-introduction in 1963 by Holmes. It is widely used in emergency medicine for distal fractures and minor operations on the upper limb and occasionally the lower.

Distension of veins and smaller vessels with local anaesthetic causes diffusion of anaesthetic solution into the nerves and produces anaesthesia for as long as the venous concentration remains high. This can be achieved by blocking the venous outflow and then filling the venous system with a large volume of a dilute local anaesthetic solution injected into a distal vein of an exsanguinated limb.

Deaths from IVRA have resulted from incorrect selection of drug (bupivacaine) and dosage, incorrect technique and the performance of the block by personnel unable to treat toxic reactions.

Advantages and indications

- Ease of administration;
- Rapidity of recovery;
- Rapid onset;
- Muscular relaxation;
- Suitable for open or closed surgical operations distal to elbow (single limb injury requiring surgical manipulation or intervention, carpel tunnel, Dupytren's contracture surgery etc.) as well as lower limb by short surgical procedure;
- IVRA is specially indicated in operations where it is desirable for the surgeon to observe movement of the hand before the end of

the operation. This may be to ensure correct tension in a tendon graft or to ascertain if adequate tenolysis has been performed.

Contraindications

- Absence of resuscitation skills or equipment;
- Unwilling or unco-operative patients;
- In conditions where the use of a tourniquet is contraindicated (sickle cell disease);
- Known allergy to local anaesthetic agent;
- Infection in the affected limb;
- Patients with large lacerations may be unsuitable because a large part of the volume injected may escape through the wound;
- Procedure lasting more than one hour.

Requirement

- Resuscitation trolley and tilting trolley;
- Pneumatic double tourniquet or two single tourniquet of adequate size for the affected limb. An automatic version is preferable;
- 40–50 mL 0.5% prilocaine is used because of its low systemic toxicity, availability in a single dose vial; and it is free of any preservative. 40 mL is the standard adult dose and this should be reduced in frail or elderly patients. Higher volume or more

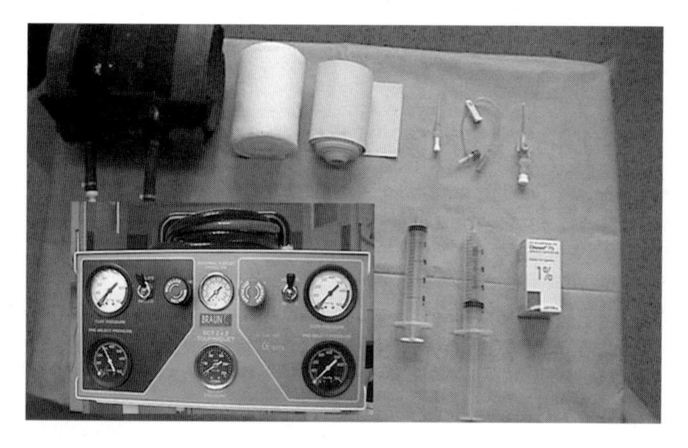

Figure 1. Essential equipments for IVRA.

concentrated solution may be used in healthy subjects with muscular, well-built forearms;
- Two intravenous cannulae.

Technique

- The procedure must be explained to the patient and informed consent must be obtained.
- Resuscitation and other necessary equipments must be checked and the patient should lie supine on a resuscitation trolley.
- Appropriate monitoring equipment must be attached to the patient. Measure the blood pressure before the procedure.
- Wrap a layer of wool padding around the circumference of the operated side above elbow or knee.
- Apply appropriate size, previously checked and properly working, double tourniquet over the padded area.
- Insert an intravenous cannula in non affected limb and check the patency. Insert a small intravenous cannula in the affected limb as distal as possible and check patency.

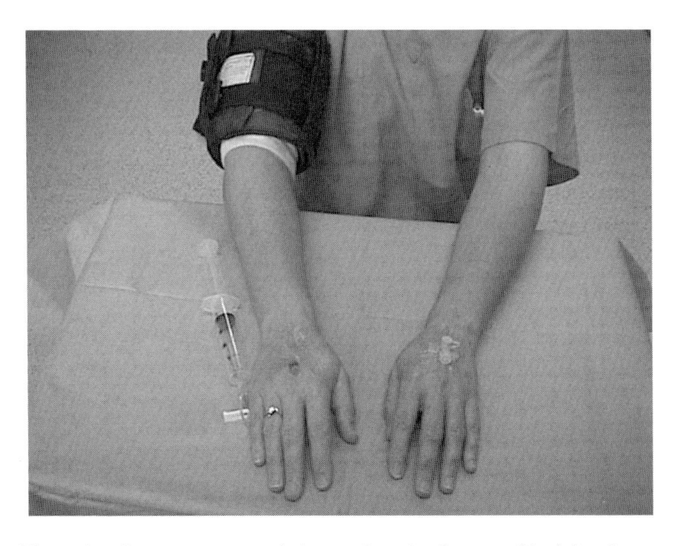

Figure 2. Intravenous cannula inserted on the dorsum of both hands (one for emergency use in non-operated hand and other on the operated side for local anaesthetic injection).

- Exsanguinate the affected limb—elevate the limb for 2–3 minutes or use an Esmarch-type bandage in a non-painful condition.
- With the limb elevated, inflate the upper or proximal cuff on the pneumatic tourniquet to 100 mm Hg above the patient's systolic pressure. Tourniquet pain may be experienced at this stage. Remove the Esmarch bandage if used and allow the limb to return to a comfortable position. Check that the distal pulse in the limb has disappeared. If it has not, then deflate the cuff and recheck the equipment and start again.
- Inject 40–50 mL of 0.5% prilocaine slowly through the cannula inserted in the affected limb.
- Check sensation in the limb over 5–10 minutes. Good anaesthesia results in 94–98% of patients. Muscle relaxation may take longer to develop.
- The patient may experience paraesthesia and the skin may appear mottled. When the patient complains of tourniquet pain, the lower or distal tourniquet, which overlies anaesthetised skin, is inflated and the proximal tourniquet is released. It is important to inform the patient that the feeling of touch is often retained.
- Patient should be monitored throughout the surgical procedure and a careful watch must be kept on the tourniquet.
- The tourniquet may be released safely after 25 minutes. Release the tourniquet pressure slowly in steps of 10 mm Hg every 30 seconds and patient must be observed closely and kept supine for 30 minutes.
- Sensation of the limb returns quickly. If surgical procedure or wound requires sutures, it is advisable to infiltrate local anaesthetic around the wound.
- Antecubital veins are best avoided because there is possibility of leakage of local anaesthetic agent under the cuff but their use has reported.
- If IVRA is used for lower limb surgery, similar principles apply but a higher volume of local anaesthetic is required and anaesthesia may not complete.

Complications

- The major problem is systemic toxicity and this is associated usually with inadvertent or premature tourniquet deflation because of failure of equipment or technique, or slow leakage of local anaesthetic agent past the tourniquet cuff. Signs of local anaesthetic agent toxicity are manifested as drowsiness, circum-oral tingling, convulsions, twitching, cardiac depression, etc. Major systemic toxicity or met-haemoglobinaemia has not been reported after the use of the recommended dosage of prilocaine;

- Tourniquet pain;
- Inadequate block can occur in 5% of patients;
- Nerve damage from tourniquet pressure is extremely rare but is more likely to occur when excessive tourniquet times are used;
- Rapid return of sensation requiring supplemental infiltration of local anaesthetic agent in case open surgical procedures.

Always

- Check the resuscitation equipment.
- Check that the tourniquet is working.
- Always have a spare patent intravenous line.
- Select an appropriate specially designed and properly maintained tourniquet for chosen limb.
- Inflate tourniquet pressure 100 mm Hg above measured systolic blood pressure.
- Keep a close eye on the tourniquet pressure.
- Never inject more than recommended volume of local anaesthetic agent.
- Monitor the patient throughout.
- Check anaesthesia.
- Inform patient that the touch sensation may be retained.
- Release the tourniquet pressure very slowly at the end of procedure.
- Look for the signs of local anaesthetic agent toxicity.

Never

- Use bupivacaine as local anaesthetic agent of choice. Always use recommended volume of prilocaine.
- Use sphygmomanometer cuffs.
- Deflate the tourniquet before 25 minutes since the initial injection.
- Use IVRA for procedures lasting more than an hour.

Further reading

1. Risdall JE, Young PC, Jones DA, Hett DA. A comparison of intercuff and single cuff techniques of intravenous regional anaesthesia using 0.5% prilocaine mixed with technetium 99m-labelled BRIDA. *Anaesthesia*. 1997;52:842–848.
2. Dunbar RW, Mazze RI. Intravenous regional anesthesia: experience with 779 cases. *Anesth Anal*. 1967;46:806–813.
3. Brown EM, McGriff JT, Malinowski W. Intravenous regional anaesthesia (Bier block): review of 20 years' experience. *Can J Anaesth*. 1989;36:307–310.
4. Henderson CL, Warriner CB, McEwen JA, Merrick PM. A North American survey of intravenous regional anesthesia. *Anesth Anal*. 1997;85:858–863.
5. Sapega AA, Heppenstall RB, Chance B, et al. Optimizing tourniquet application and release times in extremity surgery: a biochemical and ultrastructural study. *J Bone Joint Surg Am*. 1985;67:303–314.
6. El-Hassan KM, Hutton P, Black AMS. Venous pressure and arm volume changes during simulated Bier's block. *Anaesthesia*. 1984; 39:229–335.
7. Grice SC, Morell RC, Balestrieri FR et al. Intravenous regional anesthesia: evaluation and prevention of leakage under the tourniquet. *Anesthesiology*. 1986;65:316–320.

23

Central venous access

Fiona L. Clarke

The main sites used for cannulation are the internal jugular vein and the subclavian vein. A long catheter (long line) inserted in the basilic vein may also be used. The external jugular vein and the cephalic vein in the arm can be used, but these routes are less likely to be successful because of the anatomical reasons described below. Recent guidelines produced by NICE suggest that ultrasound guidance is used routinely when central venous access is obtained, although the identification of landmarks for blind central venous puncture remains a fundamental required skill.

Anatomy

The internal jugular vein and the subclavian vein are the most commonly used sites. The femoral vein (the safest in a patient with a coagulopathy) and external jugular vein are also used. A long line can be threaded up the basilic vein in the arm, or the cephalic vein.

The catheter tip should be in the superior vena cava, before this enters the right atrium.

General technique for all routes

- Explain the procedure to the patient.
- Monitor the ECG so that any ectopic beats or arrhythmias may be detected.

  Select the appropriate catheter depending on the route chosen and the reasons for insertion, for example: A 15 cm quadruple lumen catheter inserted using a Seldinger technique into the right internal jugular vein is appropriate for a patient needing multiple IV therapies on ICU but not in a patient who requires fluid resuscitation.

- Using a strict aseptic technique and wearing a gown, gloves and facemask, prepare the sterile field using an appropriate disinfectant and large drapes. You may wish to wear eye protection for this procedure.
- Position patient on a tipping trolley in a slightly head down position (negative Trendelenburg position) if using a jugular or subclavian route. If the patient is breathless, do not tip them head down until you are completely ready to start the procedure.
- Infiltrate the skin with local anaesthetic (e.g. 5 mL 1% plain lidocaine) and allow time for this to take effect (3–4 min). Remember that you are likely to be suturing the line in place and infiltrate the appropriate areas of skin.
- Identify your landmarks and identify the vein with ultrasound if available.
- Some people advocate the use of a small 'seeker needle' e.g. 23 or 18G, to locate the vein before proceeding to use the larger insertion needle.
- Attach a saline containing syringe to whichever needle you decide to use, to make it easier to confirm aspiration of blood.
- Confirm free aspiration of venous blood before inserting the guidewire.
- The guidewire should advance through the needle and into the vein without resistance. Check that no arrhythmias are caused by the irritant effects of insertion of the guidewire into the right atrium. If these occur, try to withdraw the guidewire slightly.
- A small incision (less than 5 mm) may be made with a sterile scalpel along the path of the guidewire to make insertion of the dilator easier. A large incision increases the risk of bleeding from the insertion site, may increase the risk of infection, and cause unsightly long term scarring. Remove the needle, insert the dilator over the wire, remove the dilator, then insert the catheter over the wire to the required depth, and then remove the wire. Check that venous blood can be aspirated from all lumens, and flush each lumen with sterile saline, or heparinised saline if there is likely to be a delay before the line is used. Suture the line in place, and cover the insertion site with a sterile dressing.
- Request a chest X-ray after the procedure to confirm the correct position of the line, and to rule out complications of the procedure. A chest radiograph is not required if a femoral line has been inserted unless the line is long enough to pass beyond the level of the diaphragm.

Internal jugular approach

Anatomy

The jugular bulb which, emerges through the jugular foramen, drains into the internal jugular vein. The internal jugular vein runs next to the carotid artery in the carotid sheath, initially posterior to the internal carotid artery, then lateral and finally anterolateral before joining the superior vena cava behind the sternal end of the clavicle.

Procedure

This route is the most appropriate for the ventilated patient and for a dialysis line. It should be avoided, if possible, in patients with raised intracranial pressure because of the risk of a haematoma in the neck compromising cerebral perfusion, and in patients with a suspected cervical spine injury where the neck should be immobilised.

Follow the general instructions above. The right internal jugular vein is used more often than the left. A 15 cm catheter should be appropriate for most adults for a right-sided cannulation, and a 20 cm catheter for a left-sided approach.

The landmarks for the higher approach are to identify the mastoid process and the suprasternal notch, and to imagine a line running between them. Then identify a point half way along this line, which should be at about the level of the cricoid cartilage. Feel for the carotid artery pulsations and place 2 or 3 fingers of one hand lightly on the artery. Do not press too vigorously, as this may be uncomfortable for the patient and distort the anatomy.

The patient should be asked to turn their head slightly away from the side to be cannulated. If the head is turned too far to one side, the procedure becomes more difficult and the risk of arterial puncture increases. Insert the needle at an angle of 30–45° aiming away from the artery and towards the ipsilateral nipple (or where the nipple should be). You should reach the vein within 2–3 cm in an adult. Advancing the needle more deeply will increase the risk of pneumothorax. If you do not find the vein at this depth, withdraw the needle while aspirating to make sure you have not punctured both walls of the vein, and then redirect the needle more laterally. If redirecting laterally does not locate the vein, try redirecting more medially, being aware that this increases the risk of arterial puncture. If you do accidentally puncture the artery, withdraw the needle and apply firm pressure over the artery for about 10 minutes before trying again, either on the same side, or on the opposite side.

The alternative lower approach is to identify the internal jugular vein as it runs between the two heads of the sternocleidomastoid muscle. Ask the patient to try to turn their head against the resistance of your hand to make the muscle more prominent. Aim to enter the vein at the apex of the triangle formed by the two heads and the clavicle, while palpating the carotid artery to ensure you make your puncture lateral to the pulsations. This approach is more likely to cause a pneumothorax than the higher approach.

Subclavian approach

Anatomy

The subclavian vein is a continuation of the axillary vein, and begins at the lower border of the first rib. It arches upwards over the first rib and then downwards, medially and slightly forwards across the insertion of the scalenius anterior muscle. It joins the internal jugular vein behind the sternoclavicular joint. It lies under the clavicle and anterior to and below the subclavian artery. The dome of the pleura lies behind the subclavian artery at the sternal end of the clavicle. The thoracic duct joins the left subclavian vein, which is why the right subclavian is more commonly used.

Procedure

This route is more appropriate for long-term cannulation because it is more comfortable for the patient, and insertion of temporary pacemakers or pulmonary artery catheters may be more successful using this route. The incidence of pneumothorax is higher than with the internal jugular route, and haemorrhage as a result of accidental arterial puncture is more difficult to control. It is therefore best avoided, if possible, in patients with severe lung disease or a coagulopathy. If the patient already has a chest drain in situ, use the same side for subclavian access.

The patient should be positioned on a tipping trolley, slightly head down if tolerated. A rolled towel or litre bag of fluid positioned between the shoulder blades may allow the shoulders to drop backwards into the mattress and make the angle of approach easier.

Drape the disinfected area so that you can palpate the suprasternal notch easily, and use generous amounts (e.g. 10 mL 1% lidocaine) of local anaesthetic to infiltrate the skin and subcutaneous tissue in the area just below the midpoint of the clavicle and slightly lateral to this. The best area for needle insertion is lateral to the 'S' bend of the clavicle, about 1 cm below it. Insert the needle under the skin, and initially aim upwards to place the tip of the needle under the clavicle. Then place the fingers of one hand on the suprasternal notch and redirect the tip of the needle towards your fingers, keeping under the inferior surface of the clavicle until you can aspirate venous blood into your syringe of saline. Try not to go posteriorly, as this risks entering the pleura and causing a pneumothorax. Try to palpate the subclavian artery above the clavicle so that you can direct your needle away from the artery.

- No needle should be introduced beyond 3 cm.
- Gravity will fill all central veins (head down tilt for the neck or head up for the femoral).
- Use the ultrasound to confirm your knowledge of the surface landmarks—there may not be one available when you really need to get the central line in.
- Neck veins are very collapsible—from atmospheric pressure and excessive traction/palpation of the carotid.
- If you fail twice—give up and get someone else.

Do not persist with this approach if you cannot locate the vein, as the risks of pneumothorax and arterial puncture increase with repeated attempts. If you fail to locate the subclavian vein on one side, do not attempt subclavian cannulation on the other side until you have excluded a pneumothorax by clinical examination and chest radiography.

Complications

The combined risks of major and minor complications are quoted at 10%.

Early

Technical failure
Haematoma and bleeding

Arterial puncture
Pneumothorax
Chylothorax from damage to the thoracic duct (left sided punctures)
Nerve damage—sympathetic chain causing Horner's Syndrome, brachial plexus injury
Arrhythmias
Knotting, kinking or breaking of catheters
Catheter, guide wire or air embolism

Late
Infection—local and systemic
Thrombosis
Bacterial endocarditis
Erosion of vessel wall or into pericardium, leading to tamponade
Stenosis of blood vessel wall

Further reading

1 National Institute for Clinical Excellence. Technology Appraisal Guideline No. 49. *Guidance on the use of ultrasound locating devices for placing central venous catheters*. Sept 2002. *www.nice.org.uk*
2 Department of Health. Guidelines for preventing infections associated with the insertion and maintenance of central venous catheters. *J Hosp Infect.* 2001;47(supplement):S47–S67.

24

Ultrasound and its application in venous access

Oliver Weldon

Introduction

With recent developments in ultrasound scanner design and the publication of guidelines on the use of 2-D ultrasound scanners for the placement of central venous catheters (CVCs) by NICE (National Institute of Clinical Excellence), it is now not only practicable to use 2-D ultrasound for the routine placement of CVCs but there are also medico-legal implications in not doing so.

Basic physics of ultrasound

Ultrasound is sound of a wavelength which is beyond the audible range (20–20 KHz) usually in the range of 2–15 MHz. The underlying principle is that sound emitted by an acoustic transmitter will be reflected by an object in the acoustic beam and the transmitter can also be used to detect the returning echo. This is called a transducer. Provided that the speed of sound in the medium is known, the time taken for the echo to return can be used to calculate the distance of the object from the transducer. Table 1 shows the speed of sound in different media. Echoes are

Table 1. Examples of speed of sound in different media.

Blood	$1570\,m\,s^{-1}$
Liver	$1580\,m\,s^{-1}$
Fat	$1430\,m\,s^{-1}$
Muscle	$1575\,m\,s^{-1}$
Bone	$2800\,m\,s^{-1}$
Air	$330\,m\,s^{-1}$
Water	$1480\,m\,s^{-1}$

Table 2. Examples of acoustic impedance.

Muscle	$1.64 \times 10^6 kg\,m^{-2} s^{-1}$
Liver	$1.66 \times 10^6 kg\,m^{-2} s^{-1}$
Fat	$1.31 \times 10^6 kg\,m^{-2} s^{-1}$
Bone	$5.6 \times 10^6 kg\,m^{-2} s^{-1}$
Air	$392 \times 10^6 kg\,m^{-2} s^{-1}$

generated when a sound wave meets interfaces between media with different acoustic characteristics. Different media also have different acoustic impedances (effectively resistance to the propagation of a sound wave through it). Table 2 shows the characteristic acoustic impedance for different tissues. Thus soft tissues such as muscle, fat, blood and liver all have similar speeds and acoustic impedances, but the speed of sound in bone is nearly twice as great but the impedance is four times greater. The effect of this is that bone is almost impenetrable to sound waves and will produce a characteristic 'shadow' through which nothing can be seen. Although sound passes easily through air the huge difference between the speed of sound in air and tissues results in most of the sound being reflected at any tissue/gas interface also effectively resulting in an acoustic shadow.

Another characteristic of all media is attenuation. The further the acoustic beam travels into a medium the weaker it becomes as will the returning echoes. The higher the frequency of the sound wave the greater the attenuation. Thus for deep tissue penetration a low frequency (1–2 MHz) is better. However, in order to produce good resolution of objects in the field a short wave length (higher frequency) is better (5–10 MHz). All scanners have a time gain compensation (TGC) control built into them so that the image can be made to appear of uniform brightness independent of the distance from the transducer.

Transducer design

Most ultrasound transducers use the piezoelectric (PZT) effect. When a potential difference is applied to piezoelectric material it expands: equally the application of a mechanical force to the material causes it to produce an electrical charge. Thus application of an appropriate electrical signal to the PZT will cause production of sound wave pulses and the reflected sound wave pulses will result in the production of an electrical signal by the PZT material. A linear transducer is made up of a series (128–256) of PZT elements arranged in a row. They fire in groups sequentially sending an acoustic pulse into the tissues and detecting the returning echo before the next pulse is fired, thus building up a two dimensional (2-D) image of the tissues beneath the transducer, so called B Mode or Real Time scanning.

National Institute of Clinical Excellence guidelines

In September 2002 the National Institute of Clinical Excellence (NICE) issued its Technology Appraisal Guidance No 49: Guidance for the use of ultrasound locating devices for placing central venous catheters. It contained four main recommendations:

- Two dimensional (2-D) imaging ultrasound guidance is recommended as the preferred method for insertion of central venous catheters (CVCs) into the Internal Jugular Vein (IJV) in adults and children in elective situations.
- The use of 2-D imaging ultrasound guidance should be considered in most clinical circumstances where CVC insertion is necessary either electively or in an emergency situation.
- It is recommended that all those involved in placing CVCs using 2-D imaging ultrasound guidance should undertake appropriate training to achieve competence.
- Audio-guided ultrasound guidance is not recommended for CVC insertion.

However, further in the Guidance in Section 4.3.6 '… the landmark method would remain important in some circumstances, such as emergency situations, … Consequently, the Committee thought it is important that operators maintain their ability to use the landmark method and the method continues to be taught alongside the 2-D-ultrasound-guided technique.'

Use of 2-D ultrasound for CVC placement

Equipment

Currently there are two 2-D ultrasound devices, available on the UK market, which are designed specifically for the assistance of CVC placement. These are the Site-Rite 3 (Jade Medical) and the ***i***-Look 25 (Sonosite). Both are portable battery-powered devices mountable on stands with linear transducers with small 'footprints'. Sonosite makes another scanner (180 Plus) with a choice of transducers of which the linear 38 mm is the most suitable. In addition you will need sterile transducer coupling gel and a supply of sterile covering sheaths. Otherwise you will need the same equipment that you would need for placement of a CVC by the landmark method.

Choice of technique

2-D ultrasound scanners may be used either to guide CVC placement or to assist it. With ultrasound guided placement the scanner is used to guide the passage of the needle in real time into the vein and to observe the passage of the Seldinger guide wire into the vessel and to confirm its correct placement. Ultrasound may also be used to assist CVC placement by confirming that the anatomy is normal prior to placement of the CVC using the landmark method. This does not require that the transducer is sterile and may be performed after positioning of the patient and before preparation of the sterile field for CVC insertion.

Internal jugular vein placement

- The patient should be positioned as normal for the approach being used.
- A preliminary scan is performed prior to preparing the sterile field. The scanner is switched on and the depth set to maximum. Place coupling gel on the transducer head and (gently) pass your finger over the transducer head to check the orientation of the probe right to left.
- Place the transducer orientated transversely in the midline below the cricoid cartilage and observe the shadow cast by the air in the trachea. Move the transducer to the side of planned CVC insertion and observe the circular hypoechoic (dark) structures that are the common carotid artery and internal jugular vein respectively. Adjust the near and far gain controls (if present) to obtain a satisfactory image of uniform brightness and suitable contrast and adjust the depth setting so that the vessels lie in the centre of the field.
- The artery is the round structure which is slightly pulsatile when (gently) compressed. The vein is usually ellipsoid in cross section and collapses easily with pressure from the transducer.

Try to keep the transducer pressure as light as possible or you may collapse the vein and be unable to see it separately from the artery. If the patient is awake ask him/her to perform a Valsalva manoevre and observe the substantial increase in the diameter of the vein. The vein usually lies anteriorly and laterally to the artery. If the patient is unconscious or sedated you may tip the bed or trolley head down and observe the increase in diameter.

- While keeping the transducer head in the transverse position you may move the transducer up and down the neck and observe how the relationship between artery and vein changes. You may choose to puncture at a point where there is a greater degree of separation between the artery and the vein to minimize the risk of accidental arterial puncture.
- Ultrasound guided venous puncture may be performed with the vessels imaged either transversely or longitudinally. Longitudinal scanning will permit the needle to be seen as it approaches the vein. However, this may not be possible with large transducers in patients with short necks. Transverse scanning has the advantage that a low approach to the IJV may be used and needle guides can be used. The needle may be difficult to see and the position of the needle tip must be inferred from the distortion of the tissues by the needle.
- To scan transversely, having identified the vein and keeping it in the centre of the image carefully rotate the transducer to view the vein in longitudinal axis making sure that you retain your orientation with regard to which way the transducer is pointing. You may confirm the orientation by pressing gently on the skin with your finger and observing the compression of the tissues.
- Having performed a preliminary scan you may decide that ultrasound guidance is not necessary for the procedure.
- Prepare the sterile field in the normal way having prepared your intravenous equipment.
- Prepare the transducer head: place coupling gel in the protective sterile sheath trying to avoid getting air bubbles in the gel. Carefully place the probe into the sheath and secure the sheath over the probe with an elastic band. Make sure that there is a thin covering of gel between the probe head and the sheath and place some sterile gel on the outside of the sterile sheath.
- Confirm orientation of the probe with your fingertip. Re-scan the neck as before holding the transducer in your non-dominant hand.

- If using the transverse method with a needle guide place the needle guide over the outside of the sheath or place the needle in the notches on the probe and grip with the thumb of the hand holding the transducer. Advance the needle in a series of short stabbing movements observing the distortion of the tissues to indicate the position of the needle tip while aspirating the syringe with your dominant hand. You need to be able to see the position of your hands as well as the scanner screen to make sure that the needle remains in the scan plane. If flashback occurs proceed as with your normal technique and pass the Seldinger wire though the needle. The wire should be easy to see as it lies in the vein.
- Frequently the needle transfixes the vein. The posterior wall of the vein can be seen to be tented as the needle is withdrawn until the needle suddenly flicks into the lumen of the vein and flashback occurs. Proceed as normal and confirm the position of the wire in the lumen of the vein.
- If using the longitudinal method, repeat the scan as before starting with a transverse scan and then rotating the transducer so that the vessel can be seen in long axis. Check orientation. Insert the needle at a shallow angle keeping the needle in line with the scan plane. You should be able to see the needle approaching the vessel through the tissues and obtain flashback. Again you may easily transfix the vein and observe the tenting of the posterior wall as the needle is withdrawn until flashback occurs. Continue with wire placement as normal and confirm the presence of the wire in the lumen of the vein before dilating the vessel and placing the CVC.
- If you are having difficulties look at the position of your hands not at the scanner screen. You may find the needle tip is no where near where you think it is!

> - Practice with the probe on as many normal patients before using it 'for real'.
> - If you get 'lost' look at your needle positioning not the screen.
> - Remember the landmarks.
> - Choose the site with the best visualization and separation between artery and vein.

Vascular access at other sites

Subclavian vein

Because of the acoustic shadow produced by the clavicle subclavian vein puncture under 2-D imaging will have to be performed more laterally where anatomically speaking it is the axillary vein. The vascular structures are much deeper than in the neck. Many linear probes are too bulky to fit under the clavicle and the resolution of curvilinear transducers may make it hard to separate the artery from the vein.

Femoral vein

The relationship between the femoral artery and vein changes markedly below the inguinal ligament. In one study the operators took 2.7 fewer attempts to insert a catheter using 2-D guidance although the risk of failed catheter placement and time to achieve successful catheter placement were not statistically different than using the landmark method.

Peripheral venous access

The ready availability of 2-D scanners means that peripheral veins in difficult patients can be imaged. As skills with ultrasound guided puncture develop unnecessary CVC placements may be avoided.

25

Acute pain assessment and patient controlled analgesia

Christine Sinclair

Pain assessment—general principles

Pain assessment is the most fundamental aspect in the management of pain. The use of pain assessment tools is now well recognised as a concept but the application of these to practice in the acute area is still growing.

Pain is a multi-dimensional experience and has been reported to have three major components: sensory, emotional and cognitive. The cognitive component in this context relates to the interpretation the patient makes of their pain. Therefore providing information on the nature of the pain such as wind, bruising, or the experience of phantom pain and sensation can dramatically reduce anxiety and increase tolerance if a patient has insight into what their pain might mean for them. Patient information presented preoperatively (and for chronic pain patients at a pain clinic visit) will result in realistic expectations and allow an informed choice to be made and this should therefore be included in the pain management plan.

It is important to consider the bio-psychosocial issues when dealing with patients in pain. Anxieties, lack of information and a hostile environment will create a greater perception of pain intensity; therefore the attention the patient receives on assessment of pain may significantly reduce pain perception, as inhibitory mechanisms from the cerebral cortex can result in a degree of pain gating thus reducing the need for large doses of analgesia.

Taking a pain history

It is important to document the following points in order to formulate an appropriate treatment plan

- Site of pain		a body chart is useful for this purpose

- Character of pain — descriptive words—dull, aching, throbbing, burning
- Frequency of pain — is it constant?—if not what are the frequency of attacks
- Duration of pain — how long has it been present
- Influencing factors — what makes it better or worse
- Life style issues — how is it affecting every day life
- Treatment efficacy — how has it responded to interventions

The use of assessment tools

Whilst pain assessment should be holistic and consider the broad issues, it is important to relate results with a validated tool that forms the basis of decision making in planning analgesia. The prime features of such a tool is that it is reliable when used repeatedly by the same patient and that changes in the rating of pain have precision. Inter-subject reliability is another key necessity. The subjective nature of pain does not give definitive measurements but an attempt at objectivity can be achieved through the assessment process with the use of validated tools. The tool must be appropriate to the client group and used consistently.

Visual Analogue Scale (VAS)

This concept is based on a 10 cm line where one end represents 0 = "no pain" and the other end 10 = "worst pain ever" (Figure 1). Some have 1 cm spaced markers representing categories of mild, moderate and severe pain with numerical indicators. Ideally we should aim to use the same language when passing on information of patient's pain and their responses. A pain score of 8/10 indicates severe pain. The use of the VAS may be more meaningful to patients in some visual form such as a pain ruler.

The Burford Pain Thermometer

This is used in many pain settings and incorporates numerical and verbal ratings (Figure 2). However as it only measures pain intensity it is more commonly used in the acute setting and staff should always be mindful of the factors that will affect tolerance and influence patient

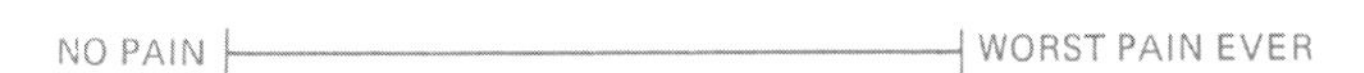

Figure 1. Visual Analogue Scale (VAS 1 to 10).

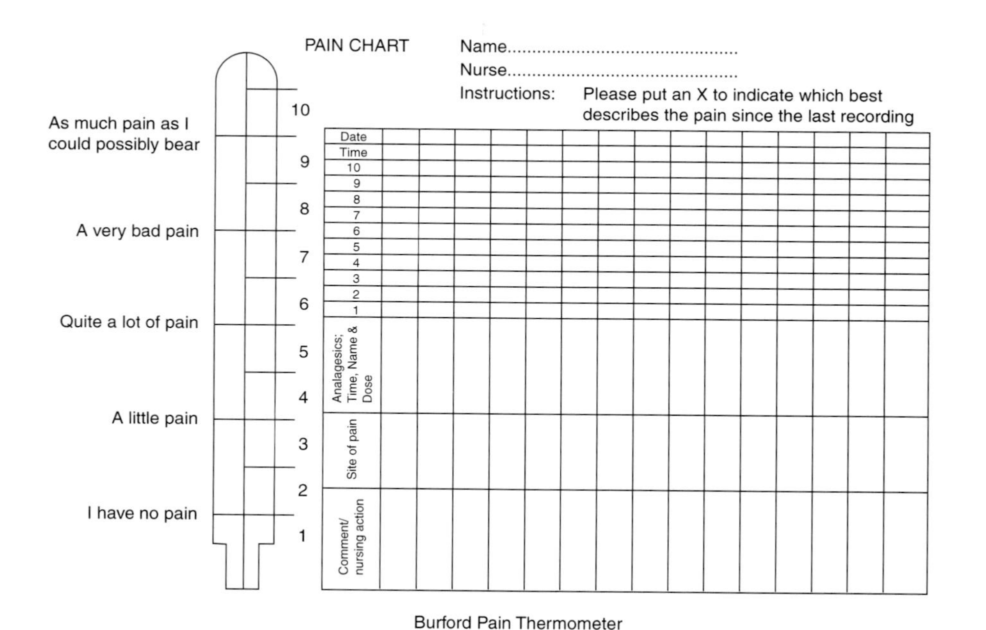

Figure 2. Typical pain chart.

perception of their pain intensity. The illustrated chart also allows trends in pain and the effects of analgesia to be recorded.

Dynamic pain assessment

Acute pain management is about optimising recovery and reducing complications. It is therefore useful to focus the assessment to function and mobility. The majority of acute pain research continues to use single evaluation measures such as pain intensity or analgesic consumption, which do not reflect the patient's wider experience.

Observing the patient's ability and behaviour on deep breathing coughing or movement will give a more accurate evaluation of analgesic requirement and effectiveness. This can then be related to a verbal rating of mild, moderate or severe pain and a numerical equivalent applied to act as a baseline for subsequent assessments and interventions.

McGill pain questionnaire

This is often used in chronic pain situations (Figure 3). However, it does have a place in acute settings where more complex pain scenarios such as ischaemic limb pain or neuropathies are often encountered. Encouraging patients to verbalise the pain experience is more valuable than focusing on numerical rating. This type of tool provides categorical descriptors and patients are asked to choose a word from a number of groups that best describes their pain. This provides an evaluation of their experience and indicates the type of pain, thus providing more reliable direction for prescribing.

Paediatric assessment tools are well developed through the use of behavioural indicators and facial expressions. In some specialist patient groups such as the unconscious there is usually an attempt to use physiological parameters as indicators of pain; however, quantifying findings is difficult with many complicating clinical factors, so the use of flow charts as a decision-making tool is a reasonable compromise.

As a handy reference observing the following principles may be useful:

Why assess:

- A professional requirement;
- Builds good patient–clinician relationships;
- Provides objective observation of the patient experience;

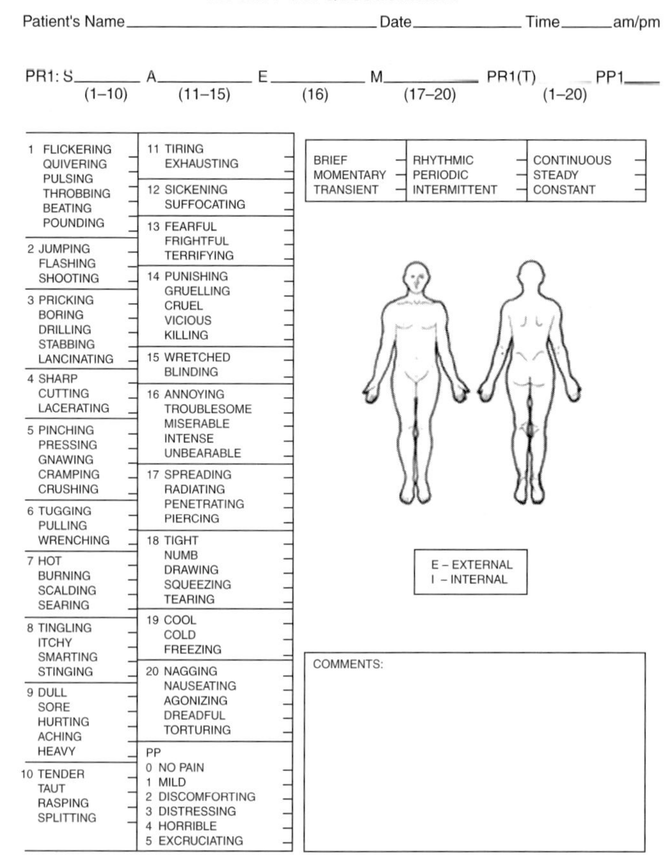

McGill Pain Questionnaire

Patient's Name____________________ Date__________ Time______am/pm

PR1: S______ (1–10) A______ (11–15) E______ (16) M______ (17–20) PR1(T) (1–20) PP1____

1 FLICKERING QUIVERING PULSING THROBBING BEATING POUNDING	11 TIRING EXHAUSTING
2 JUMPING FLASHING SHOOTING	12 SICKENING SUFFOCATING
3 PRICKING BORING DRILLING STABBING LANCINATING	13 FEARFUL FRIGHTFUL TERRIFYING
4 SHARP CUTTING LACERATING	14 PUNISHING GRUELLING CRUEL VICIOUS KILLING
5 PINCHING PRESSING GNAWING CRAMPING CRUSHING	15 WRETCHED BLINDING
6 TUGGING PULLING WRENCHING	16 ANNOYING TROUBLESOME MISERABLE INTENSE UNBEARABLE
7 HOT BURNING SCALDING SEARING	17 SPREADING RADIATING PENETRATING PIERCING
8 TINGLING ITCHY SMARTING STINGING	18 TIGHT NUMB DRAWING SQUEEZING TEARING
9 DULL SORE HURTING ACHING HEAVY	19 COOL COLD FREEZING
10 TENDER TAUT RASPING SPLITTING	20 NAGGING NAUSEATING AGONIZING DREADFUL TORTURING
	PP 0 NO PAIN 1 MILD 2 DISCOMFORTING 3 DISTRESSING 4 HORRIBLE 5 EXCRUCIATING

BRIEF MOMENTARY TRANSIENT	RHYTHMIC PERIODIC INTERMITTENT	CONTINUOUS STEADY CONSTANT

E – EXTERNAL
I – INTERNAL

COMMENTS:

Figure 3. McGill Pain Questionnaire.

- Provides a guide to prescribing;
- Provides documented evidence to underpin actions and interventions;
- A means of evaluating analgesic effect and side effects.

When to assess:

- As regularly as the clinical situation requires;
- On patient movement or physiotherapy;
- As a general observation during patient contact.

How to assess:

- Verbally, by allowing the patient the opportunity to express their experience;
- Visually, by observing patient behaviour and expression;
- Physiologically, by noting changes in heart rate, blood pressure, skin pallor;
- With reference to an appropriate assessment tool and subsequent documentation.

Guidelines following assessment

The Analgesic Ladder

Mild Pain: VAS 0–4

- Paracetamol

Moderate Pain: VAS 4–7

- Codeine/Paracetamol combinations
- Tramadol
- Anti-inflammatory preparations (NSAIDs)

Severe Pain: VAS 7–10

- Titration of intravenous opiates in 1 mg increments to comfort against side effects;
- Regular Paracetamol and NSAIDs follow immediately with longer acting agents or continue opiate therapy with the use of patient controlled analgesia.

Patient Controlled Analgesia (PCA)

PCA allows patients to self administer opiates by way of a demand system, usually a button. It allows an individual patient to respond to the enormous variation in their pain whilst the technological advances made self administration safe and practical. The patient has control of delivering small boluses which ensure that the plasma concentration of analgesic can be kept within a therapeutic range.

Indications

- Where opiates are indicated for the management of the patient's pain;
- Where oral intake is limited or not allowed;
- Where opiate therapy is required for a phase of treatment.

Table 1. Nature of pain.

Type	Meaning	Characteristics	First line recommendations
Somatic	Pain in the musculoskeletal system	Dull, aching, throbbing	Paracetamol Anti-inflammatory preparations, TNS
Visceral	Pain arising from gut or internal organs	Sharp	Codeine Paracetamol Opiates
Neuropathic	Pain arising from abnormal firing of nerves	Burning, shooting, cramping	Tricyclic antidepressants Anticonvulsant therapy (Gabapentin)
Spasmodic	Pain that is intermittent	Colicky, comes in waves, muscle tenseness	Antispasmodic agents (Buscopan, Baclofen)
Referred	Pain that is felt in another area to the primary pain due to dermatomal distribution	Tingling associated with nerve entrapment	Tricyclic antidepressants *or* simple analgesics for somatic pain
Phantom	Pain in an area that has been amputated	Cramping or crushing sensation	Tricyclic antidepressants Anticonvulsant therapy (Gabapentin)

Advantages

- Rapid onset;
- Reduces demand on nursing time and ensures more timely responses for patients with pain;
- Programmable computerised dosage delivery;
- Lock-out time interval before subsequent dose allowed;
- High degree of patient compliance;
- Low risk of over sedation and respiratory depression;
- Reduces nursing staff demands.

Guidelines

- Use dedicated equipment—a lockable pump that is designed for this purpose;
- Patient must have the cognitive and physical ability to use PCA;
- Use a dedicated giving set that incorporates a Y connection that allows the administration of IV fluids concurrently and prevents the need for extra cannulation. This must incorporate a non-return valve to prevent morphine refluxing into the fluid line;
- Morphine concentration should be standardised at 1 mg/mL;
- An adequate loading dose should precede patient bolusing in order to ensure that a therapeutic level has been established;
- It is preferable to treat any side effects symptomatically rather than add drugs unnecessarily to the syringe;
- Allow patient unrestricted use;
- Only the patient should activate the bolus device in order to ensure safety;
- Patient must have regular observations of pain score, sedation score, respiratory rate and nausea and vomiting status.

Further reading

1. Harmer M. *Patient Controlled Analgesia*. Blackwell Science Ltd.; 2002.
2. Carr ECJ, Mann EM. Pain: *Creative approaches to effective pain management*. Macmillan Press; 2000.
3. Rowbotham DJ, Macintyre, PE. *Acute pain: Clinical pain management*. Arnold; 2000.

26

Inserting a naso-gastric tube

Ian Conacher

For all its apparent simplicity, a naso-gastric tube (NGT) is a major breach of natural defences against the *milieu exterieur*. It should not be viewed lightly. Its presence is an ordeal for the conscious. It is important to recognize that, in opting to use the naso-gastric route, a NGT is likely to be present for a duration that ultimately will prove distressing. In the risk/benefit balance a NGT is an irritant: it can provoke vomiting which it is meant to prevent; and, correctly placed, it interferes with the physiological function of an intact *oesophago-gastric* sphincter, rendering it incompetent. The indications are decompression and drainage of stomach, usually as part of the care of gastro-intestinal obstruction or paralytic ileus (the 'suck' of 'drip and suck') and/or prevention post surgery. It can be used for aspiration and removal of toxic compounds (e.g. drug overdose), or enteral feeding (e.g. neuromuscular disease).

Equipment

Naso-gastric tubes are usually an 85 cm length of plastic tube. Modern ones have refinements, either of weighting to help keep position in the most dependent part of the stomach and as radio-opaque markers; or, an integral double lumen/flush system to aid and maintain patency. In addition, one laryngoscope, one Magill forceps, lubricant and Litmus paper (optional) are required (Figure 1).

Insertion

The conscious patient can be asked to swallow a NGT once it is in the oro-pharynx. However, this described insertion technique is for the unconscious, or anaesthetised, and intubated patient. In these

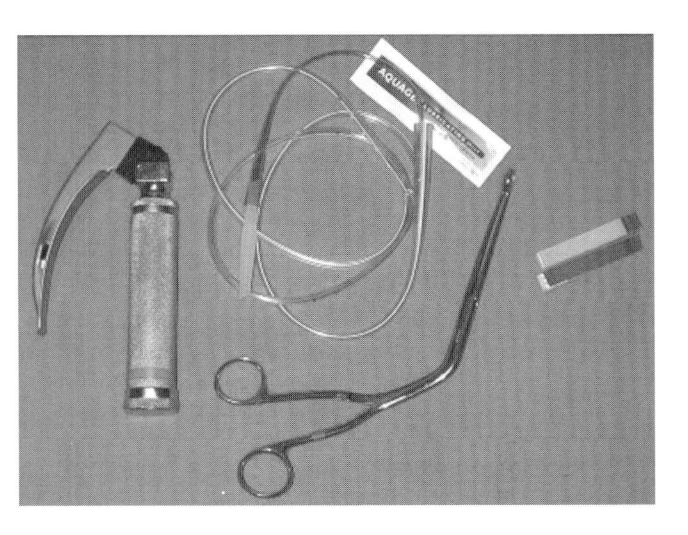

Figure 1. Equipment: *(from L to R)* Laryngoscope, nasogastric tube, lubricant, Magill forcep and Litmus paper.

circumstances, a NGT stored in a refrigerator helps reduce pliancy, making insertion easier.

- Gentle backward and upward finger pressure on the bulb of the nose exposes the *nares* and indicates the correct direction for passing the NGT.
- The tip of the well-lubricated NGT is passed, parallel to the hard palate (not cephalad into the turbinates). It is advanced without force into the oro-pharynx. It then can be seen with the aid of a laryngoscope and is grasped by the jaws of a Magill forceps, in the right hand of the operator. An upward lift of the laryngoscope exposes the top of the oesophagus, behind the endotracheal tube.
- The NGT is advanced with a 'grip and push' action with the forceps. The direction taken is more likely to be correct if the neck is extended rather than being maintained in the 'sniffing the morning air' tracheal intubation position, making the oesophagus, rather than the trachea, the natural line.
- Confirmation of placement within the stomach is by aspiration of contents, sometimes bile-stained and acid to Litmus or by injecting air and listening for 'bubbling' sounds with a stethoscope placed over the left hypochondrium. Final confirmation, essential before using NGT for feeding, is from an X-ray.

Problems

Difficulties with the basic technique may be encountered because of 'pinch points' within the nose, and with detecting the tube in the oro-pharynx—because of the presence of the tracheal tube or blood—haemorrhage easily being produced by trauma to turbinates or the nasal mucosa. Slight resistance may be encountered at the *crico-pharyngeus muscle*, but passage beyond should be without resistance. 'Tricks of the trade' can be employed for some perceived or encountered problems.

- In a planned surgical procedure, the NGT can be placed in the upper part of the oesophagus under direct vision with a laryngoscope before the airway is secured (this avoids interference from the tracheal tube, but should not be used if the risk of regurgitation is high).
- A small, plain (uncuffed, <7.0 mm i.d.) uncut endotracheal tube is first 'split' with a scalpel blade along the long axis. The endotracheal tube is passed through the *nares* and manipulated into the oesophagus to act as conduit through which the NGT is passed. The split conduit can then peeled off and extracted after the NGT is passed.
- If manipulation within the oro-pharynx is limited by, for instance a double lumen tracheal tube, the tip of the NGT can be retrieved either by touch or with a Magills forceps from the oro-pharynx and brought out of the mouth. It is then attached to a guide such as a large bore stomach tube and the combination passed back down the oesophagus, at which point the oral guide is separated from the NGT and removed from the mouth as the NGT is advanced. A variation may be required to reverse the process, that is getting a tube from the oro-pharynx (where it may have been placed retrograde at surgery from the stomach) into the naso-pharynx. Fortunately, such cumbersome manoeuvres are rarely indicated or required.

Fixation of the tube

A NGT does not lie naturally in a position that enables comfortable or reliable fixation. Tension and abrasion with consequent pain and maceration are likely around the nose irrespective of the fixation system. It may be necessary to fix at two points, at the nostril and on the forehead or the side of the face. Where the danger of aspiration of stomach contents is deemed high in a restless patient, suturing may have to be considered. Methods with adhesive strapping to the bridge of the nose are beloved of nursing staff but commercial systems of fixation with adhesives and clips are available.

Servicing and maintenance

- A chest X-ray is the final arbiter of position and confirms that the NGT does not lie in the trachea—a surprisingly common result particularly with narrow-bore tubes.
- The exit point at the nose should be regularly checked and dressed if necessary. Local infection should be treated topically.
- Flushing with saline may be necessary to clear semi-solid or particulate or faeculent material. Frequent and regular aspiration is necessary in the case of gastro-intestinal stasis and ileus. Excessive attempts should be avoided. The ability of a small tube to drain a large reservoir, like the stomach, is limited—the purpose is to decompress and reduce the amount of retained contents and pressure rather than empty it. Over-zealous aspiration may precipitate distressing hiccoughs.
- Gagging and coughing should lead to checks that the NGT has not been regurgitated, inhaled or fulfilled its usefulness.
- Decannulation can be done with the return of gastro-intestinal function, sometimes signalled by a fall off in returns from aspiration, return of bowel sounds, full return of consciousness and normal reflex activity related to swallowing and coughing.

Complications

Insertion-trauma on passage is common, usually from pushing when the tip is inappropriately pointing too far cephalad, or in the friable parts of the naso-pharyngeal mucosa. Oesophageal perforation, with the potential to cause mediastinitis, is reported. But the insertion into the trachea must be excluded.

Alternatives

Some would consider the formation of a gastrostomy as a suitable and more comfortable alternative but these are not without risk.

A percutaneous entero-gastrostomy (PEG) will serve the same function for long-term feeding.

Further reading

1 Conacher ID. Another aid for the insertion of nasogastric tubes. *Anaesthesia*. 1985;40:1246–1247.

27

Paediatric vascular access

Christopher J. Vallis

Intravenous access is a vital step in the resuscitation of children. It is also necessary for the delivery of many drugs such as inotropes and antibiotics, as well as for the delivery of routine maintenance intravenous fluids. However, it is a process that is potentially frightening and fraught with anxiety for the patient, the parents, and quite possibly the operator.

Types of vascular access include

Percutaneous peripheral vein cannulation;
Peripheral venous cut-down;
Intraosseous infusions;
Percutaneous or surgically inserted central venous access;
Arterial line insertion.

Also remember that in some situations drug administration can be achieved without venous access (see Box on page 183).

General approach to procedures in children

Explanation—The procedure should be explained to both parents and child. Talk to children in terms appropriate to their age without being patronising.

Lying to children or trying to deceive them is generally counterproductive—A child knows if a procedure is hurting.

Consent—For some invasive procedures it may be wise to obtain consent from the patient's parents or guardians even if a general anaesthetic is not involved. A 'Gillick competent' child, who understands the nature and implications of a procedure may give consent even if under 16 years.

Parents—Parents may wish to be present at minor procedures, and a parent may be very useful in calming a child during a stressful experience.

However, nervous parents should not be obliged to be present during a procedure.

Environment—Other general principles of paediatric care should not be forgotten. An exposed infant may lose heat rapidly even at normal room temperature.

Lighting—Good lighting is essential and overhead lighting in a treatment room should be supplemented if necessary by an 'angle poise' lamp. It may sometimes be found that light at an angle produces better vein visibility than bright light from directly overhead.

Restraint—Physical restraint of a young child may be essential for the successful outcome of the procedure. This should be mentioned to parents beforehand and their assistance invited but not insisted upon. There is some skill involved in holding an uncooperative child and a member of staff may be better for the job. It may be possible to sit a small child on the parent's knee whilst holding a hand out of sight behind the parent's back. A brief period of firm restraint may be less traumatic in the long term than less vigorous restraint, which leads to poorer immobilisation and the need for repeated attempts at the procedure.

Peripheral venous access

Advantages

Familiar process to most medical and nursing staff;
May be inserted without general anaesthetic;
Generally safe and free of serious complications.

Disadvantages

May be difficult in chubby infants or critically ill shut down patients (in a real emergency do not spend more than 3–4 attempts, or 90 s–2 minutes, before proceeding to alternatives);
Limb immobilisation/joint splinting may be required;
Not suitable for some drugs (e.g. dopamine) or hypertonic solutions.

Equipment

'EMLA', 'Ametop', or local anaesthetic
Skin cleaning swabs
Gloves
Needle or lancet (for initial skin puncture)

Razor (for scalp shaving)
Tourniquet
Over the needle cannulae of appropriate gauge
Splint for limb or joint immobilisation
Tape for cannula fixation
Cotton wool
Bandage for cannula concealment/further immobilisation
Syringe and normal saline to flush cannula

Procedure

1. If the procedure is not urgent, identify potential site(s) and apply local anaesthetic cream in advance.
2. Consider wearing gloves (opinions vary as to whether loss of tactile sensation has an adverse effect on success rate in small children). Consider other protection e.g. protective eye shield if necessary.
3. Wash hands.
4. Identify a suitable target vein—time spent identifying a suitable vein is well spent. Search all limbs for a suitable point. Bear in mind need for limb immobilisation if cannula inserted over a mobile joint e.g. elbow.
5. If scalp vein is chosen, shave the surrounding skin.
6. Select cannula and *very slightly* withdraw and re-insert needle to loosen cannula over needle, making later withdrawal of needle easier.
7. Cleanse skin.
8. Immobilise younger children and the limb.
9. The assistant's hands which immobilise the limb will also act as a tourniquet. Too tight a grip may easily occlude circulation entirely.
10. Stabilise the vein but avoid undue skin stretching which will tend to flatten the vein. Gentle tapping of the vein may increase its size.
11. It may be worthwhile making an initial skin puncture with another needle or lancet. (For small over the needle cannulae, e.g. 24G or 26G cannulae, there is a risk that the cannula will 'concertina' on entering the skin.)
12. Insert the cannula through the skin at an angle of about 30–40°.
13. For cannula insertion into small superficial veins, e.g. on scalp or ventral side of wrist, it is often best to enter the skin a short

distance from the target vein, and then approach the vein at a much shallower angle than the initial approach to the skin.

14 A small 'give' may be felt on entry to the vein. This may not be apparent with small cannulae. A flash-back of blood into the hub indicates successful penetration of the *needle* into the vein.

16 Holding the needle firmly; advance the cannula over the needle into the vein.

17 After insertion, flush the cannula gently with normal saline to confirm placement and fix in place.

18 The cannula should be fixed with adhesive tape or preferably with a purpose made transparent dressing. A very small piece of cotton wool under the cannula hub may improve subsequent patient comfort, and make infants less likely to try to pull out the cannula.

19 Blanching or pain on injection may indicate intra-arterial placement.

20 Fine cannulae are easy to shear if the needle is reinserted after partial withdrawal—discard and use a fresh cannula.

It is useful to also attach the giving set tubing to the skin to take the strain should the tubing be pulled rather than the tension being taken on the cannula. In small children bandaging may be necessary to further hold the cannula in place and conceal it from the patient. However, it is important to regularly inspect the site if the infusion becomes slow or infusion pressure rise, in case the cannula has 'tissued'.

There is no need to regularly replace intravenous cannulae that are working satisfactorily. However a rise in infusion pressure, or swelling, redness or pain on injection are indications for review. Small cannulae soon block unless kept open with a low rate infusion, or regularly flushed with heparinised saline.

Intraosseous fluids

This technique has been in use since the Second World War, and is again being used for rapid vascular access in emergencies.

Anatomy

Any hollow bone may be used, but the tibia and femur are most commonly used. The tibial sites are on the anterior surface, 2–3 cm below

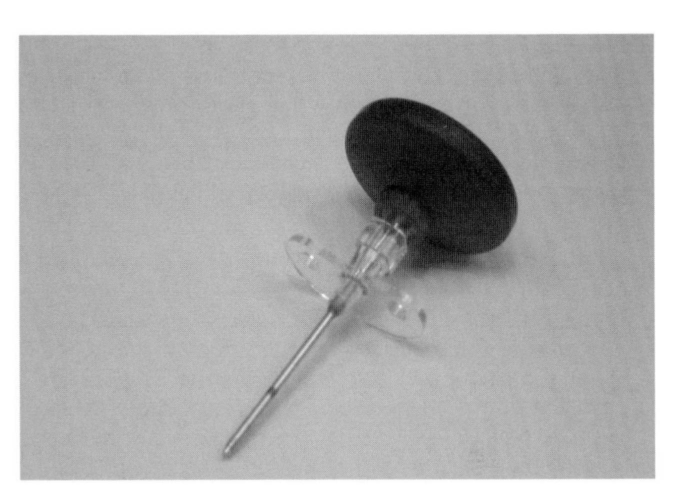

Figure 1. Intraosseous cannula.

tibial tuberosity (to avoid growth plate) and on the femur on the anterolateral surface, 2–3 cm above lateral condyle.

Equipment

Skin cleanser
Intraosseous needle
Syringes
Intravenous extension tubing with three-way tap

Procedure

1 Identify site—avoid fractured bones, as fluids will simply leak out at fracture site.
2 Clean skin.
3 Advance needle at right angles to skin with an oscillating rotating movement (some needles have a screw thread, and are screwed in).
4 As bone cortex is penetrated, a give is felt.
5 Aspirate any marrow required for analysis (see below).
6 Attach giving set.
7 Fluid will not flow by gravity—boluses of fluid should be pushed in using a syringe and three-way tap.

Notes

1. Marrow aspirated on needle insertion can be used for biochemical analysis for blood glucose and electrolytes, but inform laboratory of nature of specimen.
2. In case needle is removed or falls out of bone, re-insert in another bone (as fluid will leak out of previous hole).

- Do not be over-ambitious. Success with a 22G cannula into a small vein is better than repeated failure with a 20G.
- A common source of failure is to withdraw the needle after successful vein entry, rather than to advance the cannula over it. *After blood flashback, hold the needle exactly in place while the cannula is advanced over it.*
- Occasionally with small cannulae a flashback of blood through the needle may not occur. If you are confident of having entered the vein it may be worthwhile advancing the cannula and giving a trial injection of a small quantity of normal saline.
- Accidental transfixion is also common with veins close to the skin surface, particularly with operators more used to adults. In the event of apparent failure, very slow withdrawal of the cannula may produce a flash of blood as it is pulled back into the vein. Cautiously advancing the cannula from that point may turn failure into success.
- In the event of failure with a small cannula, use a fresh cannula.
- After two or three unsuccessful attempts, call for help. If you do decide to continue, have a brief rest and clear away the debris of previous unsuccessful attempts. It will make you and any observers feel better.

Special situations

In trauma victims try to avoid cannulation through damaged or dirty skin. However, in patients with burns, cannulation through burnt skin is possible if other sites are not available. The cannula may need to be sutured in place in this situation.

Failure in an emergency

In true emergencies do not persist for more than three or four attempts (or 90 s–2 minutes). If intravenous fluids are necessary, proceed to intraosseous access, which is quicker than venous cut down.

Epinephrine

In a cardiac arrest remember that adrenaline may be given down an endotracheal tube. The Resuscitation Council (UK) recommendations are that ten times the intravenous dose of adrenaline (i.e. 100 micrograms/kg) should be used. The adrenaline should be injected rapidly down a narrow suction catheter, beyond the tracheal end of the tube, and then flushed in with 1 or 2 mL of normal saline.

In anaphylaxis, epinephrine is given intramuscularly.

Suxamethonium

In an airway emergency, this may be given intramuscularly, and in particular may be given intramuscularly into the tongue, with rapid onset.

28

Removing a foreign body from the eye

John R. Clarke

A foreign body on the cornea or beneath the eyelid can be disabling and exquisitely painful. If the problem is managed safely and efficiently comfort may be rapidly restored without complications. Mismanagement may lead to complications and permanently reduced vision. This chapter refers to foreign bodies on the ocular surface. The possibility of ocular penetration should be considered and if likely, further investigation and ophthalmic assessment is required. Any chemical injury to the eye needs immediate irrigation. Further management of these is beyond the scope of this chapter.

Anatomy and physiology

The cornea is perfectly transparent and surfaced by a multi-layered epithelium carrying a rich sensory nerve supply of trigeminal origin. A complex tear film of mucin, aqueous and oily layers acts as a near perfect optical refracting surface and is the initial defence mechanism against minor particles in combination with the blink reflex and tearing response. Following surface injury such as an abrasion the corneal epithelial cell layers will rapidly slide to cover a small defect with a thin layer and later cell division will restore the normal five-layer thickness. Bowman's layer separates the surface epithelium from the main part of the cornea, the stroma. Injury involving the epithelium only will heal without scarring. If injury or a foreign body breaches the Bowman layer into the stroma scarring results. Such scarring in or near the central visual axis will cause loss of acuity and often symptoms of glare and photophobia. The innermost layer of the cornea, in contact with the aqueous of the anterior chamber, is the endothelium. This single layer of cells maintains clarity of the corneal stroma by active water extraction and is unable to replicate in response to injury. Repeated corneal injury may lead to endothelial failure and permanent corneal clouding.

Assessment

The history of injury is important to assess the risk of deep or penetrating injury. Windblown material or rust falling from beneath a car will not penetrate the cornea. Any high speed injury from power tools or striking metal to metal must raise suspicion of a penetrating injury and will require a dilated fundus exam and possibly radiology investigation to exclude intraocular foreign body. In children the history may not be clear and greater caution to exclude penetrating injury or intraocular foreign body is needed. This may require examination with general anaesthesia.

Foreign bodies superficially embedded in the cornea may be metal, glass, sand, wood or other organic materials.

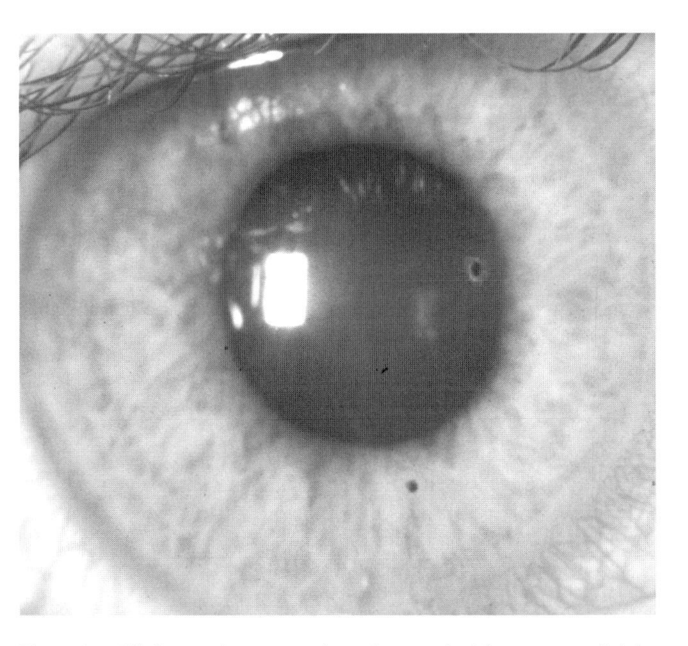

Figure 1. Slit-lamp microscope view of two typical ferrous superficial corneal foreign bodies.

The symptoms will usually be pain, watering, red eye, and a foreign body sensation. Exactly the same symptoms may be caused by corneal abrasion or corneal infective ulceration. Topical anaesthesia will relieve pain and allow easier visual acuity assessment and examination. Slit-lamp microscopy with the instillation of fluorescein may help distinguish the presence and type of abrasion or corneal ulceration. An abrasion shows brightly with the use of the cobalt blue filter. An abrasion will also be present after removal of a superficial foreign body. A particular variation is a foreign body, often a tiny piece of grit, embedded in the under surface of the upper eyelid. Blinking may be painful and a vertical linear pattern of scratches on the cornea with fluorescein is a useful clue. Such a foreign body is easily lifted off the inner tarsal surface after eversion of the lid.

Any high speed injury raises the possibility of an occult intraocular foreign body. X-ray assessment, B-scan ultrasound, CT scan of orbits are useful investigations to consider with expert fundus examination.

Indications

The only indications to remove a foreign body outside of the ophthalmic department are either a simple corneal or subtarsal foreign body.

Contraindications

All cases that would need ophthalmic advice:

- Suspicion of full thickness corneal penetration;
- Any sign of infected ulceration/infiltration of the cornea: this may require corneal scrapes for microscopy and culture before any treatment commences;
- Central visual axis involvement: advisable to seek ophthalmic expertise;
- Unexplained severe visual loss;
- Blood level visible in the anterior chamber (hyphaema);
- Pus level visible in the eye (hypopyon).

Equipment

- Slit-lamp microscope—or examination couch plus good illumination and magnification aid;

- Sterile needle;
- Visual acuity chart;
- Topical anaesthetic: Proxymetacaine and Benoxinate are good topical anaesthetics for this purpose and are available in unit-dose droppers. Proxymetacaine has the minor disadvantage of requiring refrigerated storage but stings less for most patients;
- Topical mydriatic: Cyclopentolate 1%;
- Topical antibiotic: e.g. Chloramphenicol eye ointment.

Technique

Always record the visual acuity of each eye individually, with distance glasses if worn. This should be done before detailed examination or treatment takes place and may be of medico-legal importance later. If glasses are missing or vision reduced, also record acuity with pinhole correction. A simple pinhole through a card is easy to make if needed. This may exclude simple uncorrected refractive error as a cause of reduced vision. Topical anaesthesia will reduce pain dramatically and allow eye opening for both acuity assessment and examination. The eye should be examined with good light and magnification. The slit-lamp microscope is the ideal instrument and should be available in all Accident and Emergency departments. It has a chin rest and forehead rest to stabilise the head of the seated patient combined with superb illumination and magnification. Removal of an embedded corneal foreign body by an experienced and well-trained practitioner using a slit-lamp microscope is the 21st century standard. The microscope allows the accurate assessment of the depth of the foreign body and accurate removal with minimum damage to the surrounding corneal stroma and minimal subsequent scarring. If this is not easily available removal may be achieved using a couch, good light and some magnification aid as a poor second best. The patient should be made aware of this.

A superficial corneal foreign body will not usually respond to simple irrigation. *A soft cotton bud should not be used as it will cause a large epithelial abrasion.* The best instrument is usually a sterile needle. A 25 or 21G needle is mounted on a small syringe for ease of handling. An alternative is to mount the needle on one end of a double-ended sterile cotton bud. The cotton bud end can then easily be used to gently mop up loosened particles from the corneal surface. The needle is held with the bevel facing away from the cornea and the needle in almost the same plane as the cornea. The elbow

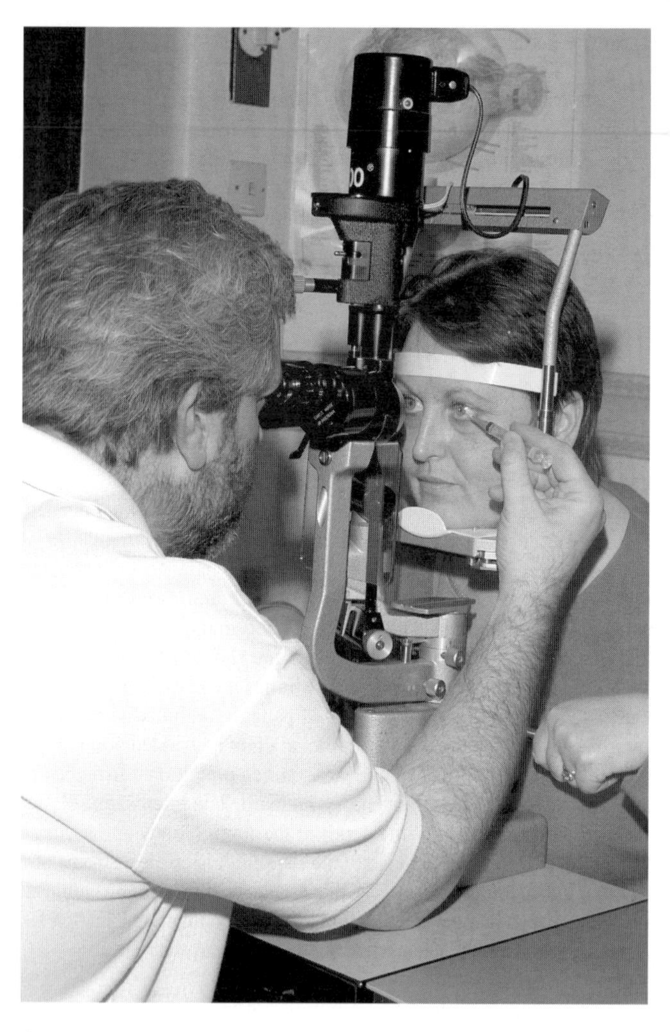

Figure 2. Method of removal of a superficial left corneal foreign body using a slit-lamp microscope plus sterile needle mounted on a disposable syringe.

of the arm holding the needle is steadied on the slit-lamp table (Figure 2). Many small particles such as grit can be lifted forwards and mobilised without creating a large abraded area. Metallic foreign bodies such as iron or steel may be firmly embedded and difficult to mobilise without surrounding dissection. These may be easier to shell out intact after waiting 24 hours for the surrounding corneal tissue to soften: with topical antibiotic cover supplied. Ferrous foreign bodies often leave a surrounding rust ring which can be shelled out with a needle or using a powered burr designed for this purpose.

Always

- Measure visual acuity of both eyes (glasses if worn)
- Take a full history of type of injury
- Have high suspicion for intraocular foreign body
- Use topical anaesthesia to allow examination if much pain
- Use a slit-lamp microscope wherever possible
- Assess the depth of the foreign body
- Consider need for examination under anaesthesia in children
- Supply topical prophylactic broad spectrum antibiotic after removal
- Consider short term topical Cyclopentolate 1% if large abrasion and much pain
- Consider other cause of symptoms if no foreign body present: dry eye syndrome, recurrent erosion syndrome, herpetic ulceration etc.
- Look beneath the lids if vertical scratch pattern with fluorescein dye
- Warn the patient of visual consequences if injury near the central visual axis
- Advise future use of protective goggles when appropriate
- Reassure patients prognosis for vision is good when a superficial foreign body does not involve central axis and infection is prevented
- Seek ophthalmic advice if serious features are present such as hyphaema, hypopyon, surrounding corneal infiltrate, profound visual loss

Never

- Forget to measure visual acuity (medico-legal imperative)
- Give topical anaesthetics for pain relief at home
- Prescribe topical steroids to reduce simple eye inflammation

- Remove a full-thickness foreign body outside of an eye operating theatre
- Fail to consider occult intraocular foreign body with high speed or metal to metal injury

Aftercare

After the foreign body is removed a small abrasion or epithelial defect is present. Deeper injury will heal with scarring which tends to fade in time. The risk of secondary infection will be reduced by topical application of an appropriate antibiotic. Chloramphenicol ointment remains very useful for this purpose as it is not commonly prescribed as a systemic antibiotic. Any suspicion of infection in the cornea evidenced by increased infiltration or opacification around the foreign body site needs urgent ophthalmic assessment. Fungal infection is rare but should be considered after injury by organic material.

If the eye is very painful Cyclopentolate 1% drops 6 hourly for 24–48 hours relieve ciliary spasm and much of the pain. If used, the patient should be warned about associated blurring and increased light sensitivity. Topical anaesthetics should not be used for pain relief beyond the examination because healing may be delayed and symptoms of serious infection suppressed. Padding the eye closed will not speed healing and most patients are more comfortable without padding. An ill-fitting pad may well cause further corneal abrasion if the eye opens beneath it.

Complications

Iron-containing foreign bodies frequently stain the surrounding corneal stroma to cause a rust ring. This may be removed gently with a needle or a special instrument with a rotating burr, by those trained in its use.

Any foreign body breaching Bowman's membrane beneath the epithelial layers will affect the corneal stroma and cause some scarring. This will fade to some extent in time but may reduce best visual acuity if central. Any deeply embedded foreign body is best managed with ophthalmic expertise and a slit-lamp microscope, especially if near the visual axis.

Secondary infection of the cornea is a serious threat to vision and is best prevented by topical antibiotic and observation until the surface epithelium is intact, as judged with fluorescein dye. Increasing injection of the eye and spreading opacification around the FB site are ominous signs. A corneal infection requires attention of the ophthalmologist to obtain corneal samples for microscopy and culture before further antibiotic treatment.

Do not use topical steroid to hasten resolution without a firm indication such as severe secondary iritis. This would require ophthalmic evaluation. Topical steroid may enhance both viral and bacterial infection in the cornea.

Do not prescribe topical anaesthesia for pain relief. Healing will be delayed and very serious symptoms may be masked.

Prevention

Repeated corneal foreign bodies cause multiple little scars on the cornea. This may lead to glare from light scatter in bright light conditions and loss of visual acuity with central corneal involvement. Secondary infection from a neglected foreign body may lead to loss of all vision if it progresses to an endophthalmitis. In most industries involving power tools, insurers now mostly insist on compulsory eye protection. Home use of power tools, hand tools with hammering and work beneath cars now probably provides the main risk. Accident and emergency staff should be prepared to recommend appropriate goggles to attending casualties.

Section 3

Respiratory Skills

29

Oxygen therapy

Praveen Kalia

Oxygen is a colourless and odourless gas, discovered by Priestley in 1771. A decrease in partial pressure of oxygen in arterial blood (hypoxia) can be treated by instituting oxygen therapy. Credit for modern oxygen therapy goes to J.S. Haldane (1917).

Role of oxygen

Tissues need oxygen and energy for survival. Mitochondrial reactions consume 90% of the oxygen and the final outcome is the production of ATP. Most of this energy is used for various active processes, such as protein synthesis, Na^+–K^+ ATPase pump, Ca^{++} ATPase pump, etc. The availability of oxygen, ADP, glucose, fats or proteins in the mitochondria regulate the production of ATP. Glucose is broken down into pyruvic acid. The citric acid cycle converts pyruvic acid into carbon dioxide and hydrogen ions. Hydrogen ions are transferred via flavoprotein—cytochrome system to a series of enzymes resulting in reduction and oxidation. Finally, hydrogen ion combines with oxygen to form water. The process of oxidation, coupled with phoshorylation of ADP by enzyme ATP synthase is called oxidative phosphorylation.

This results in production of energy which is stored as high energy phosphate bonds. The metabolism of glucose in the presence of oxygen results in production of 38 molecules of ATP. A decreased partial pressure of O_2 in tissues promotes less efficient anaerobic metabolism, resulting in production of only two molecules of ATP and lactic acid.

Oxygen cascade and transport

The partial pressure of oxygen cascades down from the inspired air to the mitochondrial level in a series of steps. The partial pressure of oxygen in the inspired air is 14.3 kPa. Addition of CO_2 and water vapour drops the partial pressure of oxygen in alveoli (PaO_2) to 13.3 kPa. The gradient between PaO_2 and venous oxygen partial pressure facilitates diffusion of oxygen across alveolar capillary junctions. The partial pressure of oxygen in the arteries (PaO_2) is 12.8 kPa, and this alveolar arterial oxygen difference is because of venous admixture and shunting. 98% of oxygen carried in the blood is attached to haemoglobin, whereas only 2% is dissolved in plasma. The dissolved fraction of oxygen is most important as this fraction facilitates the gas exchange at cellular level. Each gram of haemoglobin can carry 1.34 mL of oxygen (Hauffner's Constant).

Oxygen flux

Oxygen flux is the amount of oxygen delivered to the tissues per minute

$$\begin{aligned}\text{Oxygen flux} &= \text{Cardiac output} \times \text{arterial oxygen content} \\ &= CO \times (Hb \times SaO_2 \times 1.34 \times 10) \\ &\quad + (PaO_2 \times 0.023 \times 10)\end{aligned}$$

CO—cardiac output
SaO_2—oxygen saturation in percentage
Haemoglobin—amount in 100 mL of blood

Oxygen flux is approximately 1000 mL per minute. The amount of dissolved oxygen in plasma is proportional to partial pressure of arterial oxygen (0.023 mL/kPa/100 mL of plasma, or 0.003 mL/mm Hg/100 mL. Arterial oxygen content is 19.6 mL per 100 mL of blood. Extraction of 5 mL of oxygen per 100 mL of blood results in a venous oxygen content of 14.6 mL per 100 mL of blood.

Types of hypoxia

Hypoxic hypoxia

Inadequate oxygenation of venous blood results in decreased PaO_2, contributing to hypoxia. Clinically, the patient will show signs of peripheral and/or central cyanosis, if the reduced haemoglobin is more than 1.5 g/100 mL. Hypoxia can result from various causes.

Anaemic hypoxia

Decreased haemoglobin will decrease oxygen carrying capacity of blood. The oxygen flux would be decreased significantly, if there is a concomitant drop in cardiac output (induction of anaesthesia) and

Table 1. Causes of hypoxia.

Hypoxic
- Decreased FiO_2—high altitude, hypoxic breathing mixture
- Decreased PaO_2—diffusion hypoxia, hypercapnoea
- Inadequate ventilation (failure of pump or gas exchange)
- Central—opioids, head injury
- Neuromuscular—inadequate reversal of muscle relaxants, myasthenia gravis, Guillaine–Barre syndrome
- Musculoskeletal—chest wall trauma, kyphoscoliosis, muscular dystrophies
- Pulmonary—pneumonia, pulmonary oedema, pneumothorax, atelectasis, chronic obstructive airways disease

Cardiac—lesions contributing to shunting of blood

Anaemic—CO poisoning, iron deficiency anaemia

Stagnant—Shock, left ventricular failure

Histotoxic—Cyanide poisoning

oxygen saturation (airway obstruction). Oxygen tension is normal in this type of hypoxia. Carbon monoxide poisoning results in anaemic hypoxia. CO has strong affinity with haemoglobin and causes a reduction in the oxygen carrying capacity. Cyanosis is not seen in these patients, because of cherry red colour of carboxyhaemoglobin.

Stagnant hypoxia

Failure of oxygen delivery to the tissues, due to low cardiac output and shock states, leads to stagnant hypoxia. Arterial oxygen tension is normal in these cases.

Histotoxic hypoxia

Cells cannot utilise oxygen because of inhibition of the cytochrome enzyme systems, by various poisons such as cyanide. Arterial venous oxygen content difference is reduced.

Principles of oxygen therapy

Patients showing signs of hypoxaemia need oxygen therapy. The physiological effects of hypoxia are listed in Table 2. Airway obstruction is a common cause of hypoxia in unconscious and trauma patients. Signs of airway obstruction include intercostal and sub costal recession, paradoxical respiration, use of accessory muscles, cyanosis and stridor. The airway should be clear when oxygen therapy is instituted. The dose and duration of oxygen administered should be prescribed in the drug chart, like any other medication. Hypoventilation and inability to improve oxygenation with oxygen therapy is an indication for mechanical ventilation.

Patients requiring cardiopulmonary resuscitation need 100% oxygen. The indications of oxygen therapy are listed in Table 3. Provision of 100% oxygen results in an increased oxygen content. The amount of dissolved oxygen in plasma increases to 1.8 mL per 100 mL, but is still not adequate to meet the requirements of tissue oxygenation. Arterial hypoxaemia can be corrected by instituting oxygen therapy in patients with hypoxic hypoxia. In cases with histotoxic and stagnant hypoxia PaO_2 can be normal in spite of presence of tissue

Table 2. Physiological effects of hypoxia.

- Respiratory
  Hyperventilation, dyspnoea, tachypnoea and cyanosis;
  Hyperventilation is triggered by carotid and aortic body chemoreceptors, due to decrease in PaO_2, especially if less than 8 kPa;
  Hypoxic vasoconstriction, due to decreased potassium efflux.
- Central Nervous System
  Headache, impaired judgement, drowsiness, altered sensorium increased cerebral blood flow and coma.
- Cardiovascular System
  Tachycardia (finally bradycardia), increased stroke volume and cardiac output, decrease in systemic vascular resistance (increased $K+$ efflux), arrhythmias and cardiovascular collapse.
- Metabolic
  Lactic acidosis resulting in hyperkalaemia.

Table 3. Indications of oxygen therapy.

- Cardiac and respiratory arrest
- Hypoxaemia (Resting PaO_2 <7.8 kPa, SaO_2 <90%)
- Hypotension (systolic blood pressure <100 mm Hg)
- Low cardiac output and metabolic acidosis (bicarbonate <18 mmol/l)
- Respiratory distress (respiratory rate >24/min)
- Prevention of diffusion hypoxia
- Patients with PolyGram
- Preoxygenation before rapid sequence induction
- Carbon monoxide poisoning

Adapted from The American College of Chest Physicians and National Heart Lung and Blood Institute Recommendations.

hypoxia. Treatment should be directed towards correction to the cause of tissue hypoxia. Volume status and cardiac output needs to be normalised in the case of stagnant and administration of an antidote to cyanide in the case of cyanide induced histotoxic hypoxia.

Patients in Type II respiratory failure

Bateman and Leach have recommended an initial administration of 24% oxygen in these patients if $PaCO_2$ is more than 5.3 kPa. These patients are dependent on hypoxic drive. A high concentration of oxygen can abolish this drive leading to hypoventilation and apnoea. A stepwise increase in oxygen concentration should be introduced in 4% increments and arterial blood gas should be analysed. Falls in pH to less than 7.25 and an increase in $PaCO_2$ from the base line is an indication for not increasing inspired oxygen concentration. Higher concentration of oxygen should be used if $PaCO_2$ is less than 5.3 kPa.

Methods of oxygen delivery

Oxygen therapy can be administered in hypoxic and spontaneously breathing patients by nasal cannulae and face mask. Failure to improve oxygenation with the face mask might necessitate mechanical ventilation. Unconscious hypoventilating patients need intubation and mechanical ventilation.

The ideal device should be able to deliver accurate inspired oxygen concentration without causing rebreathing and resistance to breathing. Performance of the devices used for oxygen therapy depends on flow rate of the gas supplied, ventilatory parameters of the patient including tidal volume and peak inspiratory flow rate (PIFR) and duration of expiratory pause.

Fixed performance devices (venturi mask, ventimask)

These devices deliver accurate concentration of oxygen and are reliable. They require high flow of gases to deliver a known concentration of oxygen. These devices are also referred to HAFOE (high air flow oxygen enrichment). Fresh gas flow is always more than the peak inspiratory flow rate. This prevents re-breathing and the apparatus dead space has minimal effect. These devices work on the venturi principle. The jet of oxygen is passing through a narrow orifice results in a drop in pressure facilitating entrainment of air. Each mask is graded to give

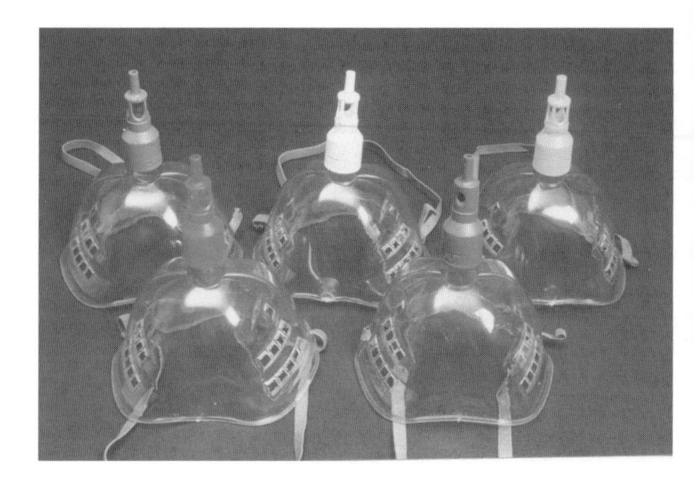

Figure 1. Ventimasks—blue (24%), white (28%), yellow (35%), red (40%) and green (60%).

a specific concentration of oxygen (Figure 1). HAFOE devices have injectors designed to deliver inspired oxygen ranging from 24% to 60%. The injector designed to deliver 24% oxygen entrains 40 litre of air with a flow rate of 4 litres per minute of oxygen. As such, high flow washes away the expired gases preventing any re-breathing. Patients are comfortable and the mask need not be a tight fit. These devices are not affected by ventilatory parameters and can provide a fixed oxygen concentration with an accuracy of ±1%.

Variable performance devices

Nasal Cannulae, MC, Hudson, Edinburgh Masks are low flow variable performance devices. Delivery of accurate concentration of oxygen cannot be assured as flow rate less than the peak inspiratory flow rate during the part of ventilatory cycle. Variable oxygen concentration is delivered because of changes in minute ventilation and duration of expiratory pause.

Nasal cannulae

These offer no dead space nor storage volume for exspired gases. There is a little variation in oxygen concentration between each breath but there is a significant variation between the patients. Approximate flow rates of oxygen and concentration of oxygen delivered are given in Table 4.

Table 4. Oxygen concentration.

	Nasal cannulae (%)	Hudson mask (%)	MC mask (%)
O_2 flow (L/min)			
2	30–35	24–38	28–50
4	30–39	35–45	41–70
6		51–60	53–74

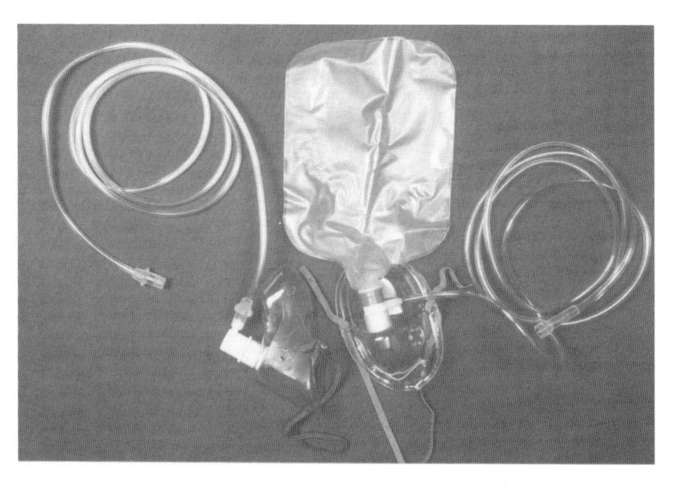

Figure 2. Hudson mask, mask with reservoir bag.

Oxygen masks

Hudson and MC Mask provide storage of gases, but increase the dead space. Many of the bags have an attached reservoir bag. The Hudson Mask can provide up to 40% of inspired oxygen at a flow rate of oxygen of 4 litres per minute. The addition of a reservoir bag can increase the delivered oxygen up to 98% (Figure 2). Most of the masks are light weight and do not provide an air tight interface or seal with the face and dilution with atmospheric air can result in decreased inspired oxygen concentration. Oxygen is supplied to the bag throughout the respiratory cycle. Patients can breath air through the vents in the mask, oxygen from the reservoir bag and expired oxygen from the mask. Relative ratios will depend upon the duration of expiratory pause, the volume of the air inspired from the vents and the relative resistance offered by the bag and air vents.

Oxygen toxicity

Oxygen can be life-saving but, at the same time, injudicious use of oxygen can cause harmful effects. Continuous use of 100% oxygen can cause absorption atelectasis, because of loss of splinting action of nitrogen. Oxygen is more soluble in blood than nitrogen. Oxygen supports combustion and can be dangerous in the presence of fire and fuel. Prolonged administration of 100% for more than 48 hours can reduce surfactant formation, increased thickening of membranes, endothelial damage, decreased mucus clearance, oedema and fibroblastic activity. The generation of free radicals, such as superoxide anion and hydrogen peroxide results in pulmonary toxicity (Lorrain–Smith effect). Administration of oxygen at more than 300 kPa (hyperbaric oxygen) can cause central nervous system toxicity, in the form of tingling, confusion, convulsions and coma. However, there is scientific evidence supporting the benefit from such therapy, in cases with carbon monoxide poisoning, decompression sickness and arterial embolism. Elevated retinal artery PO_2 can result in retinal vasoconstriction, proliferative retinopathy and retinal damage in premature babies.

Summary

Oxygen, like other therapeutic agents, should be properly prescribed, clearly indicating flow rate, route, method and duration of administration. Oxygen is useful, but harmful effects of injudicious use of oxygen should be kept in mind. Oxygen therapy should not be denied to the patients for the fear of abolishing the hypoxic drive as most patients do not hypoventilate on institution of oxygen therapy. **Hypoxia can kill the patient whereas hypercapnoea and apnoea can be managed by mechanical ventilation.**

Further reading

1 Bateman NT, Leach RM. ABC of oxygen, acute oxygen therapy. *Br Med J.* 1998;317:798–801.
2 Leigh JM. Variation in performance of oxygen therapy devices. *Anaesthesia.* 1970;25:210–222.
3 Shepherd JN, Evans TW. Postoperative intensive care of patient with respiratory disease In: Prys-Roberts C, Burnell RB (editors), *International Practice of Anaesthesia*, Vol. 1. Oxford, Butterworth-Heinemann, 1996;1–17.

30

Airway assessment

Simon Gardner and David Ryall

The ability to artificially maintain an airway and, if required, to subsequently intubate the trachea, is a relatively straightforward procedure in the majority of patients. However, in a small number of individuals, this process can be extremely problematic. These patients are said to have a difficult airway. A difficult airway can therefore be defined as 'a clinical situation in which an experienced practitioner experiences difficulty with mask ventilation, laryngeal mask insertion, intubation of the trachea, or a combination of all three.'

Formal airway assessment is essential in all patients scheduled to undergo anaesthesia or sedation. The purpose of this assessment is to allow the practitioner the best possible chance of predicting a difficult airway. Having correctly anticipated a difficult airway, the practitioner can then develop an appropriate strategy for managing the airway, utilising any of a variety of techniques which are discussed in the next chapter.

Airway assessment can be considered in two stages, i.e. clinical history and formal airway examination.

Clinical history

Wherever possible, the practitioner should undertake a pre-operative history, gathering information both from the patient and from the patient's medical notes. A well-directed clinical history will help to uncover many of the potential problems that may lead to a difficult airway. Specific areas that should be covered include;

Previous anaesthetic history

- Is the patient aware of any airway problems encountered during their previous anaesthetics?

- If previous anaesthetic charts are available, is there any record of difficulty in managing the patient's airway, and is the ease of intubation recorded?

Current medical condition

- Does the procedure the patient is about to undergo involve the airway, e.g. ENT surgery for laryngeal tumour?
- Is there infection within the airway, e.g. dental abscess, submandibular gland infection, epiglottitis?
- Is there tumour within the airway, i.e. oral or laryngeal cancer?
- Is there trauma or burns to the airway?

Past medical history

- Radiotherapy to any part of the airway;
- Pregnancy;
- Hiatus hernia or other possible risk factors for aspiration of gastric contents;
- Thyroid problems;
- Rheumatoid arthritis;
- If nasal intubation is being considered, particular attention should focus on vascular disorders e.g. haemangioma, bleeding disorders, e.g. haemophilia, and anticoagulant medication e.g. warfarin;
- Neck problems, e.g. cervical spondylosis, previous neck surgery, neck fractures, ankylosing spondylitis;
- Dentition, i.e. presence of loose teeth, caps, crowns, intermaxillary fixation, or other vulnerable dental structures;
- Congenital abnormalities affecting the airway, e.g. Pierre Robin syndrome, Treacher Collins syndrome.

Examination of the airway

The airway can be thought of as being divided into three anatomical zones—upper, middle and lower, which correspond to the supraglottic, glottic and infraglottic portions of the airway. Hence, problems in these zones can be associated with difficult laryngoscopy, intubation and ventilation respectively. Bedside assessment of the airway only allows for direct examination of the upper zone, but areas to focus on include:

- Record of the patient's height, weight and BMI, i.e. is the patient obese?
- Range of neck movements including flexion and extension of the cervical spine and movement of the occiput on the atlas;
- Mouth opening should be at least 4–6 cm;
- State of dentition, presence of buck teeth, crowns, etc.
- Is the tongue enlarged?
- Is the palate high and arched?
- Is the mandible receding or hypoplastic?
- Is the neck obviously short and/or muscular?
- Is there any other facial or jaw deformity, e.g. fractures?
- Is there any visible intra-oral pathology e.g. swelling, bleeding, foreign bodies?

It is worth noting that the presence of a beard can often hide potential anatomical difficulties and make mask ventilation difficult, as an air-tight seal is difficult to obtain.

Specific tests to predict difficult laryngoscopy

Numerous tests and measurements have been devised over the years in an attempt to predict difficult laryngoscopy and intubation. Unfortunately none of these tests are 100% reliable and therefore often generate both false positives and false negatives. It is however generally accepted that the more such tests you perform, the greater the accuracy of prediction. The actual view obtained during direct laryngoscopy is graded according to the Cormack and Lehane classification (Figure 1(a)–(d)).

Three of the most commonly described tests are considered below.

1. **Mallampati Grading**—Assesses mouth opening and tongue size.
   - Sit directly opposite the patient.
   - Ask patient to open his mouth as wide as possible and to maximally protrude his tongue.
   - Grade the resultant view of the oropharynx according to the amount of uvula and posterior pharyngeal wall that is visible.
   - The higher the score, the greater the likelihood of difficulties.
2. **Thryomental distance (Patil distance)**
   - Assesses jaw length and neck extension;

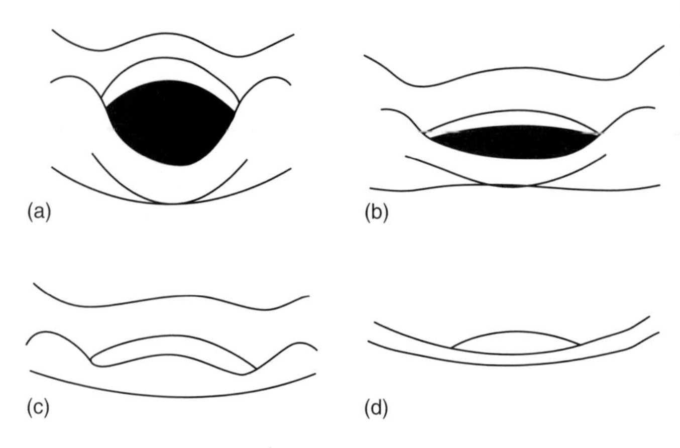

Figure 1. Cormack and Lehane classification of laryngoscopic views. (a) Grade I—full extent of vocal cords visible; (b) grade II—only posterior portion of cords visible; (c) grade III—epiglottis only visible; (d) grade IV—epiglottis not visible.

- Measures the distance between the tip of the jaw and the uppermost aspect of the thyroid cartilage;
- A distance of <6.5 cm predicts difficult intubation.

3. **Jaw protrusion**
   - Ask the patient to maximally protrude his mandible.
   - Assess the relative positions of the upper and lower teeth.
   - If the patient is unable to protrude his lower teeth anterior to his upper teeth, this may predict difficult laryngoscopy, as the jaw cannot be moved forward and there is less room for anterior displacement of the tongue.

Specific conditions which may be associated with airway problems include pregnancy and obesity.

Key questions

- Can the patient open their mouth wide?
- Can you see the back of the pharynx?
- Can they protrude their jaw forwards?
- Do they have a normal jaw?

If no to any of these or if they are obese or pregnant—seek help before starting to manage the airway.

Pregnancy

All pregnant patients undergoing general anaesthesia after the first trimester require tracheal intubation in order to minimise the risk of gastric aspiration. However pregnancy itself is associated with a 7-fold increase in the incidence of failed intubation. Reasons for this include:

- Large breasts which may interfere with insertion of the laryngoscope;
- Oral mucosal oedema may increase the size of the tongue and decrease the size of the oropharyngeal aperture;
- Cricoid pressure may distort the anatomy;
- Poor patient positioning;
- Rapid onset of hypoxia and resultant need for haste.

Obesity

The obese patient can present a particular challenge for the following reasons:

- Mouth opening and neck movement may be limited;
- Large breasts or chest wall may interfere with airway manoeuvres;
- It may be more difficult to maintain a tight seal with the facemask;
- Ventilation is harder because higher airway pressures are required to move the heavy chest wall;
- The onset of hypoxia is more rapid due to decreased functional residual capacity and increased basal oxygen consumption.

31

Drainage of a pleural effusion

Ian Conachar

The accumulation of fluid between the parietal and visceral pleura is pathological. Any pleural effusion is viewed diagnostically as either a transudate or exudate depending on the protein content of samples. Large and recurrent pleural effusions (>1 litre) are associated with malignant disease, commonly with pleural disease such as mesothelioma. As a rule of thumb, any effusion that is visible on a chest X-ray is likely to be >1 litre. Drainage is therapeutic, relieving distress, particularly that of dyspnoea. It should be considered before anaesthesia, especially if it is to involve a significant change of position like lateral for a thoracotomy, in which case the full weight of the fluid will bear on the mediastinum with haemodynamic consequences. Occasionally, the pleural space may be tapped to perform a pleurodesis. If there is a history of trauma, haemothorax is the diagnosis to be excluded. Pericardial effusion, hiatus hernia, or other abdominal viscus can be a diagnostic traps and should be considered possible in those with atypical histories. The bulk of the medium to long-term management of pleural effusions is that of chest drains and underwater seals.

Equipment

A diagnostic tap or thoracocentesis can be conducted with a large-bore needle or intravenous cannula to which a three-way tap can be attached and a rapid aspiration-drainage system rigged up to a 20 or 50 mL syringe. Off the shelf, pre-packed, sterile kits are now widely available, some with Seldinger/guide-wire systems and containing catheters for long term use which contain one-way valves and can be buried subcutaneously.

Insertion

The conscious patient should be sat up and leaning slightly forward with their arms supported on a bedside table or pillows.

- The limits of stony dullness to percussion should be defined.
- The optimal site is in the posterior axillary line. The 8th intercostal space is usually closest to the most dependent part of an effusion that can be tapped safely. Any lower and there is a risk of penetrating an abdominal viscus.
- Under sterile conditions the defined point is infiltrated with local anaesthetic to the parietal pleura. A 14G needle, with syringe for aspiration attached, is directed over the top of a rib (rather than below, avoiding the neuro-vascular bundle). For catheter insertion for long-term use an anterior approach is recommended: the patient being supine and entrance into the thorax being in the nipple line at T6 or T7.

> - Check whether there is a hiatus hernia/other viscus in the chest cavity
> - Position the patient comfortably
> - Drain slowly and gently
> - Maintain sterility throughout because infection can be difficult to treat
> - Seek radiology help if unsuccessful

Problems

Needles may get blocked with fibrinous exudate. Dry taps and haemorrhage (intercostal vessels in the intercostal groove) can occur. Effusions can be loculated and this can be a reason for a 'dry' tap. Radiological assistance may be required. Evidence of significant mediastinal shift (>2 cm toward the effusion), chylous, infected and multiloculated effusions are contraindications as is the presence of a coagulopathy.

Complications

- Early literature warns of rapid decompression and rapid re-expansion syndromes leading to pulmonary oedema. Of late, these have not featured but it remains a caveat that aspiration should be gentle and slow and not exceed 1litre at a time.

- Infection. *Empyema thoracis* is the most common complication, particularly with repeated thoracocentesis. The management of this is complex, prolonged and requires referral to specialists.
- Puncture of lung, pericardium and abdominal viscus and organs are possible but extremely rare. A mistake can be made with an enlarged liver, a hiatus hernia or a ruptured diaphragm.
- Trauma to an intercostal neuro-vascular bundle can cause haemorrhage and neuralgia.
- Mesothelioma has a tendency to grow through skin puncture and drainage holes.

Alternatives

Long-term drainage, with large bore chest drains, may be necessary, and complex systems of internal drainage into the abdomen or venous system may have to be surgically implanted. Pleurodesis, with fibrogenic irritants such as talc or tetracycline, may be required but again are specialist procedures.

32

Insertion of a chest drain

Kyee H. Han

Introduction

This is an essential skill for the management of chest conditions and a life saving procedure in a number of thoracic emergencies.

It is a means of continually draining the pleural cavity of the chest of air, blood, pleural effusion, chyle, pus, etc. This allows the underlying lung to expand and function to its maximal capacity. It is a safe procedure if performed correctly but can be life threatening in inexperienced hands. Deaths have occurred from damage to vital organs like the heart and liver.

Anatomy

Pleurae and pleural cavity

The pleura has two parts; a parietal layer which lines the thoracic cavity, and a visceral layer which completely covers the outer surfaces of the lungs and the interlobar fissures. It is important to note that the parietal layer is extremely pain sensitive. To avoid damage to the intercostal neurovascular bundle it is important that the access to the pleural cavity is gained just over the top of the rib.

Physiology

The intrapleural pressure is always negative (ranging from −4 to −6 mm Hg) in normal subjects. This is altered in conditions which require chest drain insertion. An underwater seal drainage system is required to ensure that this negative pressure is restored after the insertion of a drain.

Indications

Non trauma

- Significant pneumothorax (at least 30%);
- Lesser degree of pneumothorax when associated with respiratory distress, underlying respiratory disease which reduces the patient's respiratory reserve;
- Pneumothorax in a patient requiring mechanical ventilation;
- Recurrent or bilateral pneumothoraces;
- Drainage of haemothorax, pleural effusion, chylothorax, or empyema;
- Post-operatively after thoracotomy.

Trauma

- Any pneumothorax in a patient with multisystem trauma or multiple rib fractures or in a patient requiring mechanical ventilation;
- After needle thoracocentesis for tension pneumothorax;
- Haemothorax or chylothorax;
- With isolated low energy transfer chest trauma with no rib fracture a rim of pneumothorax <0.5 cm can be closely monitored with a repeat X-ray the next morning after admission. Any increase in size warrants insertion of a chest drain.

Procedure

The OPEN method is recommended in a patient who has not had imaging of the chest to indicate the presence of a pleural space where the drain is to be inserted.

General preparation

- Explain the procedure and reassure the patient.
- Set up necessary equipment on a procedure table.
- Position patient on bed or trolley. Sit patient at 45 degrees on the bed/trolley. Stand on the side of the chest to be drained with the patient well over towards your side of the bed. Adjust the height of the bed appropriately and raise the arm of the patient to expose the axilla where the drain is to be inserted. In patients who are supine the relevant arm is placed on top of the patients head to expose the axilla.

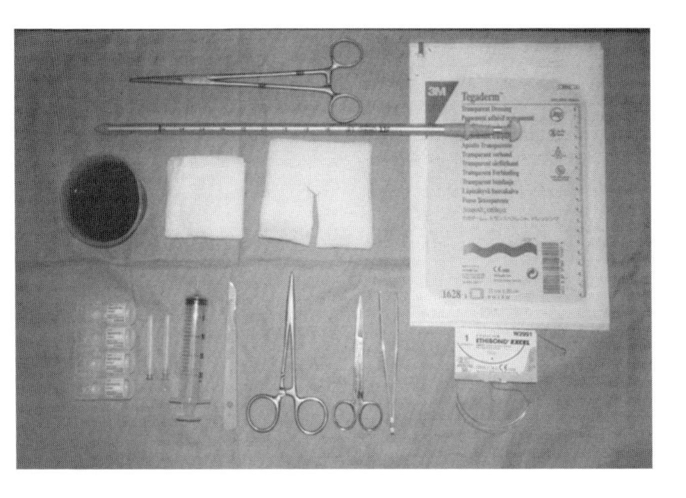

Figure 1. Equipments for chest drain.

- Ensure there is good light.
- Prepare an underwater seal bottle. The bottle is filled with sterile water up to the '0' level which is approximately 2.5 cm above the bottom of the down pipe. Sterile tubing is attached to the top of this pipe and the other end that will be later connected to the chest drain is left in a sterile wrapper.
- Scrub up and put on gown and gloves. Remember this procedure should be strictly aseptic.
- Bring the equipment tray close to the bed/trolley.

The size of the chest drain depends on the size of the patient. Generally in adults a 28–30 FG is recommended for pneumothorax and 30–32 FG is recommended for haemothorax. Drains smaller than 28 FG can block with fibrin. The drain has an outer plastic cannula and an inner trochar which has a blunt tip to prevent accidentally impaling the underlying lung.

Procedure

- Identify the safe area for chest drain insertion. This triangular area is bounded by the pectoralis major as an anterior border, mid axillary line as a posterior vertical border and a horizontal line at the nipple level. This roughly equates with the fifth intercostal space and above. Anywhere within the triangle is safe.

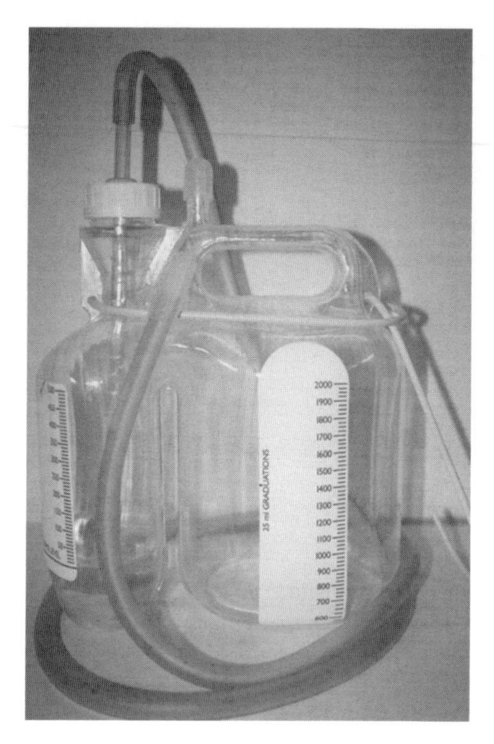

Figure 2. Underwater bottles.

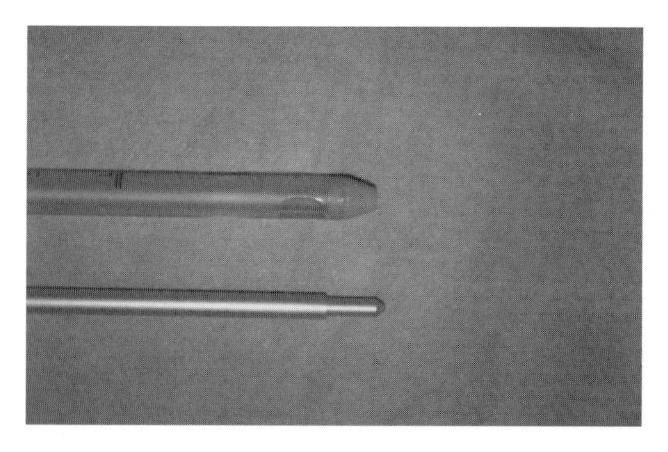

Figures 3. Introducer and trocar.

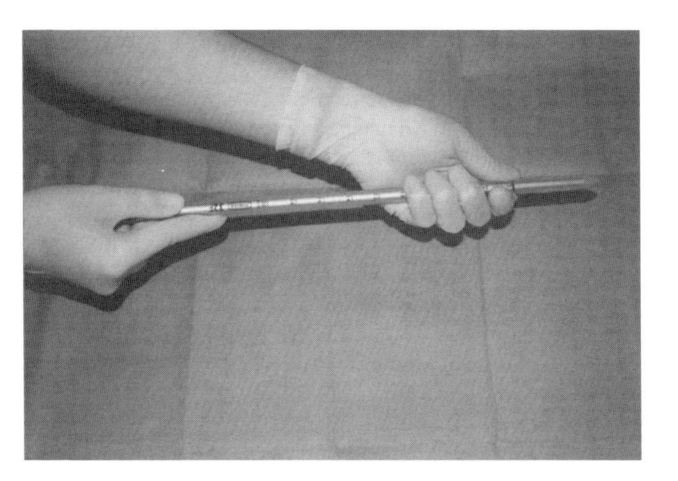

Figure 4. Assembly of introducer and trocar.

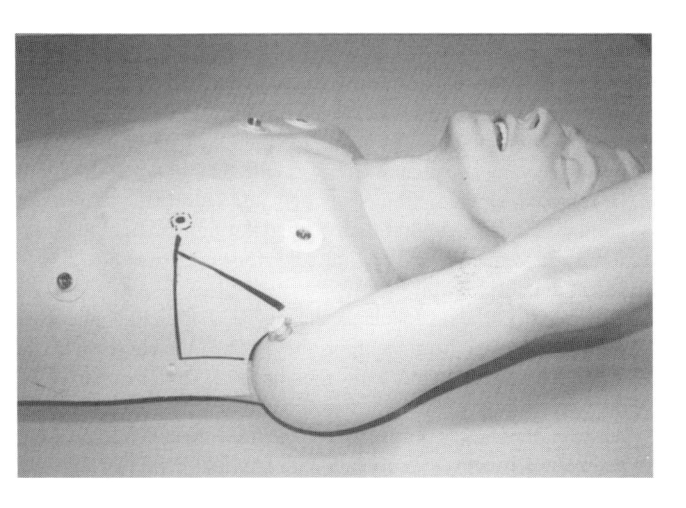

Figure 5. Anatomical landmarks for insertion of introducer and trocar.

- Wash a large area with antiseptic solution and drape the area.
- Infiltrate the insertion site with about 20 mL of local anaesthetic.
- Using a fine orange needle raise a 3 cm intradermal wheal. Then change to a green needle and infiltrating at a right angle

anaesthetize the fat and muscle layers above the rib, and aspirating in case of vascular penetration.

- Stop when the needle enters the pleural space and air or fluid/ blood is freely aspirated into the syringe. The patient may experience a sharp pain at this stage as the parietal pleura is pain sensitive. **Note the depth of the chest wall before removing the needle.**
- Local anaesthetic is now injected continuously as the needle is withdrawn from the pleural space back towards the skin. Do not be afraid to inject a large volume of lignocaine at this stage as it is important to anaesthetise all layers of the chest wall.
- If air or fluid is not aspirated the possibility of a blocked needle or an extremely thick chest wall which requires a longer needle should be considered.
- Form a tract through the chest wall. Using a scalpel blade, make a 2 cm incision through the intradermal wheal into the skin and fat staying in line with the intercostal space. Using forceps and fingers widen the tract. Next make a deeper incision through the muscle layer staying close to the superior border of the rib. The previously estimated depth of the chest wall will assist you in the depth of the incision as the aim is to partially go through the intercostal muscles and not breach the parietal pleura. Using the forceps widen the tract and enter the pleural space. You will feel a slight give as the pleural cavity is entered and air or fluid will be released. Open the forceps widely and withdraw. A finger of similar size to the drain is then pushed through the tract to check there are no unexpected pleural adhesions underneath.
- Insert the chest drain.
- Hold the trocar and cannula as shown. The left hand is placed at a similar distance from the tip as the depth of the chest wall. The cannula is gripped tightly to prevent the trocar from being inserted deeper than it is required to enter the chest cavity. Insert the drain using minimal force. Push through the tract using gentle pressure and mainly rotatory movements with the right hand placed at far end of the trocar and cannula. **If there is significant resistance — stop**; go back a step and widen the tract before trying again. As the drain enters the pleural cavity there is a small give.
- To position the chest drain. Aim the drain towards the apex of the thorax, keep the trocar stationary and advance the cannula. A rough measurement from the patient's axilla to the midclavicular line is a guide as to how far to insert the cannula. Remove the trocar completely and transiently clamp the cannula while it is

connected securely to the chest bottle tubing. Remove the clamp. There should be a free swing of fluid in the tubing, fogging of the tube and vigorous bubbling or drainage of fluid with deep breathing and coughing. If not, withdraw the drain slightly until this occurs.

- To fix the chest drain. Using a strong suture take a deep bite of skin at least 1.5 cm wide along the chest drain. Tie several throws securely encircling the drain and tighten so that the suture bites into the plastic of the drain. Make sure all the knots are secure. A second anchoring suture can be inserted on the opposite side of the drain. A purse string suture in the form of a horizontal mattress suture avoiding the drain itself is then inserted. The ends are left long and taped to the drain ready for tying when the time comes for drain removal. You should now place a small sterile dressing around the drain incision. Secure the dressing in place with two op-site transparent dressings cutting slits to fit round the drain.
- Warn the patient that after the lung expands it may be painful. Offer extra analgesia. Arrange for a chest X-ray and examine it carefully. Occasionally it is necessary to apply suction to the underwater seal bottle. Proper thoracic suction apparatus must be used which provides low pressure high volume suction at approximately 10–20 cm of water.

- Ensure all necessary instruments and equipment is available before starting procedure.
- Do not forget to identify the safe triangle and raise a large wheal to establish the exact location of drain insertion.
- Be generous with infiltration of local anaesthetic into all layers of tissue bearing in mind that the parietal pleura is extremely pain sensitive.
- The tract created for the drain should be vertical and close to the top of the rib.
- Estimate the thickness of the chest wall when infiltrating the local anaesthetic and use this as a guide when creating the tract for the drain.
- Use the open method to insert the drain. Insert a finger into the pleural space to clear adhesions and other organs.
- NEVER use force to insert the drain; use rotatory movements with steady pressure on the other end of the trocar and cannula.

Complications

- Damage to the intercostal nerve, artery, or vein. This may convert a pneumothorax to a haemopneumothorax and result in intercostal neuralgia;
- Laceration or puncture of intrathoracic and/or intra-abdominal organs with faulty technique;
- Puncture of a bullous lung cyst with the danger of creating a bronchopleural fistula with persistent air leak;
- Incorrect tube position in the extrathoracic space. If in doubt a lateral chest X-ray should also be done;
- Introduction of pleural infection, causing empyema;
- Leak around the drain if the size of the tract is larger than the drain size resulting in persistent air leak;
- Kinking, clogging or dislodging of the chest drain. Disconnection from the underwater seal system;
- Surgical emphysema at drain site;
- Recurrence of pneumothorax with incorrect technique of drain removal;
- Anaphylactic or allergic reaction to surgical antiseptic preparation or local anaesthetic;
- Sudden shortness of breath after drainage of a massive haemothorax may occur due to sudden reperfusion of the collapsed lung. It is necessary to drain it in stages clamping the drain temporarily for a few minutes between stages e.g. after 2 litres has drained. A source of significant ongoing bleeding should always be borne in mind.

33

CPAP therapy

Chris Dodds

Background

Continuous Positive Airway Pressure (CPAP) has been used successfully for nearly 20 years to maintain effective breathing in patients with a variety of respiratory and neurological disorders. However, the largest group numerically are those patients who suffer from obstructive sleep apnoea. The principle upon which CPAP works is that of delivering a pressure in the upper airway that is greater than atmospheric pressure and which maintains the patency of the airway despite the increased negative pressure caused by active inspiration. Oxygen may be administered through this system but the majority of patients simply required pressurized air to maintain their respiration.

CPAP is often used in the latter stages of weaning off ventilators in intensive care units and the systems used are both simple and reliable in the short term. These may also be used as emergency systems on wards, admission units, high dependency units and theatre recovery areas. These systems vary from the simplest where an expiratory resistance is created by lowering the expiratory limb of the breathing system under water—for example to 5 or 10 cm below the surface. Spring loaded resistors are also used and more commonly a variable spring is used. Most intensive care-based mechanical ventilators can also deliver CPAP.

The route of administration often determines the compliance of the patient, an important factor when, for many of these patients, this is a life-time treatment. The nasal route is the commonest with full face masks and oral masks some distance behind. The nasal masks may be either soft compliant silicone skins on a more rigid plastic shell or silicone plugs that fit into the nostrils. (There are

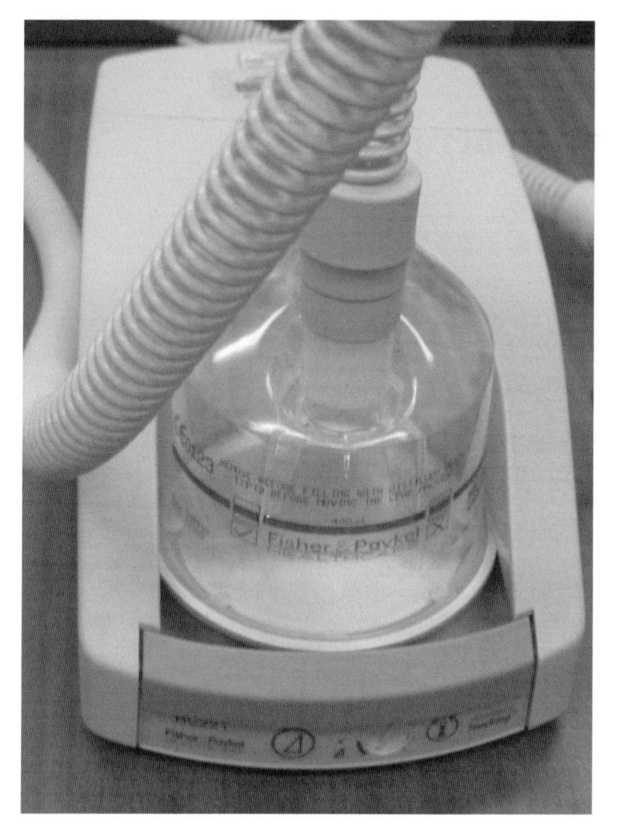

Figure 1. CPAP machine.

many manufacturers of these systems but the basic principles are consistent across them.)

The very soft skin rests on the face and moulds to nose and cheeks of the patient. It seals in a similar manner to hovercraft skirts, where the pressure differential holds the skin in place allowing the more rigid shell some movement without breaking the seal. There is a minimum pressure for this to work, and equally a maximum pressure where the skin is just forced onto the face with the risk of a poor seal (and leaks reducing effectiveness) and pressure sores on the face from the plastic shell.

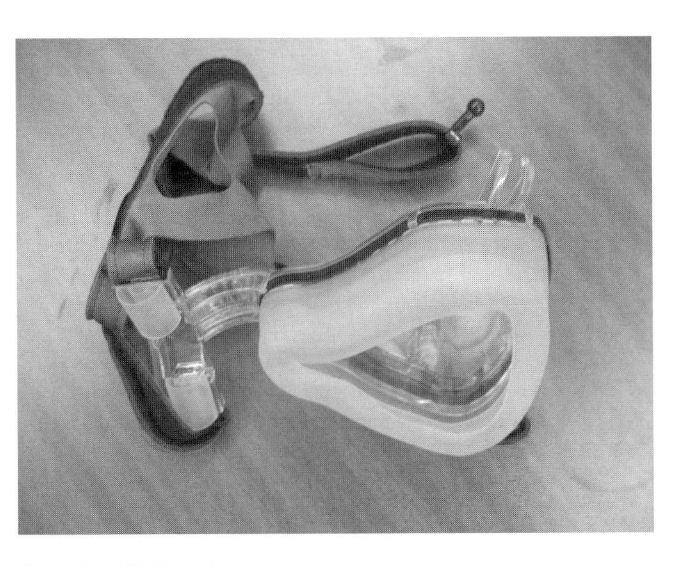

Figure 2. CPAP mask.

Practical points

- Awake patients find nasal CPAP disturbing at first—start at a low pressure.
- The mask seal is most effective at working pressures—don't worry about a leak at low pressures, and don't over-tighten the head straps.
- Positioning makes a difference—it is easier to adjust (and tolerate) CPAP if slightly propped up or sitting.
- The machines are pressure generators—they will make more noise and produce greater air flow when there is a leak.
- Humidification may be necessary from the start of treatment—check for nasal allergies/polyps/crusting.
- Sleep rebound will occur if there has been significant sleep deprivation before treatment. REM sleep is dangerous in patients with ischaemic heart disease—monitor them for the first 3–4 nights.
- V/Q changes and poor right ventricular function may cause marked falls in tissue oxygen levels—use pulse oximetry and prescribe supplemental oxygen through the CPAP system if necessary.

- Always assemble the mask away from the patient—failing to put it together in front of the patient does little to enhance their confidence in the treatment or you.
- The mask should be loosely applied—never so tight that blanching of the nose is seen (it has a watershed blood supply and pressure sores leave unsightly scars).
- The effective therapeutic pressure is nearly always above 10 cm H_2O^{-1}. If in doubt use this as the starting pressure.
- CPAP services are usually run from Sleep Clinics and, surprisingly, they work during the day—trying to get a machine at 3 am is unlikely to be successful so use a water immersion system.
- If the patient is established on a machine—do not alter it! It is set correctly.
- The first couple of nights treatment will alter V/Q and may need supplemental oxygen—monitor the patient with a pulse oximeter.
- The masks are expensive—about £80—make sure the first one is the right one.

Complications of CPAP

- Non-compliance is the commonest long-term problem and is largely determined by the expertise and commitment of the staff who initiate treatment. Having a robust support team also helps;
- Pressure damage to the face, especially the nasal bridge is a major;
- Skin infection;
- Sinusitis;
- Heart failure;
- Oesophageal reflux/gastric distension.

34

Practical guide to non-invasive ventilation

E. Sowden and Stephen Murphy

Introduction

Non-invasive ventilation via a tight-fitting facemask (NIV) is an effective alternative to invasive ventilation for respiratory failure particularly in COPD. Advantages over invasive ventilation include avoidance of intubation and its complications, easy administration by staff on a general respiratory ward rather than intensive care, and intermittent treatment facilitating patient communication and nutrition.

The main applications for NIV are ventilatory failure (hypercapnic or type II respiratory failure) due to COPD, chest wall deformities such as kyphoscoliosis, severe obesity and neuromuscular disorders. However NIV has been used successfully in hypoxaemic (type I) respiratory failure due to community acquired and opportunistic pneumonias, and cardiogenic pulmonary oedema.

Mechanism of ventilatory failure

Reduced central respiratory drive
Sedatives, COPD

Respiratory muscle weakness
Motor neurone disease,
Exacerbation of COPD, Hypokalamia

Impaired chest mechanics
Kyphoscoliosis, thoracoplasty
Obesity, COPD

Principals of NIV

The patient interface (mask) is connected via tubing (patient circuit) to the ventilator, which is sensitive to inspiration and expiration. As the patient inhales the ventilator is triggered to increase the pressure within the circuit. This inspiratory positive airways pressure (IPAP) increases airflow and tidal volume. This augments carbon dioxide elimination correcting the acidosis, and reduces the work of breathing allowing fatigued respiratory muscles to recover.

At the end of inspiration the pressure drops to just above atmospheric pressure, allowing exhalation to occur. This expiratory positive airways pressure (EPAP) keeps the airways open improving oxygenation.

Indications for NIV

Ventilation should be considered if arterial blood gases indicate acute or acute on chronic respiratory acidosis (type II respiratory failure).

pCO_2 >6 kPa and a pH <7.35

However NIV is not suitable for all patients with ventilatory failure. NIV should never be used in acute asthma and there will be situations in which NIV would be inappropriate or impractical.

Starting NIV

- Familiarise yourself with the ventilator and attachments. There are subtle differences between ventilators. Importantly there must be means for CO_2 to escape from mask and patient circuit. This may be through a simple vent in the patient end of the tubing or via a valve between the mask and tubing.
- Explain the procedure to the patient then select the best fitting mask. Determine the size with a template or by trial and error from selection of masks ensuring complete coverage of nose and mouth, and a tight seal (keeping dentures in situ will improve 'fit'). Attach nasal pressure pad (if required) and straps to mask; then connect to ventilator via patient circuit tubing.
- Set ventilator to spontaneous/timed mode. (Patient triggered ventilation, with timed backup set at 15 bpm.) Set IPAP and EPAP to

lowest settings and then switch the ventilator on. Hold the mask in position over the patient's face to enable acclimatization, and when comfortable fix the mask in position with the straps.

- Increase the IPAP by small increments (3–5 cm H_2O) up to 15–20 cm H_2O, checking for leakage of air around the mask. Allow the patient to adjust to each pressure change before increasing further. EPAP is set at 4–5 cm H_2O, and further adjustment should be unnecessary.
- Observe the patient's chest movement, listen to the ventilator, and check the LED indicators cycling between IPAP and EPAP. At the start of inspiration the IPAP LED should light up, the ventilator makes a surging sound and chest expansion occurs.
- Supplementary oxygen can be administered either through the ventilator or directly into the patient circuit or mask.
- Contingency plan. Once the patient has been stabilised a plan of action for possible treatment failure needs to be discussed and documented i.e. referral to ICU for invasive ventilation or a palliative approach to care.

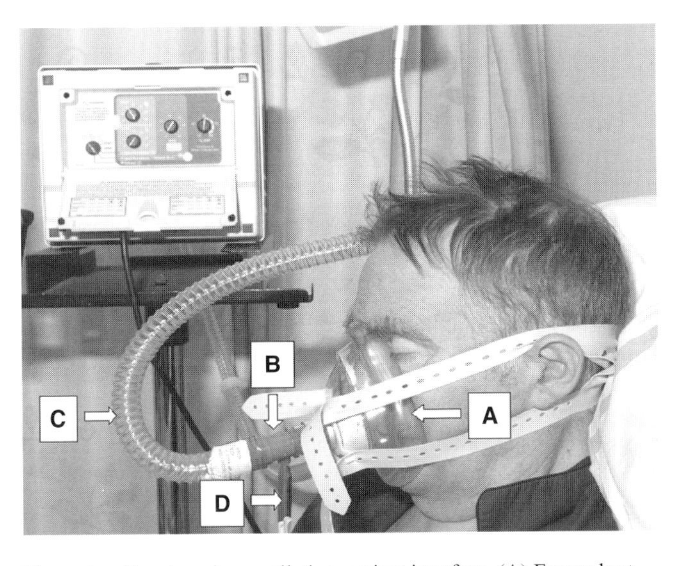

Figure 1. Non-invasive ventilation–patient interface. (A) Ensure best mask fit and minimal air leak. (B) Exhalation (CO_2) vent. (C) Patient circuit ventilator tubing. (D) Oxygen tubing.

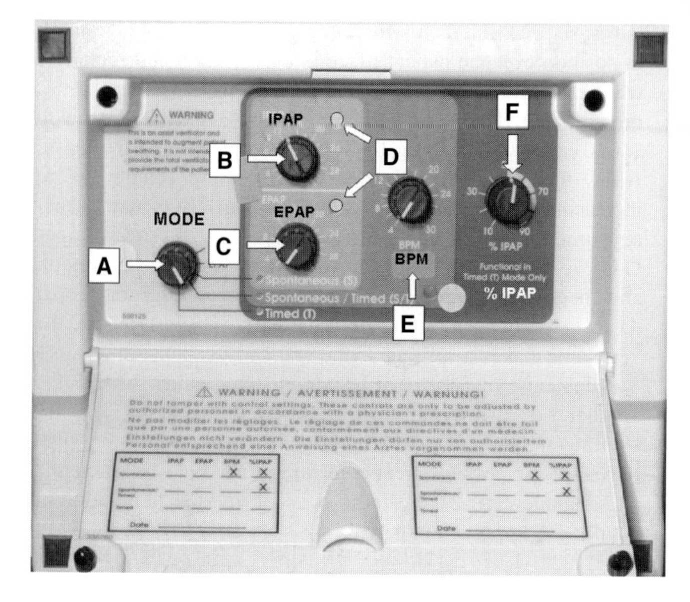

Figure 2. Non-invasive ventilation ventilator controls. (A) Ventilation mode. Set at spontaneous/timed mode. (B) IPAP. Increase gradually to 15–20 (cm H_2O). (C) EPAP. Set at 4–5 cm (cm H_2O). (D) IPAP/EPAP. Alternate blinking of LED's synchronised with patients chest movement. (E) Ventilation rate (backup in spontaneous/timed mode. Mandatory in timed (assist/control) mode (breaths per minute). (F) % IPAP or Inspiratory/Expiratory Ratio. Usually set at <50% particularly in COPD.

Monitoring

- The patient's condition should be closely monitored to assess response to NIV. Assessment is clinical (chest expansion, respiratory rate, comfort and conscious level) and physiological (pulse oximetry and arterial blood gases).
- Pulse oximetry informs on oxygenation (aim for saturation of >85%) but it is not a good measure of the efficacy of ventilation and may actually be misleading. Blood gases to determine pH and pCO_2 should be checked 1 hour after starting treatment, and again at 4 hours.
- Failure to improve should prompt you to check that adequate ventilation is being effectively delivered.

Trouble shooting

- Patient hasn't improved at 1 hour (pH and pCO_2 worse or unchanged). Reassess mask fit, tubing and connections. Check ventilator settings, ventilation mode (spontaneous/timed mode) IPAP (15–20 cm) and EPAP (4–5 cm). Is the ventilator switched on, can you hear it and feel air blowing through the CO_2 vent? Ensure CO_2 escape vent hasn't become occluded (secretions, tape). Is the patient receiving too much oxygen ($SaO_2 > 90\%$)?
- Patient is unable to trigger the ventilator. Check for air leaks, mask fit and ventilator mode. If ventilator has adjustable trigger sensitivity try reducing it. Consider increasing rate of timed backup ventilation or switching to assist/control mode.
- Patient and ventilator are not in synchrony. It is important to adjust respiratory rate of ventilator to approximate that of patients to ensure coordination between patient and ventilator. If ventilating in assist/control mode the ratio inspiratory/expiratory (IE) duration requires adjustment. Expiration is usually longer than inspiration particularly in COPD.
- Patient discomfort will lead to treatment failure. This is usually due to an ill-fitting mask. If too tight a pressure sore develops on nasal bridge and forehead. If too loose air leaks and may irritate eyes. Adjust straps and reassess. IPAP may need to be reduced temporarily.
- Ventilator alarms. Some ventilators have alarms that are triggered by high or low airflow. A high flow alarm usually indicates excessive air leak, usually at the patient interface, or disconnection of tubing. A low flow alarm suggests obstruction to airflow.

Duration of ventilation

In the first 24 hours continue ventilating for as long as the patient will tolerate, thereafter aim for a total cumulative time of 8/24 hours, predominantly overnight until pH is normal. Gradually reduce the periods of ventilation monitoring with daily arterial blood gases.

35

Pulmonary function tests

Mark Weatherhead and George Antunes

Introduction

Pulmonary function testing forms the basis of investigation into respiratory disease. Spirometry and peak flow recording are usually the baseline investigations and can easily be performed at the bedside or in clinic. More formal tests analysing lung volumes and diffusing capacity involves the need for a specialised lung function laboratory. This chapter will cover the use and interpretation of peak flow measurement and spirometry.

Peak expiratory flow

Peak expiratory flow (PEF) is the maximum airflow achieved during expiration. This occurs early in expiration and is an effort dependent procedure. Full inspiration to total lung capacity and maximal effort is essential when performing a PEF test or results are unreliable. PEF can be measured using a spirometer or pneumotachograph but hand held peak flow meters are the most commonly used instruments in clinical practice.

PEF reflects airway obstruction and is reduced in obstructive airway disease but is usually normal in restrictive lung disease (with the exception of neuromuscular weakness) as there is no limitation to airflow in these conditions. It is a less sensitive test than FEV1 and FVC and should not be used on its own in investigating lung disease. However peak flow meters are small and easy to use and provide a practical way for patients to monitor their disease at home. A single value of PEF is of limited use but serial recordings are an important tool in the diagnosis and management of asthma. PEF is also useful when upper airways obstruction is suspected as it is reduced with a relatively well preserved FEV1.

Peak flow measurement

- Before carrying out the procedure explain the test to the patient.
- The needle on the peak flow meter should be returned to zero.
- Standing or sitting position can be used.
- The patient must take a maximal inspiration to total lung capacity and then blow out as hard as possible. There should be a pause of less than 2 seconds from the end of inspiration to start of expiration. Expiration is only needed for a couple of seconds but maximal effort is essential as reduced values can be a result of only slightly sub-maximal effort rather than airways disease.
- The highest value of three correctly performed blows should be used.
- The two largest recordings should be between 40 L/min of each other (if not repeat twice more). To interpret the results always compare to predicted values for age, sex and height.
- Contraindications, problems and complications are similar as for spirometry.

Spirometry

Who to test?

Spirometry is a quick and relatively easy test to perform. Clinical applications are varied and it is indicated as a screening test in patients with breathlessness or other respiratory symptoms and also in smokers to detect Chronic Obstructive Pulmonary Disease (COPD) in early stages. It is also used in epidemiological surveys, to assess disease severity and progression, evaluate bronchodilator or bronchoconstrictor properties of the airways and in pre-operative assessment. Spirometric results however are not diagnostic and must be interpreted in conjunction with clinical history and examination.

What are we measuring?

A spirometer is a device that measures expired and sometimes inspired lung volumes over time. The reliability of results depends on the accuracy of the machine and the use of the correct technique. The measurements that are usually used in spirometry are:

- FEV1 (forced expiratory volume in one second) is the volume of air expired in the first second of forced exhalation after full inspiration. This is a measure of how quickly lungs can be emptied.
- VC (Vital capacity) is the maximum volume of air, which can be exhaled following a maximal inspiration.
- FVC (Forced vital capacity) is the vital capacity of a forced exhalation. This is often slightly less than a relaxed (or slow) VC in moderate to severe airways obstruction.
- FEV1/VC (or FVC) ratio is the FEV1 as a percentage of the VC. The ratio is usually >75% in healthy individuals but falls slowly with age.

How to do it?

Reliable results depend on patient understanding and co-operation. Most problems can be overcome with careful explanation to the patient and a demonstration of the procedure. To obtain accurate results it is recommended to avoid smoking for 24 hours prior to testing, withhold short-acting bronchodilators for six hours and not to perform testing shortly after a meal or vigorous exercise.

The patient should:

- Be sitting erect in a comfortable position. Similar results are obtained standing but forced exhalation can result in reduced cerebral blood flow and dizziness particularly in older patients.
- Breathe in fully to total lung capacity.
- Seal their lips around the mouthpiece to the spirometer. Nose clips are not usually necessary because the pressure generated with forced expiration normally opposes the soft palate to the posterior pharynx.
- Exhale for as long as possible. The FEV1 and FVC must be performed with maximal effort following inspiration but relaxed VC requires a full-unforced expiration only. Expiration should be continued for at least 6 seconds and the pause at end of inspiration should be less than 2 seconds.
- This should be repeated at least three times to obtain reliable results.

Young patients should complete expiration in 3 seconds but older normal subjects and patients with airflow obstruction may have continuous flow for 5–10 seconds and expiration may be limited by the sensation of breathlessness. Expiration may also be interrupted by chest pains or coughing.

Acceptable results should show:

- Minimum of three complete blows;
- 6 second expiration or greater;
- Less than 100 mL or 5% (whichever is greater) difference between the two highest readings for both FVC and FEV1;
- A rapid start to expiration with no interruption, coughing or hesitation.

Common problems

The most common problems are:

- Sub-maximal effort;
- Leak around mouthpiece or obstruction of mouthpiece with the tongue;
- Coughing—common in patients with COPD, asthma and pulmonary fibrosis;
- Incomplete inspiration and expiration.

Complications of spirometry

Spirometry is a very safe procedure generally but several adverse effects have occasionally been reported. These include:

- Dizziness
- Chest pain
- Coughing
- Bronchospasm
- Transmission of infection (rare)
- Syncope
- Pneumothorax (rare)

Contraindications to spirometry

Spirometry can aggravate several conditions and we would recommend avoiding in patients with:

- Pneumothorax;
- Recent thoracic or abdominal surgery;

- Acute haemoptysis of unknown cause;
- Recent myocardial infarction or large pulmonary embolus;
- Thoracic, abdominal or cerebral aneurysms;
- Known or suspected pulmonary tuberculosis (unless adequate infection control measures are provided to reduce the risk of cross infection due to contamination of the spirometer).

Interpretation of results

Once recordings are obtained it is important to interpret these in relation to the normal values for the patient's age, height, ethnic background and gender. An FEV1 of 1.5 would be significantly reduced for a 25-year-old man but could be normal for an 80-year-old lady.

Three common patterns are observed:

Ventilatory defect	Obstructive	Restrictive
FEV1	Reduced	Reduced
FVC	Normal or reduced	Reduced
FEV1/FVC ratio	Reduced	Normal or high
PEF	Reduced	Normal

Obstructive

A reduced FEV1 in relation to FVC occurs due to delayed lung emptying and is found in intrathoracic airways obstruction such as asthma or COPD. This will result in a low FEV1/VC ratio. In obstructive airways disease the FVC is often reduced as well but proportionally less than the FEV1. Other diseases that can result in obstructive pattern spirometry include bronchiectasis, sarcoidosis and endobronchial tumours.

Restrictive

A reduction of both FEV1 and FVC with a normal or high FEV1/FVC ratio is found in restrictive lung diseases. This pattern is found in interstitial lung diseases, respiratory muscle weakness and chest wall deformities. There is no obstruction to lung emptying but the patient has reduced lung volumes because the lungs are small due to increased elasticity (decreased compliance) in interstitial lung diseases or chest wall expansion is limited mechanically in respiratory muscle weakness and chest wall disease.

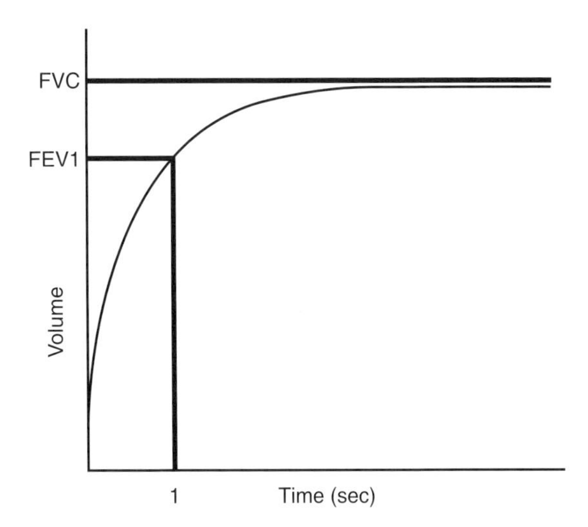

Figure 1. Normal spirometry.

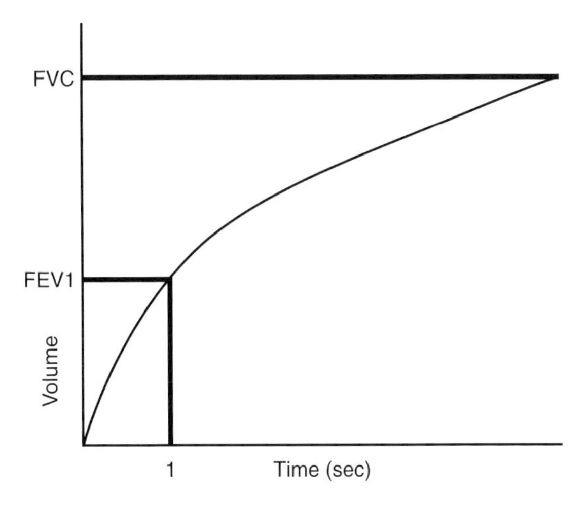

Figure 2. Obstructive spirometry.

Mixed

A reduced FVC in combination with a low FEV1/FVC ratio can occur with mixed obstructive and restrictive defects. In obstructive airways

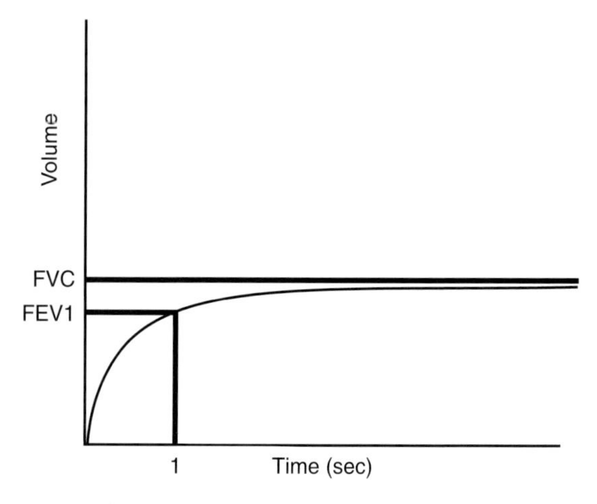

Figure 3. Restrictive spirometry.

disease the FVC can be reduced due to gas trapping secondary to airway collapse, which results in an increased residual volume rather than a true mixed defect. In these patients total lung capacity is often increased. Formal measurement of lung volumes in a lung function laboratory is necessary to distinguish between the underlying defects.

- Maximal effort and inspiration is essential for accurate FEV1 and PEF.
- A good explanation to the patient and a demonstration will overcome most problems.
- Always refer to predicted values for interpretation.
- Lung function tests *do not* make the diagnosis on their own—they *must* be interpreted with the history and examination.

36

Lumbar puncture

Roger Strachan

Introduction

Lumbar puncture (LP) is the term applied to an invasive procedure that involves the insertion of a needle into the lumbar intrathecal space to enable the aspiration of cerebrospinal fluid (CSF) for diagnostic or therapeutic purposes, or for the introduction of medical compounds into the CSF spaces. It is the easiest way to obtain CSF, and therefore is a procedure that doctors should be able to perform. It is often delegated to the more junior member of the medical team, but it may not be an easy or straightforward procedure to perform. It can be associated with complications, and where the procedure fails, this is distressing for the patient, demoralising for the doctor, and diagnostically unsatisfactory.

Anatomy

There are usually five lumbar vertebrae. The spinal cord ends at the level of L1/2, or lower in infants, which will be at risk if a lumbar puncture is performed too high. The lumbar theca tapers at L5/S1, and is not so large a target. It is therefore best to target the L3/4 or L4/5 disc space. Because of the shape of the spinous processes and the configuration of the interlaminar ligaments, access is easier just below the superior spinous process rather than above the inferior spinous process.

Technique

As in any invasive procedure, divide it into stages and always go through the procedure the same way every time. This involves:

- Explanation
- Preparation

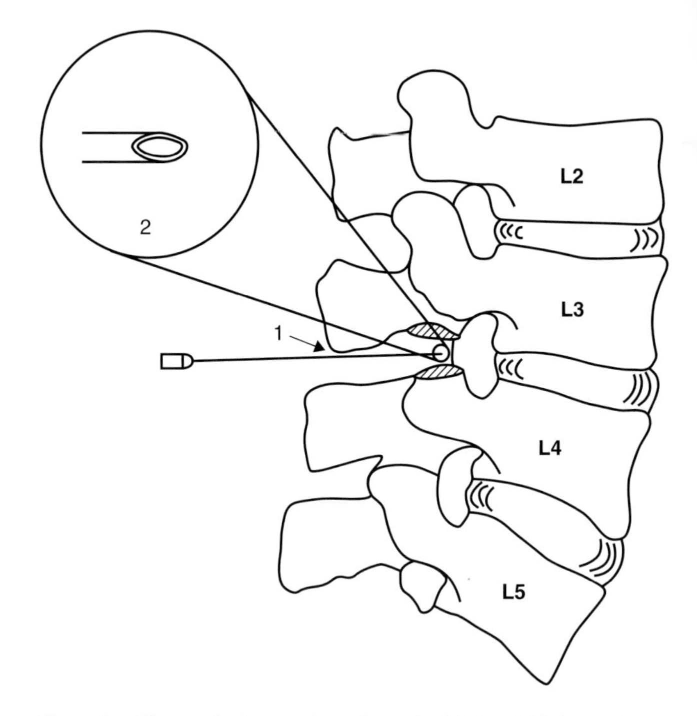

Figure 1. The needle is passed usually at the L3/4 or L4/5 interspinous space. (1) Passing the needle just below the rostral spinous process. (2) The bevel of the needle is positioned horizontally, in line with the patient's back, so that it splits the dura in the direction of its fibres.

- Positioning
- Anaesthesia
- Passing the needle
- Collecting the specimens

Explanation

It is important that the patient understands why the procedure is being done. This of course will not apply to infants, very ill or ventilated patients, but in these circumstances it is still important the parents or relatives understand the reasons behind the procedure. Explain to the patient when it will be done, how it will be done, what exactly is involved, and where it will be done (bedside, treatment room).

Preparation

Consider if the procedure is safe in this patient. Is there any evidence of raised intracranial pressure? Has the patient had lumbar surgery before? Is there a diagnosis of arachnoiditis? If the patient is very obese, consider arranging to do the procedure in the X-ray department using image intensification. You will require assistance, space, and good lighting. Ensure you have all the required materials prepared—skin antiseptic, drapes, local anaesthetic, needles, manometer (if required). The materials usually come in disposable packs. The procedure should be done with full aseptic precautions, using skin preparation, an appropriate drape and sterile gloves.

Positioning

The patient should be positioned with the spine horizontal, parallel to the bed, and the hips and shoulders vertical. A single pillow is usually sufficient. The patients back should be at the edge of the bed, and parallel to it. The knees and hips are flexed, at about 90%, sufficient to flatten out the normal lumbar lordosis. Excessive flexion (foetal position) is not required. Adjust the height of the bed so the patient's spine is at the same height as your shoulders, with you sitting on a stool or chair. Maintain patient dignity—they should be cover with a gown or sheets leaving only the lumbar spine exposed. Ensure that your trolley is to your right (if you are right handed), at an easy working distance. Do not sit too close to the patient. Palpate the iliac crest with the fingers of your left hand, and use your hand to mark out a vertical line to the lumbar spine. Your thumb can palpate the spinous processes. The iliac crest lies at the level of the L4/4 disc. Roll your thumb to either side of the spinous processes, so that you can accurately assess the midline.

Anaesthesia

Raise a small bleb of local anaesthetic (1% lidocaine) under the skin with a small orange needle. Change to a larger green needle, and enter through the bleb, injecting the anaesthetic slowly down to the interlaminar ligaments. Be careful not to enter the epidural space, or you may give the patient an epidural anaesthetic! Try to avoid using too much anaesthetic or too many punctures, as the trauma may cause bleeding and contaminate the result.

Passing the needle

Use a mid-gauge spinal needle (size 20 is ideal). Too large a needle might create a larger dural puncture, leading to post-lumbar puncture epidural leakage of CSF and postural headache. Too small a needle will bend, is more difficult to gain tactile feedback and might even break. If you have positioned the patient correctly and accurately palpated for the midline, the needle should be passed at right angles to the patient's back, parallel to the floor. The bevel of the needle should be directed vertically, towards the ceiling, so that it splits the dura in the direction of its fibres. There is a 'feel' to passing the needle, which has to be learnt. There is a give as it penetrates the interspinous ligament, sometimes a further slight give as it enters the epidural space, and a further give as the dura is penetrated. At each stage, withdraw the stylet, and inspect the needle for CSF. If none is seen, reinsert the stylet, advance further, and check again. The patient may jump a little as the dura is perforated. If you are off the midline, and irritate and hit a nerve root, the patient will express their displeasure appropriately, and report symptoms in the region of the appropriate dermatome. Withdraw slightly, check the position of the patient's back ensuring it is vertical, check for the midline, and readjust your trajectory.

Collecting the specimens

If CSF is obtained, it should not be pink or bloodstained, unless the patient has had a subarachnoid haemorrhage. Otherwise the tap is traumatic, and may no longer be diagnostic. Connect a manometer to measure the opening pressure, if this is required (e.g. in patients with benign intracranial hypertension). The CSF in the manometer can be used as you first specimen. Collect three samples, of 3 to 5 mL each. The first is for bacterial culture (the cleanest), the second for biochemistry (protein and glucose) and the third for cell count. Other specimens will depend on exactly why the LP is being done, and what the presumed diagnosis is. Do not try to aspirate CSF, by applying excessive pressure to an attached syringe. A 'dry' tap may result in patients who have significant lumbar degenerative disease making access difficult, in severe spinal arachnoiditis, in the presence of significantly sized intrathecal tumours (very rare) or where you have missed the target (too low; off the midline; against the vertebral body). Ensure that the specimens are appropriately labelled and sent to the laboratories promptly.

Complications

- Traumatic tap
- Infection (epidural abscess, meningitis)

- Epidural/spinal anaesthesia
- Root transfixion
- Implantation dermoid
- Spinal headache
- Brain herniation

Always

- Explain the procedure fully to the patient
- Take time to position the patient accurately and appropriately
- Maintain full aseptic precautions
- Take care to accurately access the midline
- Enter at the L3/4 or L4/5 intravertebral space
- Advance the needle in stages, looking for CSF at each stage
- Consider using an image intensifier in very obese patients

Never

- Perform an LP in patients with suspected raised ICP, at least without prior CT scanning
- Perform an LP in patients with suspected cord compression, at least without prior MR scanning
- Assume blood staining of the CSF is due to trauma from the LP rather than SAH, in patients where the history is suggestive of SAH

Traumatic tap/subdural haematoma

Hitting an epidural vein may lead to a heavily blood-stained CSF, or even frank blood. This usually happens if the trajectory has been off the midline, into the lateral recess, or the needle has penetrated the anterior dura. It usually ends the procedure, as the CSF will be non-diagnostic. The idea that counting a diminishing number of red cells in sequential specimens distinguishes between a traumatic puncture and a subarachnoid haemorrhage is entirely unreliable. If the clinical diagnosis is suggestive of SAH, and there is blood in the CSF, then the case requires discussion with the Neurosurgical unit, as it is likely cerebral angiography will have to be considered. Subdural haematoma causing compression is very rare, usually occurring in patients with a bleeding disorder in whom the procedure is contraindicated.

Infection

The risk of infection is remarkably small. There is a theoretical risk of meningitis, by introducing skin contaminants into the CSF. Even with indwelling spinal catheters, the risk of infection remains small. Epidural abscess is usually only seen as a result of indwelling epidural catheters.

Epidural/spinal anaesthesia

Inadvertent injection of local anaesthetic into the epidural space at the start of the procedure can cause temporary nerve root sensory blocks in the lower limb on the dependent side. As long as this is recognised, the patient can be reassured it will recover quickly. Theoretically, in small thin patients, a green 16G needle might penetrate the dura and injection of some anaesthetic may cause a temporary spinal block.

Root transfixion

Advancing the needle off the midline may lead to contact with the nerve root. Providing the needle is being advanced with an appropriate degree of caution, the patient will usually tell you if they feel any symptoms in the distribution of the nerve root, such as pain or unpleasant paraesthesia. Even in infants or unconscious/ventilated patients, the nerve root is mobile enough to make any likely damage from transfixion extremely unlikely.

Implantation dermoid

Late implantation dermoids have been rarely reported if skin cells are implanted by the needle into the deeper layers.

Spinal headache

Post-lumbar puncture postural headache is a relatively common complaint. CSF may leak from the dural puncture into the epidural space. It is one reason why larger needles should not be used, and it is best to have the bevel of the needle pointing vertically. Patients should be kept flat for a few hours after the procedure, and encouraged to drink plenty. If symptoms persist, laying flat for 24 to 48 hours may help to resolve the problem, but the evidence for this is disputed. Intravenous hydration is of no proven benefit. With persistent and debilitating symptoms, blood patching can be carried out. This is best done by an anaesthetist, who has more experience in accessing the epidural space. A needle is passed down the same trajectory and position as the original lumbar puncture and a few millilitres of the patient's own blood is injected into the epidural space. This clot helps to seal the puncture site.

Brain herniation

In patients with elevated intracranial pressure (ICP), lumbar puncture is dangerous.

The exceptions are in communicating hydrocephalus, where the intracranial CSF spaces communicate with the spinal subarachnoid space, and in patients with so-called benign intracranial hypertension. In all other cases, a reduction in the spinal CSF pressure may causes brain herniation, with compression of the midbrain at the level of the tentorium or brain stem at the level of the foramen magnum. If unchecked, this will lead to the death of the patient. Where there is ANY suggestion of raised ICP, with a reduced conscious level or symptoms of headache or vomiting, a CT brain scan should always be performed prior to any LP. In the acute situation, looking for papilloedema is NOT a reliable way to exclude raised ICP. In patients with spinal cord compression and effacement of the subarachnoid space, where there is no communication of CSF above and below the level of compression, LP can promote a sudden and significant deterioration in neurological deficits.

Section 4

Cardiovascular Skills

37

Drainage of a pericardial effusion

Robert J.R. Meikle

Percutaneous pericardiocentesis is the aspiration of fluid from the pericardial space. The fluid can be analysed for microbiological, biochemical or cytological answers. It is mainly used to relieve cardiac tamponade. This was practised as long ago as the 18th century as a blind procedure with a high complication rate and mortality. Since the development of two-dimensional echocardiography the procedure has become very safe.

Anatomy

The pericardium contains the heart and the roots of the great vessels. It lies in the mediastinum behind the body of the sternum and cartilages of the second to sixth ribs inclusively. It consists of two opposed layers of serous membrane, separated by a minimal amount of fluid. Around this is an outer sac of fibrous tissue called the fibrous pericardium. There are ligamentous attachments from the pericardium to the sternum, vertebral column and diaphragm to keep the heart fixed in place during movement. The surface markings of the heart will vary due to the age, sex, body shape, respiration, body position and disease processes of that individual. The apex of the heart almost corresponds in position to the apex beat, which can be seen and always felt below and medial to, the left nipple. It will lie in the left fifth intercostal space, slightly medial to the mid-clavicular line or about 9 cm from the midline in an average adult male.

Pathophysiology

Accumulation of fluid within the pericardial sac will produce a variable degree of cardiac compression or indeed tamponade. Pericardial pressure is normally sub-atmospheric and becomes more negative during inspiration. The pericardial sac is a closed bag and as fluid collects within it there will be an increasingly steep rise in pressure with small extra additions of fluid. A rapid increase of fluid within the pericardium produces acute tamponade with the pressure reaching 20 to 30 mm Hg. A slower accumulation of fluid over weeks will allow the pericardium to stretch and the patient to compensate and slowly develop symptoms. Both will result in a raised ventricular diastolic pressure, atrial and venous pressures. This causes a reduced stroke volume, reduced cardiac output and so reduced systemic arterial pressure. These findings of raised systemic venous pressure, reduced systemic arterial pressure and quiet heart sounds are known as Beck's triad. The x descent of the venous wave is accentuated, but the y descent is flattened or absent, as cardiac filling is severely restricted during diastole. Severe cardiac tamponade is nearly always accompanied by an accentuated decline in systemic systolic blood pressure on inspiration, called pulsus paradoxus. A decline of greater than 10 mm Hg is usually significant. In advanced cases, the pulse may disappear on inspiration. Pulsus paradoxus can also occur in COPD, bronchial asthma, pulmonary embolism and right ventricular infarction. Regional tamponade can occur with a loculated effusion following cardiac surgery, infection, or neoplasm. Clinical recognition may be difficult due to localised fluid causing left atrial or ventricular compression that fails to elevate systemic venous pressure. Two-dimensional echocardiography is needed for this diagnosis.

Indications

The main reason for therapeutic echo-guided pericardiocentesis is for the drainage of clinically significant pericardial effusions. This is defined as a patient who is symptomatic, is haemodynamically compromised and has a large effusion. The patient will usually have the following features: a tachycardia, reduced arterial pressure, pulsus paradoxus, tachypnoea, dyspnoea, peripheral oedema and distended neck veins. The main causes of cardiac tamponade are in patients following cardiac surgery (weeks), patients with neoplastic pericardial disease and patients having or who have had cardiac catheterisation especially with intervention. If an ill patient has a pericardial effusion of unknown aetiology it is useful to exclude suspected bacterial pericarditis, tuberculous pericarditis and malignant pericardial effusion by pericardiocentesis. In all other effusions with stable patients it is usually not indicated, as the diagnostic yield is low, about 6%.

Contraindications

- No pericardial effusion on CT scan or echocardiography;
- Thrombocytopaenia of less than 80×10^9/L;
- Uncorrected coagulopathy;
- Infection of the skin or soft tissue at the planned needle site;
- An uncooperative and restless patient;
- High-risk situations would be those with small effusions, effusions only lying posterior or which are loculated. Also high risk would be an acute traumatic haemopericardium that re-accumulates faster than it can be drawn off.

Patient preparation

The problem, technique and risks are discussed with the patient to obtain a written consent. The patient should be fasted for six hours. A premedication may be used, either a benzodiazepine or an injection of opiate with hyoscine or atropine to minimise vagal responses as the pericardium is punctured. A recent chest X-ray, ECG, coagulation screen, platelet count, and potassium level should be reviewed and cross-match is made. A large peripheral cannula is inserted into a vein with an IV drip. A high-risk case may require a cardiothoracic team to be rapidly available.

Equipment

Full emergency airway and resuscitation equipment must immediately be available. This must include a defibrillator and a standard tray of emergency drugs.

A source of oxygen and suction equipment must be present.

Monitoring equipment must include an ECG, BP cuff or invasive arterial line, pulse oximeter and a two-dimensional echocardiography machine.

Skin prep pack with alcoholic Betadine, sterile gloves and gown. 1% lidocaine with syringes and needles. A 16 to 18G 9 cm long sheathed needle, with a 50 mL sterile syringe and three-way tap.

Anaesthetic drugs such as propofol, suxamethonium, atracurium and fentanyl would be useful if a resuscitated patient has to be kept under intravenous anaesthesia for the rest of the procedure.

Techniques

Monitoring is established and the vital signs are recorded. The patient is placed in a supine position with the head raised at 20° to 30°. An experienced echocardiologist locates the effusion. The ideal entry site, the point at which the distance from skin to maximal fluid accumulation is minimised, without any important structures in the way, is identified. The area is cleaned, draped and infiltrated with 1% lignocaine. The needle can be placed for a subxiphoid (subcostal) or an apical (anterior chest wall) approach. The American Heart Association recommends the subxiphoid. This reduces the risks of coronary artery, internal mammary artery or pleural surface laceration. In using echocardiography as the standard method of needle localisation, a number of centres have found that the majority of approaches are apical. It is not possible to continuously monitor the needle tip by echocardiography so the placement can be checked by injecting a small amount of agitated saline that will be visualised with the echo. Some resistance is felt as the pericardial surface is encountered. A 'pop' may be felt as the needle enters the sac. Prior to the use of echocardiography, an ECG lead was connected to the pericardial needle to allow contact with the myocardium to be recognised. Once in place, the needle should be firmly held beside the skin to prevent further entry. Fluid is withdrawn until the echo demonstrates that there is minimal effusion left. A J-type guidewire can be passed through the needle into the sac, the needle withdrawn and a plastic catheter threaded into the sac if extended drainage is required. This may be left in place for 48 hours with minimal risk of infection.

Recurrent effusion due to neoplastic pericardial invasion may be treated with sclerosing or chemotherapeutic drugs via the pericardial catheter or surgery. Surgery carries a high periopertive morbidity and mortality in this group of ill patients.

Continue to monitor the patient's vital signs for four hours and depending on the aetiology a repeat echo may be planned. Many centres report a success rate of 95–99% in removing fluid or relieving tamponade using echocardiography.

Complications

Death due to any event below.

- Acute haemopericardium due to myocardial laceration or puncture;

- Puncture of ventricular chambers may require surgery, but atrial puncture tends to settle itself;
- Laceration of a coronary artery requiring surgical repair;
- Injury to the intercostal or thoracic artery requiring surgical repair;
- Pneumothorax requiring observation or a chest drain;
- Haemothorax due to intercostal artery or pulmonary laceration;
- Puncture of peritoneal cavity or abdominal viscera;
- Self-limiting ventricular tachycardia or progression to a cardiac arrest;
- Vasovagal bradycardia;
- Air embolism.

The rate of complications is about 1% for major events requiring intervention. It is 3–4% for minor events which require no specific treatment but should be followed up with appropriate monitoring.

Always

- Use a two-dimensional echocardiographically guided technique
- Use an experienced echocardiologist
- Use cardiac laboratory facilities
- Check coagulation and platelet count first
- Establish IV access before the procedure
- Have full airway and resuscitation equipment ready which includes a defibrillator and emergency drugs
- Monitor the patient throughout the procedure
- Use agitated saline as a contrast agent to identify the needle tip placement
- Use extended catheter drainage for patients at high risk of re-accumulation
- Be prepared to carry this procedure out on an emergency basis

Never

- Use blind needle pericardiocentesis
- Leave samples for cytology or microbiology in the fridge overnight
- Leave a pericardial catheter for more than 48 hours

38

Pulmonary artery catheterization

Emilio Garcia

The pulmonary artery catheter (PAC) was first designed by Professors Swan and Ganz in 1970, since then there have been several modifications of the original design, although the general principle remains the same. The PAC is a flow directed balloon-tipped catheter that allows simultaneous measurement of right atrial pressures and pulmonary artery pressures, and can be used to estimate cardiac output (Figure 1).

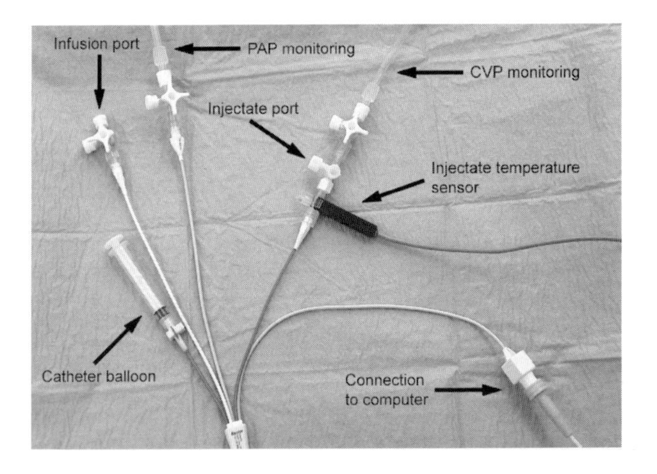

Figure 1. Pulmonary artery catheter.

Despite multiple trials and meta-analysis attempts to prove the advantages or disadvantages of the PAC it remains a useful and reliable tool in intensive care units.

General characteristics

- 120 cm length;
- Balloon up to 1.5 mL;

- Proximal opening 30 cm from tip;
- 10 cm marks;
- 50 cm marks;
- Thermistor 4 cm from catheter tip.

Indications

Assessment of cardiac filling in situations when CVP measurements are unreliable;
Assessment of cardiac output and its optimisation;
Investigation of cardiac shunts;
Measurement of mixed venous oxygen;
Pulmonary angiography;
Peri-operative monitoring of high risk patients.

Contraindications

Absolute contraindications

Absence of skilled personnel or equipment;
Lack of patient consent.

Relative contraindications

Coagulopathy;
Permanent pacemaker;
Artificial valve.

Direct measurements

Temperature;
Atrial and pulmonary artery pressures;
Cardiac output;
Oximetry.

Necessary equipment

Monitor with two invasive pressure recording channels;
Compatible transducer system connected to a pressure bag × 2;
PAC introducer;
Pulmonary artery catheter;
Sterile trolley;

Protective sheath;
Tilting bed or trolley;
ECG monitor;
Full resuscitation facilities;
Cardiac output module for monitor;
Temperature transducer.

Technique for floating

Having obtained patients consent or documenting in the patient notes that benefits outweighs the risk in the case of an unconscious patient, check all equipment and connections are available and compatible.

Then under full aseptic technique the first step entails in gaining central intravenous access using a Seldinger technique as demonstrated in Chapter 23. The route used is not important; however the left subclavian or right internal jugular veins are easier because they follow the normal curvature of the catheter.

After passing the wire through the needle, the needle is removed and the introducer and dilator mounted together are inserted after making a small incision at skin level with a small scalpel blade (failure to make an incision may result in damage to the introducer or the PAC).

Preparation of pulmonary artery catheter

- Follow the manufacturer's instructions.
- Check expiry date and correct size and catheter type.
- If using an oxymetric PAC calibrate the oximeter without removing the end from the black cover.
- Once that is done follow normal procedure.
- Inspect catheter.
- Attach syringe to balloon port. Inflate to 1.5 mL. The inflated balloon should have a donut-shape and the catheter should be in the middle (Figure 2). Ensure that the balloon inflates and deflates easily.
- Offer all other ends to your assistant. All ports should be flushed and filled to ensure patency and transducers attached to pulmonary artery and CVP ports. Calibration should be made referring to patients mid-axillary line. All other ends (thermistor/oximeter/heating element) should also be attached.

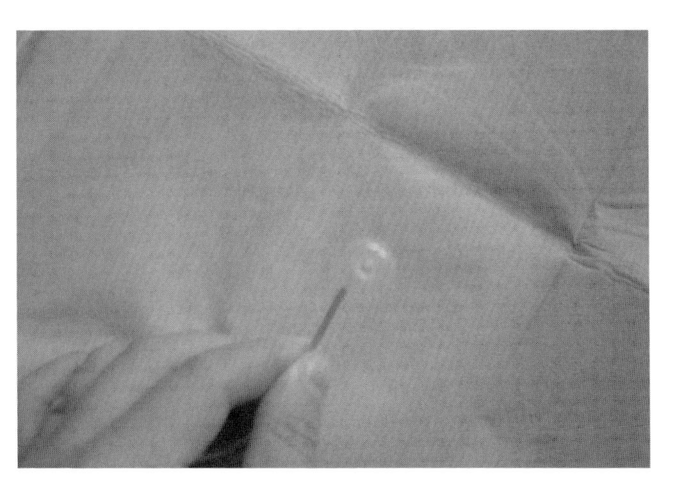

Figure 2. Inflated balloon of pulmonary catheter.

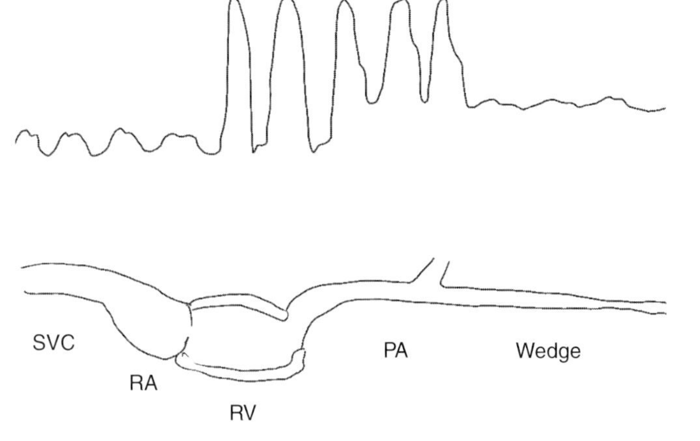

Figure 3. Different waveforms obtained during pulmonary artery catheterisation.

- Connect the protective sheath before inserting catheter.
- Insert catheter to 15 cm and then inflate balloon. The catheter is then outside the introducer.
- Always advance with balloon inflated.

- Always withdraw catheter with balloon deflated.
- Inflate balloon once in right atrium.
- Advance catheter 3 cm at the time looking carefully at monitor for arrhythmias and pressure curve (Figure 3).
- Once the balloon is wedged there is at the end of diastole a column of blood between L ventricle and catheter.
- By convention measurement of PAOP is done at the end of systole and at end expiration.

Complications

- Coiling/knotting of catheter;
- Damage to valves/myocardium;
- Valve regurgitation;
- Arrhythmias;
- Pulmonary artery damage/rupture;
- Pulmonary infarction;
- Catheter sepsis (PAC should not be left in for more than 72 hours).

Normal values

	Range
R atrial pressure	3–6
R ventricular systolic pressure	18–30
R ventricular diastolic pressure	2–8
PA systolic pressure	18–30
PA diastolic pressure	5–15
PAOP	5–14

PA 15–30/4–12 mm Hg; RV 15–30/0 mm Hg;
PAOP 2–10 mm Hg; CI 2.8–4.2 L/min/m^2.

Parameters measured

Right heart pressures; this is measured continually as the catheter is advanced. Once the catheter is in position the catheter will allow simultaneously monitoring of both pulmonary artery and R ventricular pressures. In the absence of pulmonary valve stenosis or an atrial myxoma PA systolic and RV systolic should be the same.

Pulmonary artery occlusion pressure

Wedging of the pulmonary artery catheter is dangerous and should only be performed by trained personnel. Before performing a wedge change the screen mode of your monitor to 'wedge'. Ensure that there is no residual air in the balloon, and then gently inflate balloon till wedging occurs. Note that full inflation of the balloon is not necessary and can be dangerous. The pulmonary artery diastolic pressure is close to pulmonary artery occlusion pressure, the latter normally 1–3 mm Hg lower. When this correlation exists data can be estimated from PADP, but when the relationship is different by >5 mm Hg, for instance in pulmonary hypertension, pulmonary fibrosis or pulmonary embolism, data derived from PADP could be misleading.

Always

- Use aseptic technique
- Pre fill all lumens with normal saline
- Record pressures during insertion
- Confirm position on CxR
- Remove after 72 hours
- Use pacing if bifascicular block
- Always transduce distal lumen pressure to alert if accidental wedging occurs
- Refloat catheter if patient ventilatory situation changes

One must remember

- Pulmonary oedema is likely to develop if PAOC is greater than patients oncotic pressure.
- Trends are more informative than single readings.

Never

- Overinflate the ballon
- Do not leave ballon inflated
- Do not just act on single readings
- Do not leave catheter in for more than 72 hours

39

Cardiac output measurement

Khalid J. Khan

Introduction

The cardiac output (CO) is the amount of blood pumped by the ventricles every minute. This is one of the most important factors that determines the supply of oxygen and other nutrients to the tissues. Cardiac output varies enormously under different states in health and disease, e.g. body surface area, rest, exercise, following major surgery, sepsis and various heart diseases. The Fick principle described in 1870 was the first method used for cardiac output estimation and remains the gold standard. However, cardiac output was first measured in the clinical setting in 1970s, with the introduction of pulmonary artery floatation catheter using thermodilution technique and rapidly gained popularity. Recently, non-invasive methods of cardiac output estimation have become possible.

Anatomy

The right and the left atria are the receiving chambers from the systemic and the pulmonary venous circulation respectively. Blood then enters the respective ventricles during diastole and is then ejected during systole into the pulmonary and systemic circulation. Since the right and the left ventricles are connected in series, the output of the two ventricles is identical under normal circumstances. However, it may differ in cases of abnormal connection between the chambers or isolated ventricular failure.

Physiology

Cardiac output is the product of heart rate and stroke volume.

Heart rate

The adult untrained heart produces its optimum output in the range of 70–90 beats per minute, while it falls at either extreme. However, a trained athlete's heart can produce a large output at much slower rate owing to large stroke volume while a neonatal heart is very much more rate dependant since its stroke volume is largely fixed.

Stroke volume

Stroke volume is the amount of blood pumped every beat. It is dependant on the preload, contractility and the afterload.

Preload

Preload is defined as the initial stretch of the myocardium before contracting and the force of contraction is directly proportional to the amount of that initial stretch. In normal subjects preload translates into the volume of blood in the ventricle prior to systole. Although preload is a measure of volume it is related to the chamber pressure. This relationship between volume and pressure is called *compliance.* As pressure is much easier to measure than volume in routine clinical practice, preload of the right and left ventricles is measured as right atrial or central venous pressure and left atrial or pulmonary artery occlusion pressure respectively. However, these pressures do not reflect volume or preload accurately under various disease states, when compliance is abnormal.

Contractility

It is the measure of the force of contraction during ventricular systole. It is also a measure of the inotropic state of the heart. It is measured as the rate of rise of ventricular pressure (dp/dt). The contractility increases as a result of endogenous or exogenous inotropic agents.

Afterload

This is the resistance against which the right and left ventricles contract, namely the pulmonary and systemic vascular resistance respectively.

Indications

Cardiac output measurement is an essential component of haemodynamic monitoring. In critically ill patients clinical assessment is unreliable and the indirect indicators of cardiac output (filling pressures and systemic blood pressure) may also be inaccurate due to the altered compliance of the ventricles and the peripheral circulation. The commonest clinical dilemma is hypotension, which could be due to extremes of heart rate, reduced preload, reduced myocardial contractility or systemic arterial vasodilatation. Certainly in the last two, measurement of cardiac output is essential to pursue the correct therapy. Hence the common indications are:

- Assessment of cardiac function;
- Management of hypotension;
- Assessment of the need for and response of inotropic therapy;
- Oxygen consumption studies.

Cardiac output measurement

There are various methods of CO measurement in use in the laboratory and clinical bedside settings that require varying degree of invasive procedures and hence carry potential for complications. There is constant search for an ideal method but currently none exists.

Table 1. Classification of cardiac output tests relating to the degree of invasiveness of the procedure.

Highly invasive	Moderately invasive	Minimally invasive	Non-invasive
• Direct Fick • PAC based methods	• Indirect Fick • PiCCO system doppler	• LiDCO/ pulseCO system • Oesophageal echo • Transoesophageal echo • NICO system	• Clinical • Bioimpedence • Transthoracic

Table 2. Characteristics of an ideal cardiac output method.

- No contraindications for use;
- Non or least invasive;
- Easy to use;
- Minimally operator dependant;
- Accurate;
- Reproducible;
- Minimal side effects and complications;
- Validated by appropriate studies.

Current commonly used methods of cardiac output measurement:

1. Indirect Fick principle
   - CO_2 rebreathing method
2. Indicator dilution
   - Dye
   - Thermodilution
   - Heat transfer
3. Ultrasound
   - Oesophageal Doppler
   - Transthoracic echocardiography
   - Transoesophageal echocardiography
4. Combination methods
   - PiCCO system
   - LiDCO system

I. Indirect Fick method

The blood flow through lungs is calculated using the Fick principle and is based on CO_2 elimination.

$$Q = \frac{V_{CO_2}}{C_{vCO_2} - C_{aCO_2}}$$

where Q is cardiac output, V_{CO_2} is the volume of CO_2 elimination in ml/min, C_{vCO_2} and C_{aCO_2} are arterial and venous CO_2 content in blood, respectively.

CO_2 concentration is estimated in the expired volume, venous and arterial CO_2 are estimated from measurements made at the mouth using CO_2 rebreathing methods.

II. Indicator dilution

(a) Dye dilution (see Figure 1)

This is rarely used clinically but provides the basis for the other 'dilution' methods currently used.

(b) Thermodilution (see Figure 2)

This requires a pulmonary artery catheter (PAC) and is the most commonly used method in the haemodynamic management of patients in the ICU and peri-operative setting. This can be used to provide intermittent or continuous CO.

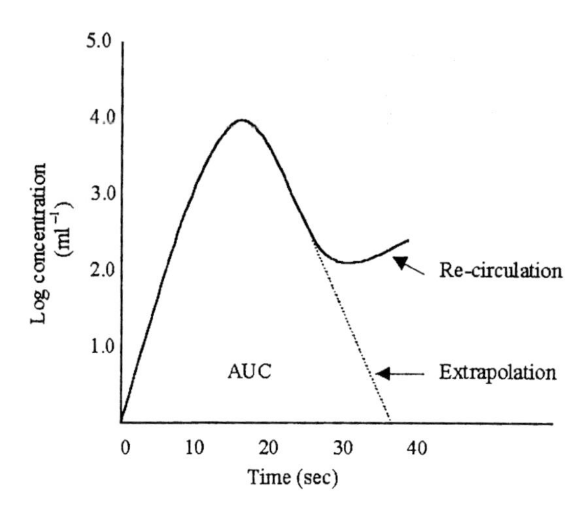

Figure 1. Dye dilution curve.

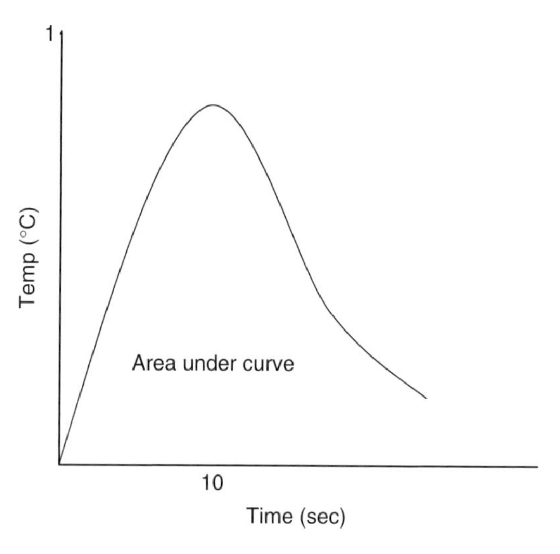

Figure 2. Thermodilution curve.

(c) Intermittent bolus injection

This requires a PAC, a CO computer and uses cold normal saline as the injectate. The cold solution should be injected into the right atrium through the proximal port of the catheter just proximal to the injectate

- Confirm correct position of PAC
- Make sure no warm fluids being administered during measurements
- Confirm computer constant
- Inject fast and steady
- Inject during the same respiratory phase
- Reject abnormal looking curves
- Average at least three readings

temperature sensor, as fast as possible and at the same point of the ventilatory phase, preferably end expiration. This leads to a drop in temperature of the blood near the tip of the catheter that is proportional to the blood flow. The temperature change is plotted as a function of time and the resultant curve is called thermodilution curve. An average of three readings, within 10% of each should be obtained.

Advantages

- Considered as the gold standard in clinical setting;
- Repeated measurements possible;
- Widely used.

Disadvantages

- Invasive;
- Operator dependant;
- Intermittent.

Continuous method

Recently several products have been developed that use temperature gradients to provide a continuous estimate of cardiac output.

(a) CCO/CCOmbo (Edwards Lifesciences)

These are special pulmonary artery floatation catheters that have a heating filament and a temperature sensor near the tip of the catheter. The filament is heated in a random sequence and a thermodilution curve obtained.

(b) TruCATH (BD Medical system)

This is based upon the principle of mass heat-transfer and uses a special pulmonary artery catheter that has two thermistors, one in the right atrium and the other in the pulmonary artery. Cardiac output is calculated from the amount of energy required to maintain the thermistor in the right atrium, 1°C above the blood temperature measured in the pulmonary artery.

III. Doppler Ultrasound

2D and continuous wave Doppler echocardiography and oesophageal Doppler can provide relatively non-invasive, continuous, real time estimation of cardiac output. The velocity of the moving blood (red cells) is estimated from the Doppler shift

$$v = \frac{c(Fs - Fr)}{2Fr(\cos\theta)}$$

where v is velocity, c is speed of sound in blood, $Fs - Fr$ is change in frequency and θ is the intercept angle between the ultrasound beam and the direction of blood flow.

Stroke volume is calculated as the velocity time integral (VTI) times the cross sectional area (CSA) of the region of flow. The region of flow for this purpose is the descending thoracic aorta in case of oesophageal Doppler and left ventricular outflow tract in echocardiography.

$$\text{SV} = \text{CSA} \times \text{VTI}$$

Limitations of this technique are:

- Assumption that the descending aorta and LV outflow tract are tubular;
- Accurate echocardiographic measurements depend upon good quality picture acquisition and alignment with blood flow;
- Considerable mathematical derivations;
- Operator dependency.

IV. Combination methods

These two methods are minimally invasive and provide continuous measurement of stroke volume.

(a) PiCCO System

This system combines the thermodilution and arterial pulse contour analysis. A central venous catheter and a proximal arterial line are required. The system is calibrated by performing transcardio-pulmonary thermodilution. Cold saline is injected in the central venous catheter and the temperature difference sensed by the thermistor in the arterial catheter. The arterial waveform is then analysed to derive ejection systolic area. Beat to beat calculations are averaged over 30 second cycles.

(b) LiDCO System

This combines dye dilution and arterial pulse contour analysis. It requires venous access and a lithium sensor attached to a radial arterial catheter. Injecting a small dose of lithium chloride into a central or peripheral vein and acquiring a lithium dilution curve (see Figure 1) calibrates the system. Continuous, real-time, beat-to-beat stroke volume is calculated by pulse contour analysis (PulseCO).

Both methods may encounter problems with abnormal waveforms, for instance during intra-aortic balloon counter-pulsation or atrial fibrillation, otherwise the available data suggests a good correlation with thermodilution methods.

40

Intra-aortic balloon counter-pulsation

James Park

The intra-aortic balloon pump is a mechanical cardiac assist device. Its underlying principle is that if afterload could be reduced by removing blood from the femoral artery during systole and replacing it during diastole, cardiac output could be augmented. The concept was developed during the 1960s by using a balloon placed in the descending aorta to displace blood by inflating and deflating at the appropriate time of the cardiac cycle. Ten years later percutaneous insertion became possible along with the ability to measure aortic pressures via an integral lumen. Timing algorithms and microprocessor control have progressed and transport devices have become available.

Theory

A basic understanding of the cardiac cycle is required in order to make sense of the theory of intra-aortic balloon counter-pulsation.

A thin polyurethane balloon mounted on a catheter is inserted into the descending aorta with its tip positioned just distal to the origin of the left subclavian artery. Catheters are available with balloon volumes from 2.5 to 50 mL. Our adult cardiac centre currently stocks 34 mL and 40 mL balloons with an 8FG profile.

The balloon is attached to a pump console. The console consists of an input section, a user interface, an electronic centre to control the gas mechanics, a gas reservoir and back up batteries.

The balloon is timed to fill during diastole when the ventricles are relaxed and the aortic valve is closed. Diastolic pressure is augmented and blood is displaced away from the balloon. Immediately

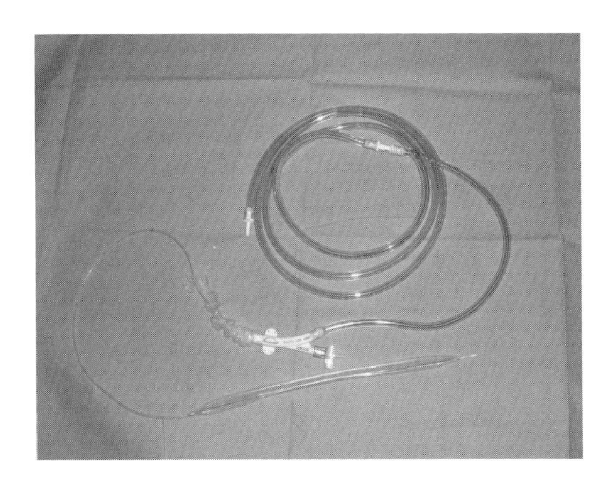

Figure 1. An adult intra-aortic balloon catheter.

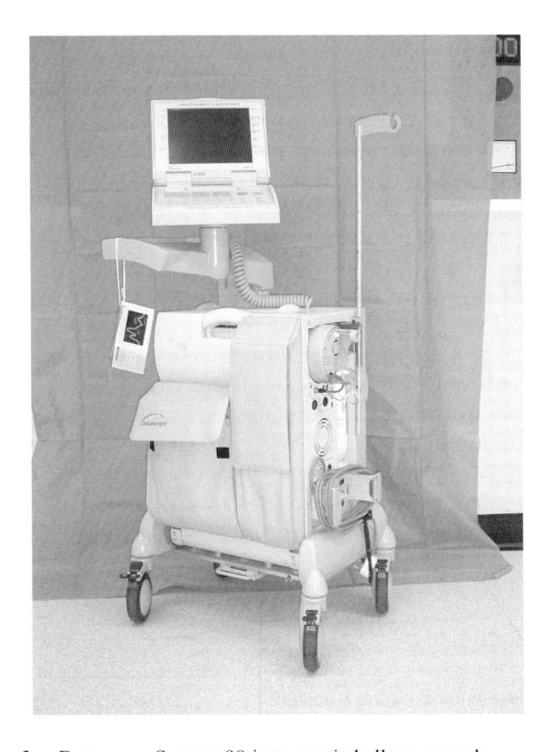

Figure 2. Datascope System 98 intra-aortic balloon console.

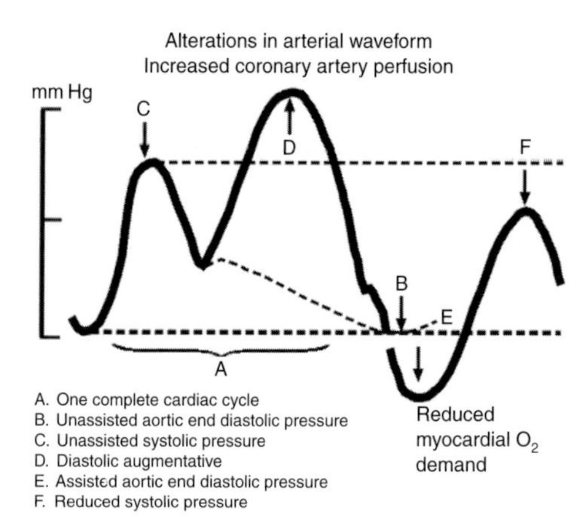

Figure 3. Alterations in arterial waveform associated with intra-aortic balloon counterpulsation.

before the next ventricular contraction the balloon is deflated which reduces the aortic end diastolic pressure and hence the afterload. Thus intra-aortic balloon counter-pulsation would appear to increase myocardial oxygen supply (especially to the left ventricle) by diastolic augmentation and decrease myocardial oxygen demand by reducing afterload.

Following insertion of an intra-aortic balloon pump heart rate commonly decreases, cardiac output increases, systemic vascular resistance decreases, left ventricular end diastolic pressure decreases and mean arterial pressure increases. It is not clear whether diastolic augmentation or afterload reduction is responsible for these effects; it is probable that in some patients afterload reduction is the predominant beneficial effect and in others diastolic augmentation is relatively more important. Some workers have failed to demonstrate an increase in coronary blood flow with intra-aortic balloon counter-pulsation.

Indications

Intra-aortic balloon counter-pulsation was originally developed as a therapy for cardiogenic shock, but indications have grown to encompass most instances where there is a need to restore the balance

Table 1. Indications.

Cardiogenic shock or left ventricular failure	Myocardial infarction Myocarditis Cardiomyopathy Myocardial contusion Pharmacological
Mechanical complication of myocardial infarction	Ventriculoseptal defect Papillary muscle rupture
Unstable angina refractory to medical therapy	
Procedural support	Coronary angiography Coronary angioplasty Off pump coronary artery bypass surgery High risk non cardiac surgical patient
Arrhythmia	Post myocardial infarction ventricular irritability
Cardiac surgery	To support weaning from cardiopulmonary bypass Low output state following cardiopulmonary bypass Myocardial stunning Bridge to transplantation

between myocardial oxygen supply and demand. However the wide variation in the frequency of intra-aortic balloon counter-pulsation in different institutions reflects a lack of good quality outcome data; the optimum use of the intra-aortic balloon pump has yet to be defined.

Contraindications

Contraindications to intra-aortic balloon counter-pulsation may be relative or occasionally absolute. Often a decision has to be made based on the balance of perceived risks versus potential benefits.

Insertion

Insertion is usually via the femoral artery using a modified Seldinger technique. Insertion should be carried out by trained or appropriately supervised personnel working in a suitable clinical area such as an operating theatre, intensive care unit, coronary care unit or cardiac

Table 2. Contraindications.

Absolute	Aortic dissection Brain stem death or do not resuscitate order
Relative	Aortic regurgitation Aortic aneurysm Severe peripheral vascular disease Chronic end stage heart failure without the potential to recover Massive trauma

catheter laboratory with or without radiological control. The patient should be appropriately monitored. If the patient is conscious the procedure should be carefully explained and the consent obtained. A balloon of the size appropriate to the patient's height is chosen according to the manufacturers instructions. Both inguinal regions are carefully painted with a suitable surgical preparation and the patient draped from head to toe. Both femoral arteries are palpated. The side with the greater pulse is chosen if this is identifiable. If the patient is conscious the puncture area is carefully and thoroughly infiltrated with local anaesthetic solution. The femoral artery is then punctured and the supplied guidewire advanced cephalad until the J-shaped lies in the ascending aorta near the origin of the left subclavian artery. The puncture needle is then removed.

The distance from the femoral arterial puncture site to the origin of the left subclavian artery is approximately the distance from the puncture site to the manubrio-sternal angle. The length of balloon to be inserted can be estimated by placing the tip of the wrapped balloon catheter at the angle of Louis and noting the distance to the femoral artery puncture sight using the balloon catheter as a measure. Fluroscopy can be used to aid positioning. The femoral artery is then gently dilated to accept the supplied sheath/dilator combination then the dilator is removed leaving the guidewire in the sheath. The delicate balloon catheter is carefully unwrapped to avoid perforation. It is then threaded over the guidewire and advanced to lie in the previously estimated position. As the balloon catheter enters the sheath blood will escape via the longitudinal folds which form channels in the tightly wrapped balloon.

The guidewire is then removed and the sheath pulled back and connected to the leak proof cuff on the balloon catheter hub. It is preferable to remove the entire sheath from the femoral artery as this is likely to reduce the incidence of ischaemic complications. The catheter is then sutured into place and a clear sterile dressing applied.

Counter-pulsation is now initiated. The console is switched on and the balloon catheter is attached to the gas line. The pressure transducer is connected and zeroed. The patient ECG electrodes are attached or the ECG input slaved from the patient monitor. The source from which the cardiac cycle is derived is chosen. The gas reservoir is filled and pumping initiated. Maximum effect is derived from a 1:1 augmentation ratio but some workers prefer to augment every other cardiac cycle initially. This allows them to compare assisted cycles with unassisted cycles and facilitates adjustments to timing.

The radial pulses are checked and should be equal and reflect the augmented pulse waveform. A chest X-ray or hard copy from radiological screening is obtained to check the position of the balloon catheter tip. This should be visible at the level of the second to third intercostal space on an anteroposterior film. The right size of balloon correctly positioned will end proximal to the renal arteries. Systemic heparinisation is initiated to achieve an activated partial thromboplastin time of 50–84 seconds or an activated clotting time of 180–220 seconds.

Triggering

Balloon activity is timed according to the patient's cardiac cycle. This is usually derived from the R wave of the patient's ECG. Alternatively the cardiac cycle can be derived from the arterial pressure waveform from the lumen of the balloon catheter, from an external pacemaker or, in certain incidences, an intrinsic pump rate. Triggering from the arterial pressure waveform may be particularly useful during tachyarrhythmias, cardiac pacing or in patients with poor identification of R waves on the ECG monitor.

Timing

Accurate timing of inflation and deflation is essential for maximum augmentation. Automatic timing is becoming more successful as algorithms become more sophisticated but some manual adjustment

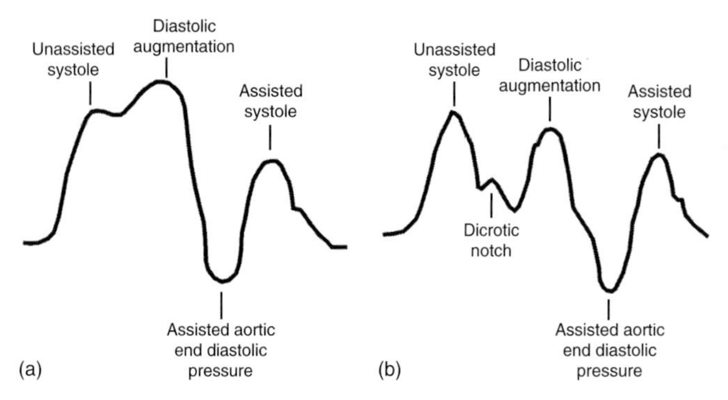

Figure 4. Timing errors (Redrawn from an original courtesy of the Datascope Corporation). (a) Early inflation. Inflation of the intra-aortic balloon prior to aortic valve closure. Waveform characteristics: Inflation of the intra-aortic balloon prior to the dichrotic notch; diastolic augmentation encroaches onto systole (may be unable to distinguish). Physiological effects: Potential premature closure of the aortic valve; potential increase in left ventricular end diastolic volume, left ventricular end diastolic pressure and pulmonary artery occlusion pressure; increased left ventricular wall stress or afterload; aortic regurgitation; increased myocardial oxygen demand. (b) Late inflation. Inflation of the intra-aortic balloon markedly after closure of the aortic valve. Waveform characteristics: Inflation of the intra-aortic balloon after the dichrotic notch; absence of sharp V; sub-optimal diastolic augmentation. Physiological effects: Sub-optimal coronary artery perfusion.

of timing may be required. Failure of automatic timing tends to occur during arrhythmias or when timing is affected by balloon position.

Balloon inflation is timed to commence at the beginning of diastole.This usually occurs at the dichrotic notch of the arterial pressure waveform (which coincides with aortic valve closure). Balloon deflation is timed to occur at the end of diastole immediately prior to the beginning of the arterial upstroke which occurs when the aortic valve opens. This is found by adjusting the deflation timing to find the lowest achievable diastolic pressure. This will also lower the peak systolic pressure in most instances.

If balloon inflation happens too early left ventricular strain and aortic insufficiency could result, if inflation occurs too late the anticipated increase in coronary perfusion pressure may be reduced. If

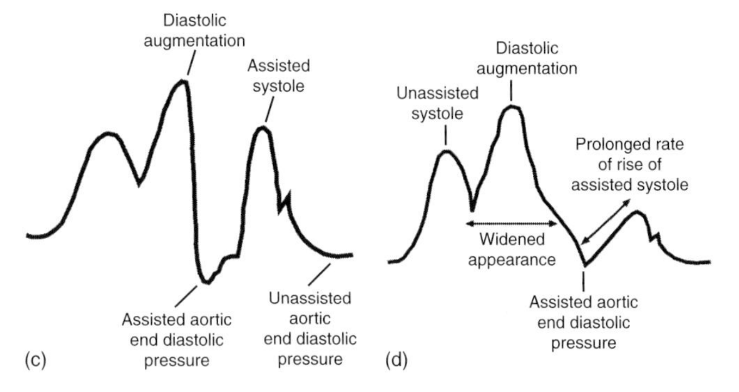

Figure 4. (*continued*)
(c) Early deflation. Premature deflation of the intra-aortic balloon during the diastolic phase. Waveform characteristics: Deflation of the intra-aortic balloon is seen as a sharp drop following diastolic augmentation; sub-optimal diastolic augmentation; assisted aortic end diastolic pressure may be equal to or less than the unassisted systolic end diastolic pressure; assisted systolic pressure may rise. Physiological-effects: Sub-optimal coronary perfusion; potential for retrograde coronary and carotid blood flow; angina may occur as a result of retrograde coronary blood flow; sub-optimal afterload reduction; increased myocardial oxygen demand.
(d) Late deflation. Waveform characteristics: Assisted aortic end-diastolic pressure may be equal to the unassisted aortic end diastolic pressure; rate of rise of assisted systole is prolonged; diastolic augmentation may appear widened. Physiological effects: Afterload reduction is essentially absent; increased myocardial oxygen consumption due to the left ventricle ejecting against a greater resistance and a prolonged isovolumetric contraction phase; intra-aortic balloon may impede left ventricular ejection and increase the afterload.

balloon deflation is too early the magnitude of afterload reduction is reduced and if deflation is too late afterload and left ventricular work is increased.

Weaning

The decision to wean support is based on evidence of an improved cardiac performance. It may be necessary to discontinue support following various complications or following a decision that further active management is inappropriate.

The frequency of augmentation (augmentation ratio) is reduced from 1:1 to 1:2, 1:3, 1:4 and sometimes 1:8 at appropriate intervals guided by assessment of the patient's response to reduction of support. The degree of augmentation may also be reduced. When it is clear that the patient is able to progress without further mechanical support the balloon catheter is removed.

Removal

Removal may be open (surgical) or closed. Adequate time for anticoagulation to be reverse is allowed. During closed removal the femoral artery distal to the insertion point is manually occluded and the balloon is withdrawn. Allowing about five seconds of bleeding may prevent any accumulated clot from passing distally. Pressure is then applied to the puncture site for at least 20 minutes either manually or by using a mechanical compression device.

Complications

Various complications associated with intra-aortic balloon counter-pulsation have been described.

Table 3. Complications.

Vascular	Equipment related	Miscellaneous
Peripheral embolisation	Incorrect positioning	Haemolysis
Femoral artery thrombosis	Incorrect timing	Thrombocytopenia
Compartment syndrome	Leak in gas line	Bleeding secondary to anticoagulation
Late claudication	Occlusion of pressure lumen	Infection
Major puncture site bleeding	Console failure	Paraplegia
Minor puncture site bleeding	Tear during insertion	Spinal cord necrosis
Femoral venous cannulation	Rupture during operation	Left internal mammary occlusion
Femoral artery pseudoaneurysm	Gas embolisation	
Aortic perforation	Inadvertent removal	
Aortic dissection	Entrapment	
Visceral ischaemia		

The most common complication of intra-aortic balloon pump therapy is limb ischaemia. Frequent, careful observation of peripheral perfusion is mandatory and intra-aortic balloon catheter removal may be necessary. Balloon pumps are supplied with a Doppler device to assist in this assessment. Other vascular complications are less frequent but may present dramatically and may require surgical intervention.

Balloon related complications generally require removal and reinsertion or repositioning. In the rare event of balloon rupture a leak detector on the gas circuit prevents further gas escape and sounds an alarm. Clinically significant gas embolism is usually prevented.

Conclusion

Intra-aortic balloon counter-pulsation is increasingly used in cardiac centres as a means of temporary mechanical cardiac support. It is carried out in a high risk population and may have life or limb threatening complications. Its optimal role is yet to be defined. With the availability of transportable devices it is possible that in the near future intra-aortic balloon counter-pulsation will be initiated in secondary centres prior to transfer to a cardiac unit. In the author's view this technique should only be used in specialist centres by appropriately trained personnel. However, as the role of the intra-aortic balloon pump becomes better defined it is likely to be seen in referring secondary centres. It is imperative that the clinicians and nursing staff involved have appropriate training and their expertise is maintained.

41

Temporary pacing

Deepak Kejariwal and Basant K. Chaudhury

Anatomy and physiology

The sinoatrial node (SAN) is situated at the junction of the superior vena cava and right atrium. The atrioventricular node (AVN) is situated in the right atrium, at the lower end of the interatrial septum. The annulus fibrosus (fibrous ring) separates the atria from the ventricle. From the AVN the His bundle passes through the annulus fibrosus and divides into right and left bundles. The left is subdivided into anterior and posterior hemibundles, and all His fibres radiate out as the Purkinje network.

SAN is the origin of the impulses responsible for heart rhythm under normal conditions. The impulse travels through the AVN and His bundle into the myocardium.

Table 1. Indications for temporary transvenous cardiac pacing.

Emergency/acute

Acute myocardial infarction (Class I: ACC/AHA):

- Asystole;
- Symptomatic bradycardia (sinus bradycardia with hypotension and type I 2nd degree AV block with hypotension not responsive to atropine);
- Bilateral bundle branch block (alternating BBB or RBBB with alternating LAHB/LPHB);
- New or indeterminate age bifascicular block with first degree AV block;
- Mobitz type II second degree AV block.

Bradycardia not associated with acute myocardial infarction

- Asystole;
- 2nd or 3rd degree AV block with haemodynamic compromise or syncope at rest;
- Ventricular tachyarrhythmias secondary to bradycardia.

Situations where temporary pacing may offer benefit after acute myocardial infarction; placement of transcutaneous electrodes may be more appropriate than transvenous pacing (class II ACC/AHA)

Class IIa	RBBB with LAFB or LPFB (new or indeterminate) *RBBB with 1st degree AV block* *LBBB (new or indeterminate)* *Recurrent sinus pauses (>3 seconds) not responsive to atropine* *Incessant VT, for atrial or ventricular overdrive pacing (transvenous pacing required)*
Class IIb	Bifascicular block of indeterminate age New or age indeterminate isolated RBBB

Situations where temporary pacing is not indicated

Acute myocardial infarction (Class III ACC/AHA)

- First degree heart block;
- Type I 2nd degree heart block (Wenckebach) with normal haemodynamics;
- Accelerated idioventricular rhythm;
- Bundle branch block or fascicular block known to exist before acute MI.

Bradycardia not associated with acute myocardial infarction

- Sinus node disease without haemodynamic compromise or syncope at rest;
- Type II second degree or third degree heart block (constant or intermittent) without haemodynamic compromise, syncope or associated ventricular tachyarrhythmias at rest.

Procedure

Temporary pacing has two components: obtaining central venous access and intracardiac placement of the pacing wire.

Obtaining central venous access

There are arguments in favour of and against all the major venous access sites (internal and external jugular, subclavian, brachial, femoral).

Table 2. Abbreviations.

Class I:	Conditions for which there is evidence and/or general agreement that a given procedure or treatment is beneficial, useful, and effective.
Class II:	Conditions for which there is conflicting evidence and/or a divergence of opinion about the usefulness/efficacy of a procedure or treatment.
Class IIa:	Weight of evidence/opinion is in favor of usefulness/efficacy.
Class IIb:	Usefulness/efficacy is less well established by evidence/opinion.
Class III:	Conditions for which there is evidence and/or general agreement that a procedure/treatment is not useful/effective and in some cases may be harmful.
ACC:	American College of Cardiology
AHA:	American Heart Association.

Femoral placement probably offers the least stable wire position and limits patient mobility more than other routes (see Chapter 23).

Current recommendation from the British Cardiac Society is that the right internal jugular route as most suitable for the inexperienced operator; this offers the most direct route to the right ventricle, and is associated with the highest success rate and least complications. In patients receiving or likely to receive thrombolytic treatment, the femoral, brachial or external jugular are the routes of choice. It is also generally best to avoid the left subclavian approach if permanent pacing may be required, as this is the site most used for permanent pacing.

Intracardiac placement of the pacing wire

- A sheath (usually 7F) is inserted, through which the pacing wire is inserted. The sheath may be left in the vein, as it makes the repositioning of the wire easier, if needed.
- The wire is advanced into the right atrium through the sheath and passed through the sterile plastic cover that accompanies the sheath.
- Crossing the tricuspid valve is done most easily by pointing the lead tip downwards and towards to the left cardiac border and advancing across the valve. The lead is then advanced to a position at the right ventricular apex.

- If it fails to cross, an alternative is to create a loop in the right atrium by pointing the lead tip to the right cardiac border and then prolapsing the loop across the valve by rotating the lead. The lead tip may then require manipulation to the apex; this is often performed most easily by passing the lead tip to the right ventricular outflow tract, gently withdrawing the lead, and allowing the tip to drop down into the apex.
- Connect the wire to the pacing box and a stimulation threshold should be determined. With continuous ECG monitoring, begin pacing at a rate 10 beats faster than the patients intrinsic heart rate with output set at 5 mA. The output is gradually reduced until capture fail to occur. This is the pacing threshold and should be <1 mA normally. The pacemaker output should be set at 3–5 times the pacing threshold.
- In an emergency, pacing is used in a fixed mode. If the pacemaker is to be used in a demand mode, it is important that there is adequate sensing of the endocardial sensing of the endocardial electrogram. To ensure good sensing, the pacing rate is set slower than the patients intrinsic rate, and sensitivity of the pulse generator is set at its most sensitive level and then is decreased (higher numbers) gradually. The setting at which the pacemaker fails to sense and begins pacing competitively with the patients intrinsic rhythm is the sensing threshold. For demand pacing, the sensitivity is set at a more sensitive level than the sensing threshold.
- Check for positional stability—with the pacing in fixed mode—ask the patient to take some deep breaths, cough forcefully, and sniff. If failure of capture occurs, the wire would need to be repositioned.
- The wire is covered with the plastic sheath and the sheath with the wire is sutured to the skin.

Post-insertion care

- Obtain a CXR—to check proper positioning of tip of the wire and to exclude complication particularly pneumothorax.
- Baseline 12 lead ECG—to document the QRS morphologic features with the wire in proper position. (A change in the morpholog of the paced QRS may be the first sign of electrode displacement.)
- Continuous ECG monitoring is essential.

- Daily evaluation should include—inspection of entry site, cardiac auscultation, threshold determination and evaluation of intrinsic rhythm.

Complications

- Failure to gain venous access, pneumothorax or haemothorax.
- Infection and thromboembolism: Routine antibiotic treatment is not required, but any sign of infection indicates the need to change the wire. Antibiotic prophylaxis should be considered with the femoral route. Also thromboembolism is more common when the femoral route is used.
- The mechanical effects of the lead: Arrthymias and perforation. Ventricular ectopic activity and occasionally prolonged ventricular arrhythmias occur as the wire crosses the tricuspid valve but usually resolve once manipulation has ceased—only occasionally removal or repositioning is required.

The pacing lead may penetrate and occasionally perforate the RV. This is usually manifested by raised pacing thresholds and sometimes by pericarditic pain and a pericardial friction rub. The lead can usually be withdrawn back into the ventricle and repostioned without problem. Rarely this may result in cardiac tamponade and will require treatment. Echocardiogram is needed after repositioning under these circumstances.

- Failure to pace: if the pacemaker suddenly fails, the most common reason is usually wire displacement. Remedy - increase the pacing output of the box and check all the connections of the wire and the battery of the box. Try and move the patient to the left lateral position until the wire can be repositioned.

Always

- Choose the right internal jugular for pacing;
- Choose the femoral, brachial or external jugular, if thrombolysis is an option;
- CXR and 12-lead ECG after pacemaker insertion;
- Check daily for pacing thresholds, evidence of infections around the venous sites, integrity of connections, and battery status of the pulse generator;

- Continuous cardiac monitoring;
- Consider antibiotic prophylaxis, if femoral route is used.

Always seek advice from Registrar/Consultant.

Never

- Choose left subclavian route;
- Do transvenous pacing before thrombolysis in a bradycardic patient with acute myocardial infarction.

Further reading

1 Ramraka PS, Moore KP. *Oxford handbook of acute medicine*. Oxford, Oxford University Press 1997.

2 Gammage MD. Temporary cardiac pacing. *Heart* 2000;83: 715–720.

Section 5

Anaesthetic Skills

42

Checking an anaesthesia machine

Nigel Puttick

Introduction

Anaesthesia is often likened to flying. While this is not always a good analogy, the pre-flight check of an aircraft is indeed very similar to checking the anaesthetic machine. As a novice pilot, I was once impatient to get in the air, and breezed through my pre-flight inspection. My instructor pulled me up sharply and told me that the pre-flight was my last chance *not* to fly, and proceeded to regale me with instances of pilots who took off in defective aircraft, for example with control surfaces locked or fuel not turned on, and in some cases didn't live to tell the tale. Similarly, with an anaesthetic machine, the pre-use check is your last chance *not* to use it, rather than a mundane chore to go through at the start of the list. Your patients' lives, and also potentially your career, may be at stake. While there is no single generic checklist applicable to all machines (or aircraft), there are general principles which will guide you in performing a thorough check relevant to the particular machine you are about to use, and which if applied to a new or unfamiliar machine will enable you to learn about its essential features and safe operation.

The basis of the User Test

We should first consider what minimum functions of our machine are essential. Most importantly, we need to know that there is a proven supply of oxygen (with an adequate reserve and a failure alarm), and that we can ventilate the patient's lungs with a correctly-functioning, leak-free breathing system (also with a back-up). We must be able to ensure continued safe anaesthesia, and we need suction and scavenging. Together, these form our first line of defence against equipment failures, and while there are many other potential problem areas to consider, will provide the basis of our machine check—the User Test.

The basic, fully manual and mechanical 'Boyle's machine' now rarely exists in operating theatres, but is still common in the anaesthetic induction rooms widely used in the UK. Most modern anaesthetic machines are highly integrated and incorporate complex automated self-test routines at power-on. In many cases, these must be completed before the machine can physically be used, and it is both usual and acceptable for these to be carried out by the anaesthetic assistant before the operating session. However, it is important that you have read the operating manual and understand the nature and limitations of the self-test, as none comprehensively address the issues identified earlier. You should know how to perform it yourself, and just as importantly, how to establish that it has indeed been done—and when. These details may differ greatly between models and manufacturers. You *must* still perform a User Test, as this will test functions not usually covered by the self-test and assure you that the machine is indeed ready to use safely. It is essential to perform a User Test before the start of each session, and again if the machine is disconnected and moved during the list (this may also require a self-test). If you use a separate machine for induction, that must also be tested. If the machine is unfamiliar to you, it is wise to ask a senior colleague for training in its use. However, a generic User Test has added value in that it will help you to familiarise yourself with the machine, and to find the features and controls which are critical for safety. These many safety-critical components and processes are identified below with an asterisk—you need to know where they all are and how they work, in case you have to find and use them in a critical situation. The User Test will ensure that you find them, and with practice it should take very little time to carry out: five minutes at most. If any step does not produce the expected result, you should identify and correct the fault if possible, or reject the machine.

Oxygen supply

- Before starting, the white oxygen pipeline Schrader connector* should be plugged in to the correct outlet* on the wall or pendant, and the reserve O_2 cylinder* turned off (by handwheel* or key*). Turn all gas flows off.
- If there is an Air/N_2O selector*, set it to N_2O.
- Check that the O_2 pipeline pressure gauge* shows 4 bar.
- Set the gas flows to 4 L/min O_2, 4 L/min N_2O.

- Disconnect the pipeline, and press the oxygen flush* button: this fails the oxygen supply rapidly.
- As the supply pressure drops, the O_2 flow* will first drop, followed by both an audible O_2 failure alarm* and interruption of N_2O flow*.
- Turn on the reserve O_2 cylinder, and note that the alarm is cancelled, and flows of both O_2 and N_2O are restored. Note the contents on its pressure gauge*, and consider whether this is adequate* to continue in event of pipeline failure.
- Now turn off the reserve O_2 cylinder, press the flush to fail the oxygen (O_2 failure alarm sounds and N_2O is interrupted).
- Reconnect the O_2 pipeline, which should cancel the alarm and restore the flows, and check the pipeline pressure.
- You have now established the following; the oxygen pipeline is at the correct pressure, and is connected internally to the O_2 flow control; the O_2 failure alarm works; the N_2O cut-off works; there is an adequate back-up cylinder supply of O_2 which is now turned off; and finally the pipeline is indeed connected and supplying O_2 to the machine.
- You have avoided the trap of leaving the cylinder turned on: in the event of a pipeline failure this would (in many machines) prevent the O_2 failure alarm from sounding until it was empty, leaving you with no reserve.
- Importantly, you now know exactly what to do in the event of an O_2 pipeline failure (but please do find out where additional cylinders are kept).
- Optionally, you could also check the air pipeline and N_2O pipeline (and reserve cylinder if fitted) using the same principles.
- This leaves a final step—ensuring that it is actually 100% oxygen that is being delivered. This requires an oxygen analyser, which should be present in some form on all machines. It is often suggested that the oxygen analyser* should be located at the Common Gas Outlet (CGO)*: frequently they are not, by design, and some new machines do not even have a CGO as such. The appropriate location depends primarily on the type of breathing system in use, and partly on the type of O_2 sensor in use. In the case of a basic anaesthetic machine with a standard 22 mm CGO and a simple breathing system* such as a Bain or T-piece which will be used at high flow, a fuel cell sensor can be located between the CGO and the breathing system. This is described as a 'mainstream' position for the O_2 analyser—what comes out of the CGO is what is delivered to the patient. This type of analyser

is passive, in that it doesn't extract a sample of gas. As a result, the sensor will only measure the O_2 concentration at that point, and so could read 100% even if the flow has been turned off and no oxygen is actually being delivered to the patient. Another example of the mainstream position is in the inspiratory limb of a circle system, close to or mounted on the absorber. For your User Test, you should first remove* the sensor from its housing* and see that the display* reads 21%* in room air, then replace* it and turn on O_2 at high flow: the display should rise rapidly to 100%*. A better solution is to use a 'sidestream' O_2 analyser, which is normally part of the anaesthetic gas monitor. This extracts a continuous sample of gas from the breathing system, and the connector* (usually a male Luer lock) should be located as close as possible to the final connection to the patient, for example at the patient filter, where it will measure what the patient is actually breathing. A similar technique applies; turn on the O_2 analyser and see that it reads 21% while sampling room air, then turn on the O_2 at high flow, and place the sample tubing connector at or within the end of the breathing system, and watch the display which should rise rapidly to 100%. In doing this, you have also checked that the analyser is calibrated* correctly. You should of course read the manual and learn how to operate and calibrate the O_2/gas analyser you use, and consider the possible causes of a displayed O_2 concentration of less than 100%.

Breathing System and ability to ventilate

- Does your machine have switchable or alternative gas outlets? If so, ensure that you know how to switch* between them, that the one you intend to use is selected*, and that the desired breathing system* is fitted to the correct outlet*.
- Examine the breathing system visually for correct assembly*.
- In the case of a Bain system, you must check that the inner* coaxial tube is connected proximally in order to prevent rebreathing, and that it is not obstructed by kinking. To do this, press the oxygen flush; the high velocity gas flow causes a reduction in pressure inside the outer tubing by the Venturi effect, sucking the bag flat. If the inner tube is disconnected, this will not happen; if kinked, you will hear the machine pressure relief valve* open.
- With a circle system, check visually that both one-way valve discs are present, and that there is sufficient fresh soda lime present. Set

the controls (expiratory valve* and manual/spontaneous* or bag/ventilator switch* if fitted) for manual ventilation.

- Now check that you can ventilate manually. This requires a leak-free, unobstructed breathing system. Close the expiratory valve*, occlude the patient end with your thumb (or an obturator), fill the bag* using the O_2 flush* and squeeze the bag to check for leaks. It should be obviously gas-tight*. Next, keeping the breathing system occluded, let the bag fill until it is distended, then release the occlusion: there should be obvious rapid deflation* through the end of the breathing system. This is a dynamic test of the patency of the entire breathing system up to the patient connector, including the filter and angle piece or catheter mount if fitted, and is important in the light of recent reports of accidental blockage of components by extraneous objects such as IV infusion set caps.
- If there is a leak, you must find and eliminate it. Among the many possible sources of leaks, the commonest include a hole in the bag, split corrugated tubing, cracked O_2 analyser housing, missing cap from gas sampling port, particles of soda lime on CO_2 absorber* O-ring seals, and missing or damaged O-ring seals elsewhere. CO_2 absorbers are particularly prone to leaks; one type has a water drainage port that can be left open.
- Particular attention should be paid to vaporisers*, as they can be the source of large leaks. With interchangeable vaporisers, an O-ring can be retained in a vaporiser when removed, so it is missing when the next one is fitted leading to a leak of the entire fresh gas flow (you would be wise to recheck for leaks whenever a vaporiser is changed). Such a leak is usually audible at high flow rates, occurs whether the vaporiser is on or off, and disappears when the vaporiser is removed. Alternatively, if the filler port is left open, a smaller leak will occur only when the vaporiser is turned on; it may or may not be audible but should be detectable by smell. When troubleshooting leaks, check with vaporisers fitted, first turned off then turned on, then removed—look for the O-rings. Other leaks occurring before the CGO can be hard to pinpoint and are not amenable to correction by the user.
- If you find a leak that you cannot eliminate, you must reject the machine. Note that some automated self-tests check for leaks, and may give you an indication of the size of leak and where in the system it is: read the manual.
- Finally, there must be an alternative means of ventilation in the event of an unforeseen failure of the breathing system.

A self-inflating bag* should be physically located on the machine—find it and check that it is assembled and functions correctly.

Continued safe anaesthesia

- You must establish that you can deliver the desired anaesthetic agents, that respiration can take place without rebreathing, and that in the event of a power failure you can still maintain both anaesthesia and respiration. Suction and scavenging must be functional.
- If you intend to use a vaporiser, check that it is present, correctly latched* in place, adequately filled*, and that the filler* and drain* ports are closed. If using a machine with two or more vaporisers, ensure that all have an interlock* device that prevents them being turned on simultaneously. If one without an interlock is fitted (e.g. Tec 3), it must be used as a single vaporiser, any others being removed.
- If an Air/N_2O selector is fitted, set it appropriately before starting.
- The two commonest causes of rebreathing—misconnected Bain inner tube and insufficient fresh soda lime—have already been covered. Be particularly careful about the type of indicator* used (white → purple or pink → white) and know that 'regeneration' of colour occurs. If in doubt, change the soda lime, as it can be awkward to do so during a case.
- Power failure can range from simple, such as the plug being pulled out of the socket, to unexpected loss of mains supply followed by generator failure. In the event of power failure, what happens to the machine you are using? If it is dependent on electrical power to function, as with many newer machines, it must have a battery backup* or uninterruptible power supply (UPS)*. You should establish how to check that this is charged* and functional, how long it will last*, and that you are indeed running on mains* power at the start of the session! You may consider testing this (not during anaesthesia, of course) by disconnecting the power supply at the wall—no damage will occur and you will discover many of the answers for yourself. In addition you should read the manual.
- If the machine does not have battery backup, consider how you will ventilate manually* and understand that you will lose monitoring.

- Many theatres have essential* and non-essential* power outlets. Ensure that the machine is plugged into the essential supply, which will have generator* or high capacity UPS* backup, or sometimes both. Check what type of backup power supply is fitted in your theatre and what happens in the event of a power failure or generator test. What would your course of action be in the event of a total loss of power? This may not seem to be part of a User Test, but it is essential knowledge, and may well differ between locations. Find out *before* you need to know.
- Suction is essential at all times during anaesthesia, not just induction and emergence. Check that it is present, connected, has the correct aspirator (preferably Yankauer) fitted, and that it works *before* the patient regurgitates. Do not let the scrub staff use your suction for the surgical team—you could need it at any time.
- Scavenging is mandatory to ensure anaesthetic gas mixtures do not pollute the operating theatre atmosphere. Check that it is connected and working—this may require a visual check.

Incorporating all the above into a generic User Test is actually quite straightforward and can be easily developed into a checking routine specific to a particular manufacturer and model. The process of performing the User Test identifies and locates the safety-critical components and prepares the user for quick and correct reaction to equipment failure. Potentially lethal faults can be quickly identified and eliminated before use on a patient. With this understanding of the critical systems, you can perform thought experiments—how would you know if a particular failure had occurred, and how would you deal with it? Such scenarios can be simulated mentally as learning exercises during quiet periods of clinical anaesthesia, or played out realistically on a simulator.

Example for a specific type of anaesthetic machine

As an example, Table 1 reproduces a locally developed User Test for a Drager Cato anaesthetic machine. This machine carries out a self-test at power-on, which requires some user involvement. It tests correct electronic and software function of the ventilator control system and patient monitors, then tests the functioning of the breathing system. It first checks the internal pneumatically actuated valves, then tests the compliance of the breathing system, and finally checks for leaks in both manual/spontaneous and IPPV modes. It will only return to standby mode and allow clinical use if the test is completed successfully and within strict limits for measured leakage. The time of

Table 1. User Test for Drager Cato.

Power ON, pipelines IN, self-test DONE, in STANDBY mode

General Visual Check
- Pipeline pressure gauges read 4 bar
- CGO: fresh gas hose fitted and tight
- Air/N_2O selector set to N_2O
- Vaporiser—fitted, latched, filled, filler tightened
- Absorber—sufficient fresh soda lime (check colour)
- Scavenging—connected, operating
- If machine has UPS, check all four green lights are ON
- Check self-test performed on 8050 from standby, press knob then "Config", check three ticks

Gases
- Turn on flows of 4 L/min O_2 and 4 L/min N_2O
- Disconnect O_2 pipeline, press O_2 flush hear O_2 failure alarm, see both flows interrupted
- Turn on O_2 cylinder—check contents >50 bar O_2 alarm cancelled, O_2 and N_2O flows restored
- Turn cylinder off, press flush check O_2 failure alarm sounds again
- Reconnect O_2 pipeline check alarm cancelled, flows restored
- Turn flows off
- (Optionally, check N_2O and Air supplies)

Breathing system etc:
- Flip expiratory valve to MAN, occlude Y-piece
- Fill bag using O_2 flush and squeeze hard
- Machine should switch to MAN/SPONT mode (auto wake up)
- Squeeze bag again, should now be leak free
- Allow bag to distend, release occlusion, bag deflates freely
- Check self-inflating bag present and functional
- Check suction connected and functional (vacuum)

Monitors
- Should now both be ON (after auto wake up)
- 8050 (gases/ventilation)
  - check O_2 sensor reads 21% (sample room air)
  - check time (<24 hrs) and results of self test (page 284)
  - place sample tube in Y-piece
  - turn on high flow O_2
  - check O_2 sensor reads 100%
- 8040 (CVS monitor)
  - select 'erase data' to reset default alarm limits

test, leakage and compliance are displayed for the user. However, the self-test does not address several of the key elements identified above, as these are not under the control of the machine, and so we must perform a User Test.

- Always test the anaesthetic machine before clinical use.
- Remember it is your last chance *not* to use it.
- Don't omit to test the machine in the induction room.
- Understand the basis of the User Test: integrity of oxygen supply, ability to ventilate, and provision of safe continued anaesthesia.
- Use the test to familiarise yourself with your machine and its safety-critical controls and components.
- Understand your machine: ask for training, and read the manual.
- Mentally rehearse your responses to equipment, gas, or power failures.

Conclusion

You should now understand the need for a User Test performed before clinical use of an anaesthetic machine. If you do not have checklists locally, you should be able to construct one for your department. Consider whether you should document that a self-test and User Test have been performed. Some further issues remain; for example, what to do if you reject a machine, what you should do in the event of a machine failure in use, and how Critical Incident Reporting is carried out in your department or Trust.

43

Monitoring and anaesthesia

Stephen Bonner

The origin of the word monitor is from *monere*, to warn. The purpose of monitoring during anaesthesia is to detect physiological abnormalities, abnormal trends or warn of potential errors that may cause harm to the patient. Early detection of abnormalities leads to early correction, which usually is more effective in preventing harm. Recently anaesthetic monitoring has included monitoring of depth of anaesthesia, in order to avoid awareness under anaesthesia. It must be stressed that the most effective monitor is the continued presence and vigilance of the anaesthetist throughout anaesthesia. Monitoring exists to aid the observation of the patient, not to replace it.

Monitoring anaesthetic equipment (see Chapter 42)

Alarms

All alarms must be correctly set, checked by the anaesthetist and enabled once anaesthesia commences. In particular airway pressure alarms should be used when the patient is artificially ventilated.

Table 1. Minimum monitoring guidelines during anaesthesia (AAGBI).

Induction of anaesthesia	Maintenance of anaesthesia	Recovery from anaesthesia	Local anaesthesia ± conscious sedation
Pulse oximetry	Pulse oximetry	Pulse oximetry	Pulse oximetry
NIBP	NIBP	NIBP	NIBP
ECG	ECG		ECG
Capnography	Capnography		
	Vapour analyser		

In addition to patient monitoring: (*1*) *Monitoring Anaesthetic Equipment:* Oxygen supply; Breathing Systems; Alarms; Vapour analyser; Infusion devices. (*2*) *Immediately available:* Nerve stimulator if muscle relaxants used; Temperature monitoring; ECG and capnography in recovery.

Oxygen supply

An oxygen analyser with an audible alarm must always be used during anaesthesia in order to prevent the administration of hypoxic gas mixtures being delivered to the patient.

Patient monitoring devices

Electrocardiography (see Chapters 9 and 10)

The ECG is essential during anaesthesia to monitor cardiac rate, detect arrhythmias, monitor conduction defects, pacemaker function and detect peri-operative ischaemia. Standard lead II is the best lead for monitoring arrhythmias, conduction defects and inferior ischaemia (right coronary artery territory) whereas the chest leads detect anterolateral ischaemia (anterior descending and circumflex artery territories).

Non-invasive blood pressure measurement

Blood pressure measurement is an important indicator of blood flow and perfusion. It may be measured indirectly via automated sphygmomanometers and is standard monitoring during anaesthesia as well as recovery and throughout the peri-operative period.

Invasive blood pressure measurement (see Chapter 4)

Blood pressure may be monitored invasively using an indwelling intra-arterial catheter, giving accurate beat to beat blood pressure

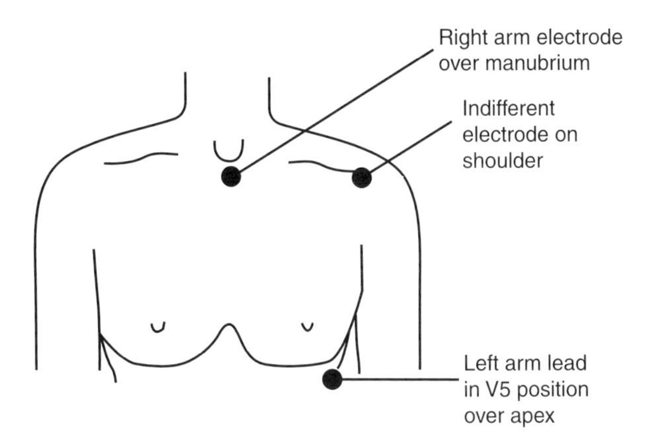

Figure 1. CM_5 ECG monitoring configuration.

measurement. This is indicated if cardiovascular instability is predicted, from either patient factors, such as cardiac disease, surgical factors, such as massive blood loss and requirements for continual blood pressure measurement and regular blood gas estimation peri-operatively.

Peri-operative intra-arterial blood pressure measurement

Indications

- Expected major blood loss
- Cardiothoracic surgery
- Neurosurgery
- Induced hypotension
- Critically ill patients
- Patient factors, e.g. LVF
- Frequent blood gas analysis

Contraindications (all relative)

- Positive Allen's test
- Raynaud's syndrome
- Severe peripheral vascular disease

Complications

- Peripheral ischaemia
- Thrombosis
- Embolisation of clot/air
- Infection
- Misinterpretation of readings
- False aneurysm formation (rare)

Pulse oximetry

Pulse oximetry is described under basic monitoring and also forms an essential part of standard monitoring during anaesthesia, in recovery and throughout the peri-operative period, particularly for high risk patients and those with respiratory disease. Generally intra-operatively the lower alarm limit should be set for 94%, which approximately corresponds to a PaO_2 of 10 kPa.

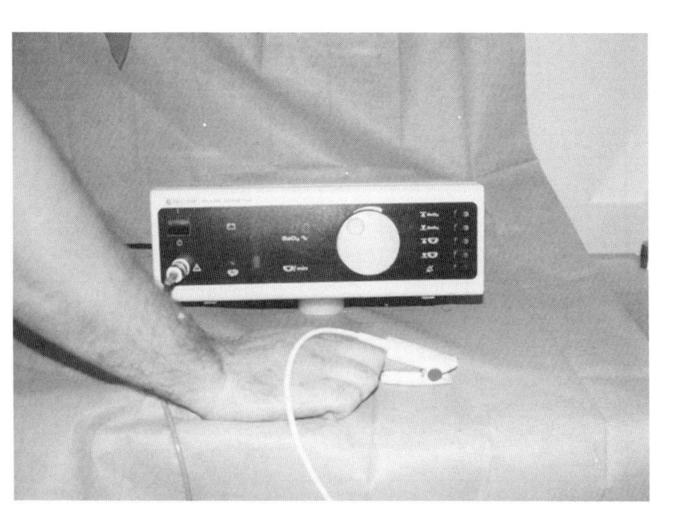

Figure 2. Pulse oximeter.

- Move oximeter probe hourly during long cases.
- If not working with a vasoconstricted patient, try an ear lobe.

Temperature monitoring

Hypothermia (<35°C) is associated with shivering, increased myocardial oxygen consumption, myocardial depression, VF below 28°C, decreased cerebral blood flow, hyperglycaemia, abnormal clotting and poor wound healing. Equally an increased temperature increases metabolic activity, causes hypotension through vasodilatation. Intra-operative temperature monitoring guides active warming. This is particularly important for children, who lose heat rapidly due to a high surface area despite a high metabolic rate and for long procedures since heat production is decreased during anaesthesia.

Temperature monitoring also gives important information about peripheral perfusion if the core/peripheral temperature gradient is measured, since peripheral vasoconstriction, e.g. in hypovolaemia,

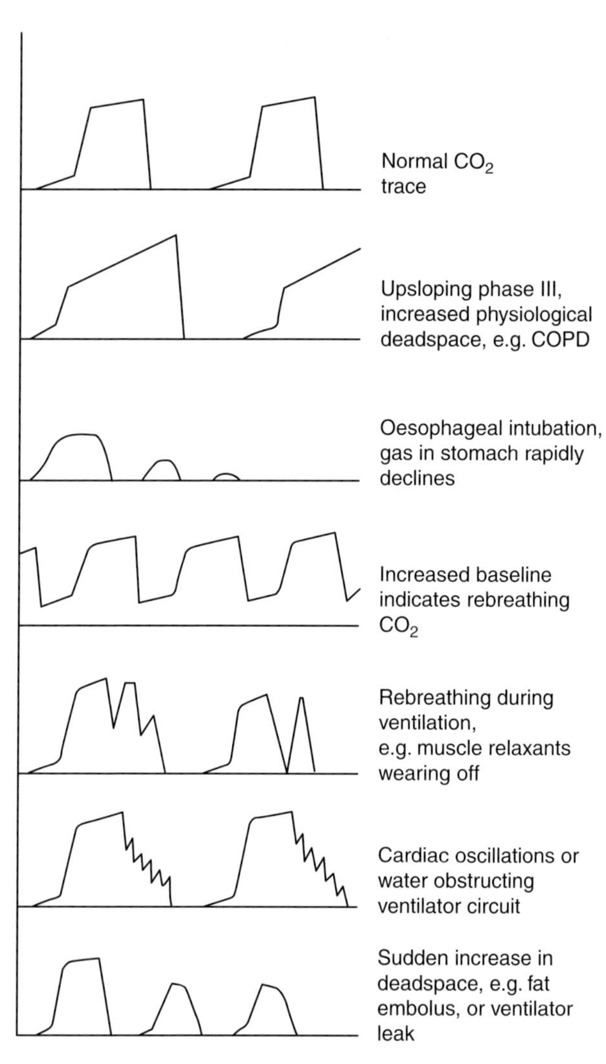

Figure 3. Some typical end tidal CO_2 traces.

leads to peripheral cooling. Sepsis, allergic reactions, head injury may all cause high temperatures under anaesthesia. However, a rapidly rising temperature up to 2ºC per hour should lead to a suspicion of malignant hyperthermia.

The commonest methods of intra-operative temperature measurement currently used are thermocouples and thermistors. Commonly used routes intra-operatively include nasopharyngeal, rectal and thermistors incorporated onto urinary catheters for central temperature measurement and skin for peripheral measurement.

End tidal CO_2 monitoring

Capnography, end tidal CO_2 monitoring (Pet_{CO_2}), is an essential monitor that indicates correct placement of endotracheal intubation, the adequacy of ventilation and sudden changes intra-operatively in dead-space, such as fat embolus. The major advantage is that monitoring is breath by breath gives real time data, which may be acted on immediately, e.g. to detect disconnection of the ventilator circuit intra-operatively (see Figure 3).

Volatile agent monitoring

Inspiratory and expiratory volatile anaesthetic vapour monitoring ensures that anaesthetic vapour is being delivered to the patient. Most instruments use infrared absorbtion spectophotometry and give breath by breath monitoring.

Neuromuscular monitoring

Neuromuscular monitoring should be used whenever muscle relaxants are administered. This can be used to indicate whether adequate relaxation has been achieved for the surgical procedure or that the drug effect is wearing off toward the end of anaesthesia and can be safely reversed.

- Three common patterns of stimulation may be used.
- The commonest pattern is a *Train of Four* (TOF), where four twitches are delivered at 0.5 sec intervals. This assesses non-depolarising block. The TOF ratio is the ratio of the fourth contraction to the first. In clinical practice the TOF count is more useful. If surgical muscle relaxation is required, this usually necessitates no more than a TOF count of one or two. Muscle relaxation may be reversed if one twitch is present.

- If there is no response to a TOF, it may still be possible to reverse non-depolarising blockade, and this is assessed using a *post tetanic count*. A tetanic stimulus is given, 50 Hz at 5 seconds, followed by stimulation at 1 Hz. The number of palpable muscle movement, e.g. finger twitches is the post tetanic count. If the post tetanic count is more than 10, the block may still be reversed with neostigmine.
- A twitch–tetanus–twitch pattern is useful in distinguishing the sort of block, in particular a partial depolarising, i.e. suxamethonium block, from a non-depolarising block. This is particularly useful if both drugs have been administered, there is concern over suxamethonium apnoea or repeated doses of suxamethonium have been administered which can give a 'dual' block, imitating a non depolarising block.

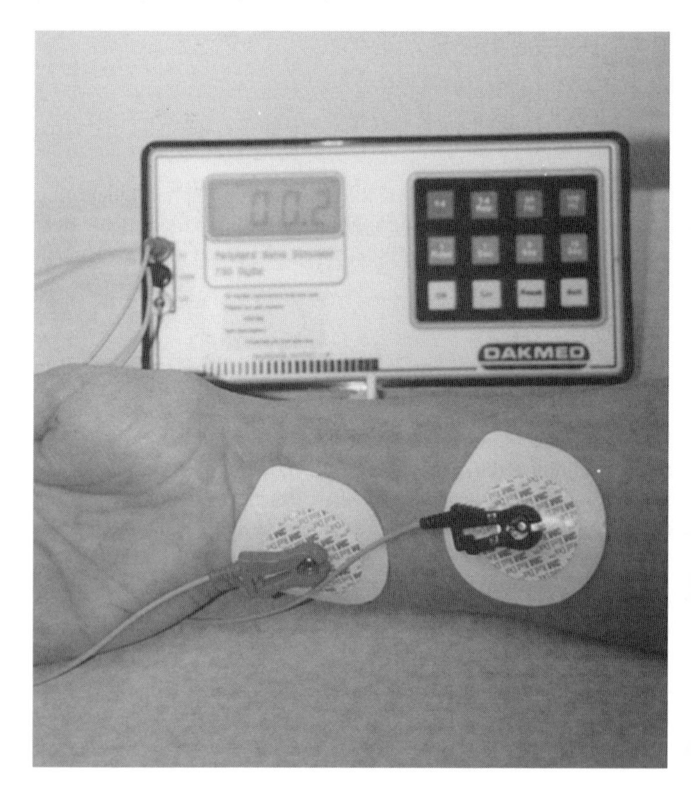

Figure 4. Ulnar nerve stimulation.

- In twitch–tetanus–twitch, a train of single stimuli at less than I every 3 secs, is followed by a tetanic burst at 50 Hz for 3 secs, then the single stimuli repeated.
- In a partial non-depolarising block, weak muscle twitches are followed by a non sustained contraction on the tetanic burst, followed by increased muscle contraction during the post tetanic train. This is called post tetanic potentiation. This is similar to the block seen in myasthenia gravis.
- In a partial depolarising block, the twitches are weak, the tetanic burst gives a weak, but sustained contraction and the post tetanic twitches are similar to the first, with no post tetanic potentiation.

Depth of anaesthesia monitoring

Awareness of events under anaesthesia is rare (current studies suggest less than 0.1% of cases) and historically usually due to faulty technique, but is occasionally due to unforeseen equipment failure. Monitoring of depth of anaesthesia/sedation can be either by clinical monitoring or using depth of anaesthesia monitors. Clinical monitoring of depth of anaesthesia includes spontaneous movement and a fast respiratory rate in the non-paralysed patient, but for the paralysed patient one needs to rely on signs of stimulation of the sympathetic nervous system.

Equipment used to monitor depth of anaesthesia relies on EEG activity, auditory evoked potentials or oesophageal contractility. One monitor currently entering clinical practice measures the Bispectral index.

Bispectral index monitoring

General anaesthesia is associated with a decrease in the average EEG frequency and an increase in the average power. Bispectral Index

Table 2. Signs of 'light' anaesthesia in a paralysed patient.

Lacrimation
Sweating
Flushing
Pupillary dilation
Tachycardia
Hypertension

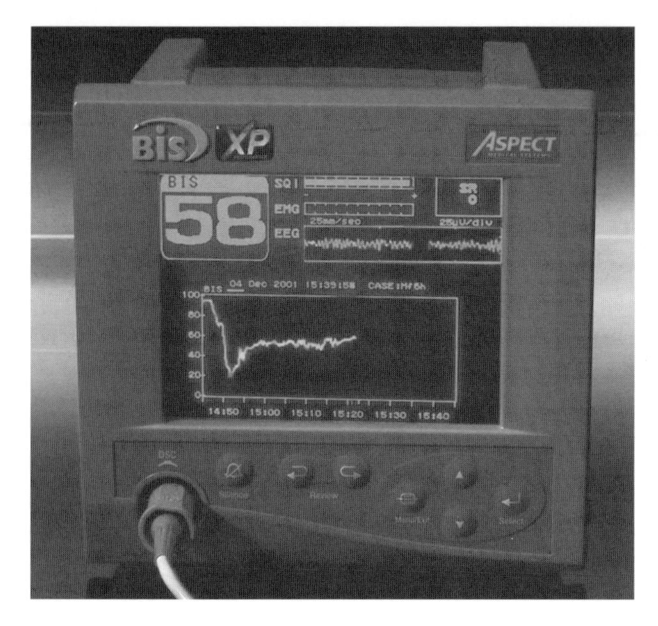

Figure 5. BIS traces.

Analysis (BIS) is a computer generated number derived using both EEG power and frequency information together with bispectral analysis, which quantifies the synchronisation of the underlying frequencies in the signal. The result is a number between 100, representing an awake patient and 0, representing a flat line EEG. BIS values of 65–85 are recommended for sedation and 40–60 for general anaesthesia (Figure 5).

Magnetic resonance imaging

General anaesthesia may occasionally be required in the magnetic resonance unit and this has special requirements for monitoring. Problems relate to both the strong magnetic field rendering most monitors useless or dangerous since they may be hurled by the strong magnetic field, together with limited access to the patient making monitoring even more vital. All monitoring used must be special MRI compatible equipment, labelled *MR safe* or *MR compatible* and this includes special cables. Padding must be placed between the cables and the skin of the patient. Standards of monitoring during anaesthesia, sedation and recovery must equate to standards expected elsewhere. MR compatible monitors include ECG, NIBP, oximetry, capnography, inspired oxygen concentration and volatile agent monitoring. These may be monitored outside the scanner if appropriate.

Patient transfer

Any critically ill intubated patient being transferred either to another hospital, or even in the hospital, must be assumed to be anaesthetised and warrants appropriate monitoring, particularly cardiovascular, with ECG and invasive blood pressure monitoring, but also airway monitoring, in particular disconnect alarm, high airway pressure alarm and capnography.

44

Difficult intubation

Simon Gardner and David Ryall

Intubation may be defined as being difficult when three or more attempts are made or when greater than ten minutes has been spent on the process. As we have already discussed (Chapter 6), pre-operative assessment greatly increases the chances of predicting airway difficulties, and therefore allows adaptive measures to be taken before the patient is anaesthetised.

If a difficult intubation is anticipated, immediate consideration should be given to the following points.

Is general anaesthesia necessary?

Many surgical procedures can be conducted under regional or local anaesthesia. The majority of infra-umbilical operations can, if necessary, be performed under spinal or epidural anaesthesia. Regional anaesthesia can also be used in the upper limb, the eye and areas of the face. Certain patient populations will not tolerate regional techniques i.e. children and the elderly or confused. Also certain operations will by their very nature demand general anaesthesia e.g. complex cardiac surgery.

Is intubation necessary?

If general anaesthesia is deemed appropriate, one must then determine if it is essential for the trachea to be intubated. Various factors will influence this decision but it is worthwhile remembering that many of the conditions that make intubation difficult may also make it difficult to maintain a patent airway once the patient is asleep.

- Does the type of operation necessitate intubation e.g. cardiac, neurosurgery or upper GI surgery?

- Does the patient's medical condition necessitate intubation e.g. hiatus hernia, pregnancy, extreme obesity?
- What is the probable duration of anaesthesia? It is prudent to intubate all cases lasting three hours or longer
- Can the patient be allowed to breathe spontaneously during anaesthesia? Laryngeal mask airways are ideally suited for spontaneously breathing patients and in certain well-chosen cases, intermittent positive pressure ventilation can be instituted via an LMA.

Does attempted intubation pose too high a risk of airway obstruction?

Patients with severe upper airway obstruction, particularly those with laryngeal tumours may obstruct their airway completely if any attempt at intubation is made. The safest option in many cases is to perform a tracheostomy under local anaesthesia.

Once the decision to proceed with intubation has been made, the following considerations should be satisfied.

- Appropriate place—An operating theatre, anaesthetic room or similarly equipped area;
- Adequate assistance—The presence of two anaesthetists is often helpful, as it allows one to monitor the patient, while the other concentrates on securing the airway;
- Adequate equipment—All equipment which might prove necessary should be immediately available and checked at the start (Figure 1);
- Adequate monitoring should be attached to the patient.

Where difficult intubation is anticipated, attempts at intubation may be made with the patient anaesthetised or prior to the induction of anaesthesia. The latter has the advantage of minimising the risk of losing control of the airway. However it requires a co-operative patient, an experienced anaesthetist, and is not suitable for many patients (children, dementia).

Attempting intubation in the awake patient

The commonest method of achieving an awake tracheal intubation is by the use of a fibreoptic laryngoscope (Figure 2). A fibreoptic scope,

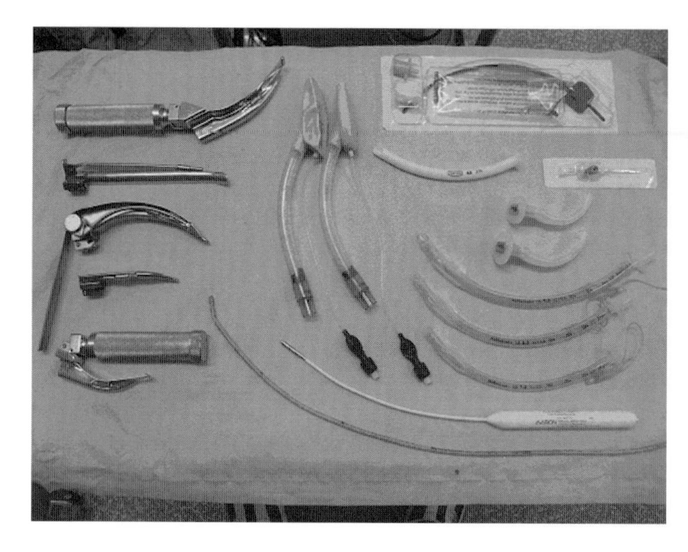

Figure 1. A selection of equipment used for airway management.

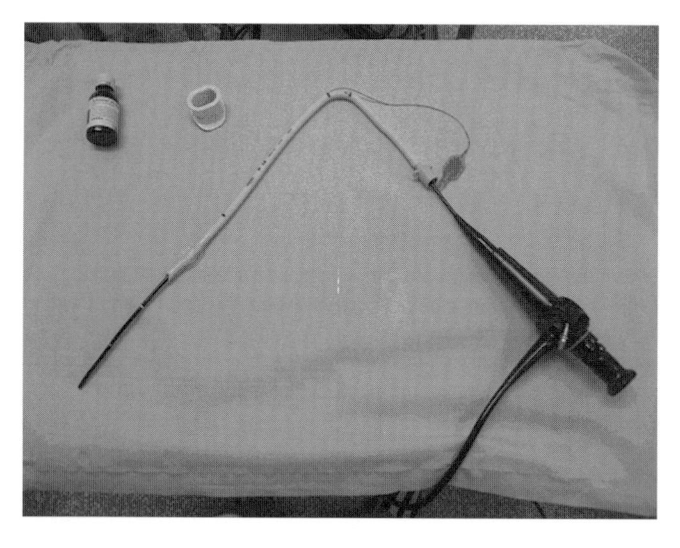

Figure 2. A fibreoptic laryngoscope with a nasal endotracheal tube mounted.

with a tracheal tube mounted on it, is passed through the mouth or nose into the trachea, and the tube is then slid over the scope into the trachea. The exact technique of awake fibreoptic intubation is beyond the scope of this book, but will require the following as a basic minimum.

- A calm and co-operative patient;
- Detailed pre-operative consent;
- An anti-sialogogue to decrease secretions;
- Provision of supplementary oxygen during the procedure;
- Local anaesthesia to the whole of the airway including the mouth, nose, pharynx and the entire larynx.

Attempting intubation with the patient anaesthetised

In the majority of patients, general anaesthesia is instituted prior to attempting tracheal intubation. Particular attention should always be given to maintaining adequate oxygenation throughout. Nitrous oxide should not be administered until the airway has been secured. Under no circumstances should a muscle relaxant be given until one is certain that the patient's airway can be maintained and manual ventilation can be performed.

Various devices and techniques have been developed to assist in securing endotracheal intubation. These can be broadly classified as follows.

- Laryngoscopes;
- The view of the laryngeal inlet obtained at direct laryngoscopy may vary considerably (see Cormack and Lehane Grading). Substituting a conventional curved Macintosh blade for a straight bladed laryngoscope e.g. Magill may improve the view, particularly in children. Alternatively, a McCoy blade, which has a moveable tip, may assist in moving the epiglottis anteriorly, thus allowing better access to the larynx;
- Devices over which an endotracheal tube can be threaded;
- Whilst performing laryngoscopy, it may be possible to guide a small diameter gum elastic bougie under the epiglottis and then anteriorly through the vocal cords. Once within the trachea, an endotracheal tube can be railroaded over the top of the bougie. An intubating stylette is a semi-rigid device which fits inside a conventional endotracheal tube allowing it to be moulded in such a way as to provide a better angle of approach to the larynx,

i.e. the tip can be curved anteriorly. An intubating light wand is effectively a bougie with a light source at the tip. The light can be seen through the skin as it passes through the larynx;

- Fibreoptic devices;
- Fibreoptic laryngoscopes can be either flexible or rigid. They are passes either orally or nasally into the trachea under indirect vision. Once again, the endotracheal tube is fed over the top of the fibrescope;
- Laryngeal mask airways (LMAs);
- Small diameter endotracheal tubes can be threaded through a conventional laryngeal mask into the trachea. More recently, a specially adapted laryngeal mask known as the intubating laryngeal mask (ILMA) airway has been developed. This device lacks the bars found on the aperture of a conventional LMA, allowing a larger sized proprietary endotracheal tube to be passed.

Retrograde intubation

- An introducer needle is directed transdermally into the trachea between the cricoid cartilage and the first tracheal ring (or alternatively through the cricothyroid membrane). Once the needle is correctly positioned, a Seldinger wire is threaded through the needle and is then directed cephalad towards the oropharynx. The wire can then be pulled out through the mouth, and an endotracheal tube can be railroaded backwards over the wire, into the trachea.

Management of failed intubation in the anaesthetised patient

In a small number of patients intubation of the trachea may prove impossible, and when this occurs unexpectedly, it can be extremely alarming. However, a rational approach to airway management should ensure patient safety. Important points to remember if intubation proves difficult, include:

- Do not persist with attempts to intubate the trachea. The most important part of management is to maintain oxygenation;
- Get senior assistance.

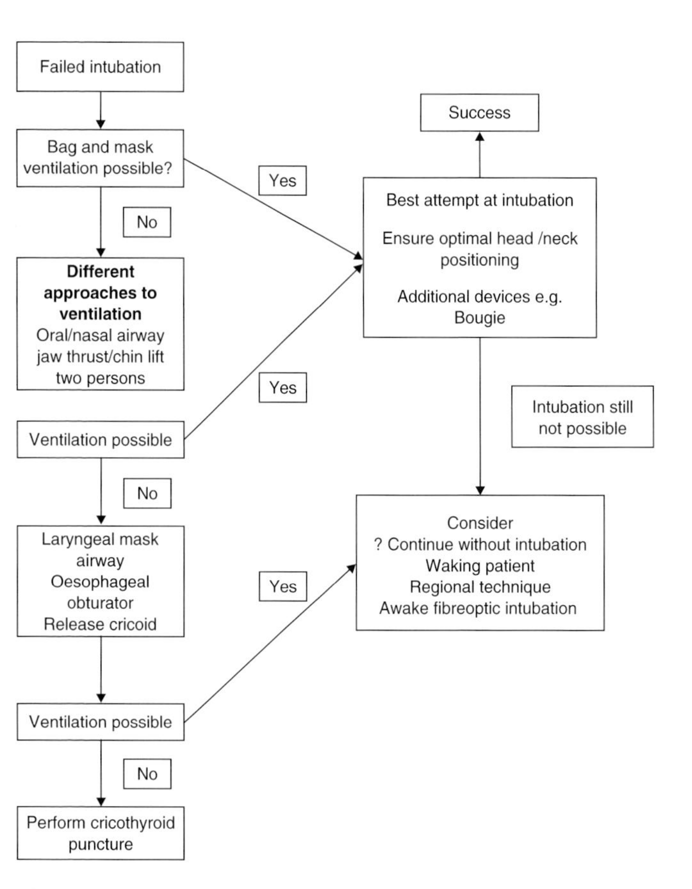

Figure 3. A protocol for failed intubation and ventilation during anaesthesia.

45

Spinal anaesthesia

Tim Meek and John Hughes

Introduction

Spinal anaesthesia is a means of achieving excellent surgical anaesthesia, without resorting to general anaesthesia. It is the commonest form of anaesthesia for caesarean section, and is also used in urological and lower limb surgery. It relies on placing a small quantity of local anaesthetic agent in direct contact with the spinal nervous tissue in the subarachnoid space to produce a dense blockade of nerve conduction. Spinal anaesthesia is a complex procedure, which you would only undertake in a supervised situation. What follows should therefore be considered as an outline guide to aid your understanding. Note however, that the skills of accessing the subarachnoid space are those required to perform lumbar puncture to obtain a sample of cerebro-spinal fluid (CSF).

Anatomy (see Chapter 36)

- In spinal anaesthesia, local anaesthetic is injected into the cerebro-spinal fluid (CSF), where it acts directly on the nervous tissue.
- The important anatomical relations are shown in Figure 1.
- In adults, the spinal cord commonly terminates at the L_1 vertebra or L_{1-2} interspace. However, in a significant proportion, it may reach the L_2 vertebra.
- The thecal sac contains the cauda equina (the nerves below the termination of the spinal cord) and CSF, and terminates at about the level of S_2.
- To avoid damage to the spinal cord, the spinal needle should not be inserted above the level of L_3.
- Spinal anaesthesia is not suitable for children because the spinal cord terminates at a lower level (L_4 in the infant) and is at risk of being damaged, and because adequate patient cooperation is difficult to obtain.

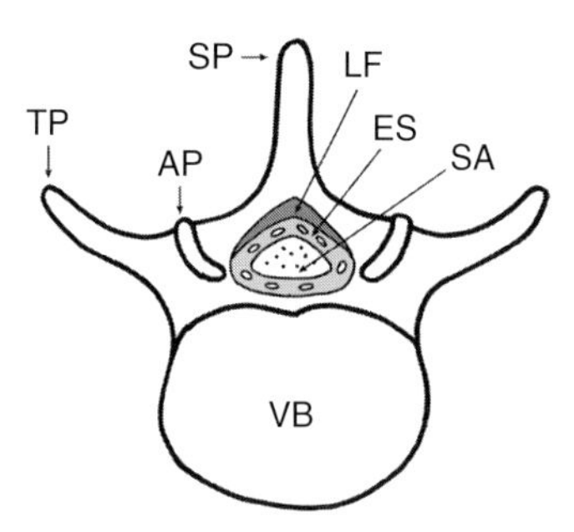

Figure 1. A schematic drawing of a lumbar vertebra, viewed from above, to show the important anatomical structures and relations. TP— transverse process; SP—spinous process; AP—articular process; LF—ligamentum flavum (running perpendicular to page); ES—epidural space (containing fat and veins); SA—sub-arachnoid space (enclosed within the meninges (dura and arachnoid mater), containing cerebro-spinal fluid and cauda equina); VB—vertebral body.

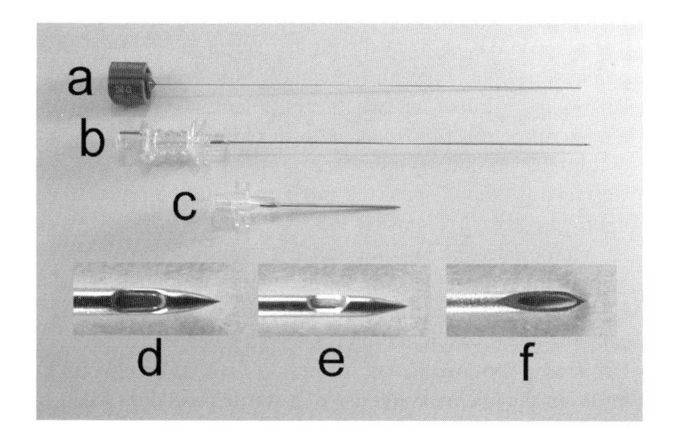

Figure 2. Components of a spinal needle. (a) Obturator for needle; (b) spinal needle (note clear hub); (c) introducer for spinal needle; (d) Sprotte tip; (e) Whitacre tip; (f) Quincke tip.

Special equipment

- The spinal needle is long, flexible and of small gauge (22–26G) and comes with an introducer needle (Figure 2).

- There are three types of needle tip (Figure 2):
  - Quincke ('cutting' tip—similar to ordinary hypodermic needle);
  - Sprotte ('pencil point');
  - Whitacre (also pencil point, but hole is smaller and more distal).
- The pencil point tip parts the fibres of the meninges, rather than cutting them, which is said to reduce CSF leak after removal of the needle. This reduces the incidence of post-dural puncture headache (see below).

Procedure

- The procedure and its complications are discussed with the patient and consent is obtained.
- Large bore IV access is required.
- Standard monitoring (ECG, pulse oximetry, blood pressure) during placement is good practice.
- The procedure is performed with the patient in either the sitting or lateral position; operator preference is the deciding factor.
- Positioning is important: whether sitting or lateral, the patient's lumbar spine must be adequately flexed to overcome the natural lumbar lordosis (Figure 3).
- Correct positioning opens the gap between the vertebral spines, improving access (Figure 4).
- An appropriate vertebral interspace is identified by palpation. A straight line drawn between the iliac crests is at the level of the L_{4-5} interspace most often, but may be as high as L_{3-4}. Thus, care must be taken in interpreting this landmark.
- Full sterile precautions are mandatory: hat, gown, gloves and mask for the operator, and use of a sterile procedure pack.
- The patient's back is cleaned aseptically; many studies now suggest that chlorhexidine in alcohol solution has better antimicrobial properties than iodine-containing solutions.
- Local anaesthetic is infiltrated into the skin and underlying tissues.
- A spinal needle is used to locate the sub-arachnoid space and to inject local anaesthetic (the steps are illustrated in Figure 5) as follows:
  - The introducer needle is inserted first, followed by the spinal needle.

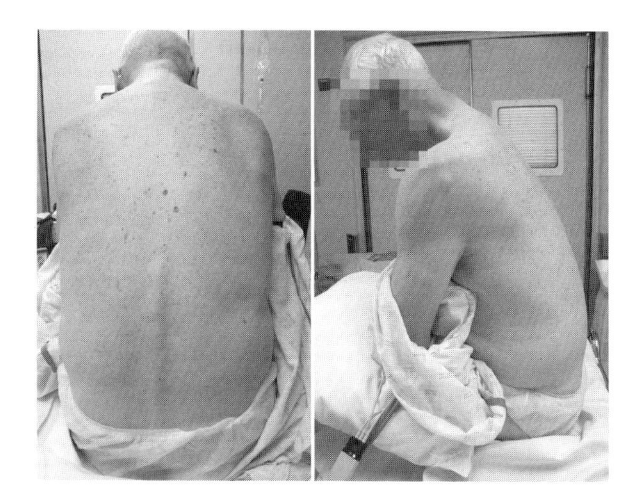

Figure 3. Positioning for spinal anaesthesia. The lumbar spinous processes are clearly visible in this patient (left) and the lumbar lordosis has been flattened (right). The same result can be achieved with the patient in the lateral position.

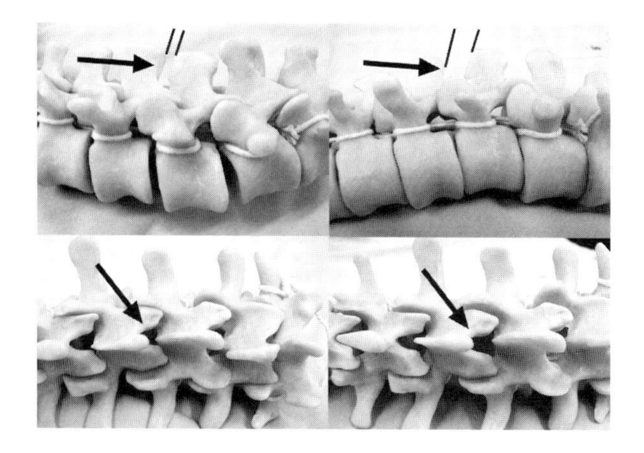

Figure 4. A model spine demonstration, showing the differences between the flexed and extended positions. In the lateral views (top), the gap between the spinous processes can be seen to increase upon flexion, whereas in the posterior views (bottom), the available aperture between articular processes can be seen to increase (The L2/3 interspace is indicated in each photo for comparison).

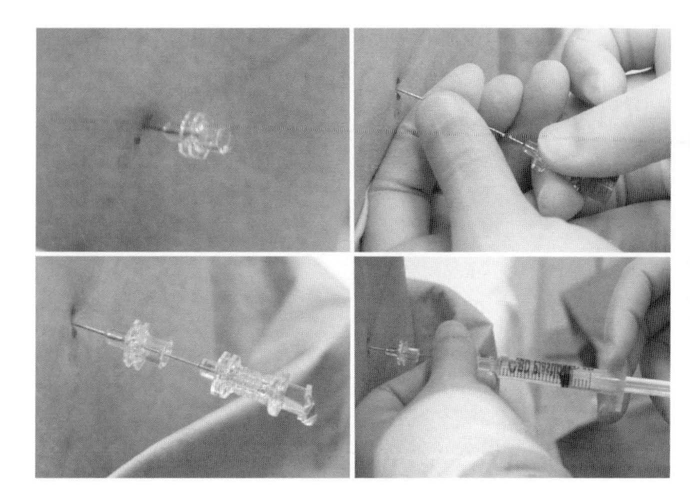

Figure 5. Administering a spinal anaesthetic. Top left: Placement of introducer needle. Top right: The spinal needle is passed through the introducer to an appropriate depth. Bottom left: when the obturator is removed from the spinal needle, cerebro-spinal fluid (CSF) fills the hub and drips out. Bottom right: following confirmation of aspiration of clear CSF, local anaesthetic is slowly injected.

- The needle direction should be as close to perpendicular to the skin as is possible—cranial angulation increases the risk of contacting the spinal cord above.
- A faint 'pop' is sometimes felt as the meninges are breached.
- On removing the obturator from the spinal needle CSF should be seen flowing into the hub.
- The local anaesthetic solution is injected slowly—there should be no pain.
- The needle and introducer are removed together.

Local anaesthetic solution

- The most common local anaesthetic used for spinals is bupivacaine 0.5%, which is long lasting and potent. A typical volume would be 2.5–3.0 mL.
- It is most commonly used in its hyperbaric form, which contains dextrose 8%. This makes it heavier than CSF, which means the

patient's position can be used to control and/or limit its spread within the subarachnoid space.
- It is becoming increasingly common to add an opiate to the local anaesthetic. This is intended to improve intra- and/or post-operative analgesia. Fentanyl 10–25 μg, or diamorphine 200–400 μg are commonly used.

Assessing the block

- The height of block required depends upon the operation to be performed.
- For example, for caesarean section, a level of T_4 is required, whereas for a knee replacement, T_{10} is adequate.
- It is common to test the level using cold or pinprick. Recent opinion suggests that, for caesarean section at least, loss of light touch is a better predictor of adequate analgesia.
- Adequate block should be ensured before the surgeon is given permission to start.

Management of block

- If the patient is to remain awake, regular verbal contact and reassurance is important.
- The patient may prefer to receive sedation:
  - Midazolam in 0.5–1 mg increments is commonly used;
  - Over-sedation should be avoided—the patient should remain rousable.
- If the block wears off before surgery is complete, it is important to have a plan:
  - Analgesia can be supplemented by inhaled entonox or IV opioids;
  - General anaesthesia may be necessary;
  - If combined spinal-epidural (CSE) has been used (see below), the epidural component can be used to extend the block.
- Combined spinal-anaesthesia is increasingly common:
  - An epidural is placed at the same time as the spinal;
  - The epidural can be used to extend the duration of surgical anaesthesia;
  - The epidural may also be used to provide post-operative analgesia.

- Correct patient positioning is central to success.
- To reduce risk of nerve damage:
  - A vertebral interspace at or below L_{3-4} is used.
  - Cranial angulation of the needle is avoided;
  - Pain on needle insertion or injection should be viewed as suspicious.
- Sedation should always be used cautiously.
- A plan of action is needed in case the block wears off early or fails.

Complications

- Hypotension is the commonest problem:
  - It happens because the local anaesthetic blocks the sympathetic nerve fibres, leading to temporary sympathectomy and thus vasodilatation;
  - Treatment is with vasopressor (e.g. metaraminol, phenylephrine) and adequate fluid loading.
- Headache complicates under 1% of spinals:
  - It is caused by CSF leakage, resulting in a low pressure headache;
  - Pencil point needles reduce the incidence of headache.
- High spinal or total spinal blockade are rare. They occur when the local anaesthetic spreads unusually high. Symptoms include: severe hypotension, bradycardia (cardiac sympathetic efferents are at T_{2-4}), difficulty breathing, coughing or phonating and unconsciousness. Treatment is supportive, including: vasopressors, anti-muscarinics, fluids, respiratory assistance, including intubation and ventilation if required.
- Severe or permanent neurological damage is very rare. A prospective study showed an approximate 6:10000 risk of neurological injury following spinal anaesthesia. The injury usually recovered, and was most commonly a radiculopathy. The risk of injury can be reduced by careful technique and by choosing an appropriate vertebral interspace.

46

Epidural anaesthesia

Tim Meek and John Hughes

Introduction

The 'epidural' is a versatile regional anaesthesia technique. It relies upon placement of a small plastic catheter into the epidural space (literally the space outside the dura), through which local anaesthetic or other drugs can be injected. Epidurals are used in the thoracic or lumbar regions, depending upon the site of surgery.
They can be used:

- As a sole means of providing surgical anaesthesia (e.g. caesarean section);
- As intra-operative analgesia during general anaesthesia;
- To supplement or prolong spinal anaesthesia (as part of combined spinal epidural technique—see Chapter 45);
- For post-operative analgesia in any of the above situations;
- As the most effective form of analgesia during labour.

Placing and using an epidural is a complex procedure, which you would only undertake in a supervised situation. What follows should therefore be considered as an outline guide to aid your understanding.

Anatomy

- The important anatomical relations are the same as those for spinal anaesthesia (Figure 1, see Chapter 45).
- The epidural space is a potential space, which lies between the inner aspect of the bony vertebral canal and the meninges. Laterally it extends some distance with the spinal nerve roots. It contains fat, and a plexus of veins.
- The epidural space extends from the foramen magnum superiorly to the sacro-coccygeal membrane inferiorly.

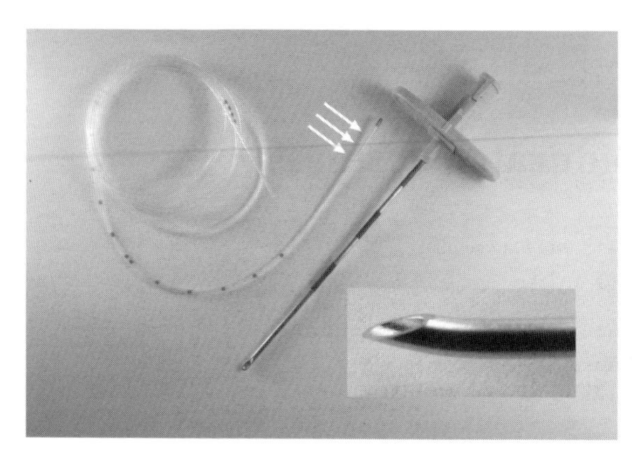

Figure 1. A typical Tuohy epidural needle. The centimetre markings on the needle and catheter can be seen. The 'wings' used to hold and guide the needle can be removed according to operator preference. The three small orifices at the end of the catheter are indicated. Inset: close up of the end of the needle, demonstrating the Huber point.

Special equipment

- The Tuohy needle (Figure 1) is used to locate the epidural space and to pass the epidural catheter through. It has:
  - Centimetre markings;
  - A gently curved cutting tip, known as a Huber point;
  - Detachable 'wings', which can be used to grasp the needle firmly whilst advancing it.
- The epidural catheter (Figure 1) has:
  - Centimetre markings to allow the correct length of catheter to be left in the epidural space;
  - No distal end orifice, but multiple (often three) side orifices in the last 2–3 cm of the catheter.

Procedure

- Preparation and patient positioning for the procedure are the same as for spinal anaesthesia.
- An appropriate vertebral interspace is identified by palpation. It is not necessary to limit the technique to below L_{3-4}.

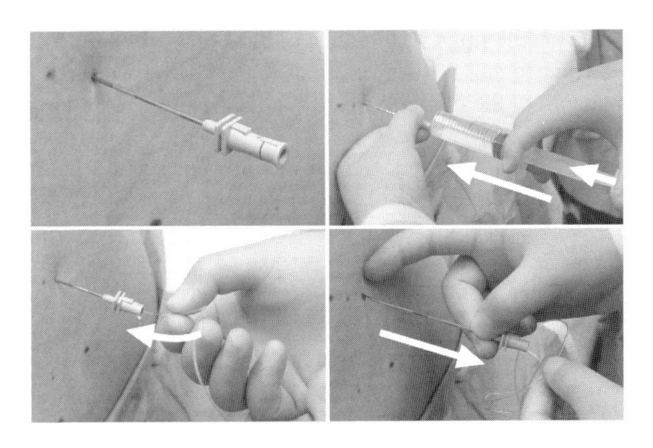

Figure 2. Insertion of an epidural catheter. Top left: the Tuohy needle is inserted into the intervertebral space (the 'wings' have not been used by this operator). Top right: a syringe containing normal saline is attached and both syringe and needle are advanced in unison until breach of the ligamentum flavum is signalled by loss of resistance. Bottom left: the catheter is passed. Bottom right: the needle is removed over the catheter, which is held firmly to prevent withdrawal.

- The interspace chosen is dictated by the operative site, for example:
  - Upper thoracic—T_{4-5}, lower thoracic/upper abdominal—T_{10-11}.
- The patient's anatomy may require use of an adjacent or nearby space (the 'best' space).
- The Tuohy needle is inserted into the interspace, and its obturator removed.
- The epidural space is located using a 'loss of resistance' technique (Figure 2). Loss of resistance to saline is the most common (although some operators use air):
  - A syringe containing normal saline is attached;
  - Both needle and syringe are advanced in unison;
  - Constant pressure is applied to the syringe plunger;
  - When the needle tip is within the tough ligamentum flavum, its orifice is occluded and there is great resistance felt in the plunger;
  - As the needle exits the ligamentum flavum, resistance is suddenly lost;

    - The needle tip is now in the epidural space; it should not be advanced any further, or the dura may be punctured.
- The depth of the epidural space is noted, using the markings on the needle.
- The syringe is detached, and (providing no CSF flow is noted), the catheter is passed until 5–7 cm is protruding into the space.
- The needle is removed, taking great care not to withdraw the catheter at all.
- The catheter is then withdrawn until 4–6 cm remains in the epidural space.
- The Luer connector is attached and two tests are performed:
    - Aspiration—no CSF or blood should be seen in the catheter;
    - Siphon—when the catheter is held vertically upwards, any fluid within should siphon downward into the low pressure epidural space. If the fluid level rises, this suggests higher pressure and raises the possibility of placement within the CSF;
    - If these tests are satisfactory, the filter is attached and the catheter secured according to local protocol.

Test dose

- The purpose of the test dose is to exclude intravenous and sub-arachnoid placement of the catheter, both of which could have serious consequences.
- A common test dose is 3–5 mL of 0.5% bupivacaine, administered rapidly.
- Following administration, the patient is assessed for signs or symptoms suggestive of catheter misplacement:
    - Intravenously (circumoral tingling or numbness, twitching);
    - Sub-arachnoid (profound and rapidly occurring spinal blockade and/or hypotension).
- If negative, the catheter is deemed safe to use.

Intra-operative management

Surgical analgesia during general anaesthesia is most commonly achieved using:

- Strong local anaesthetic solution (e.g. 20–40 mL of laevo-bupivacaine 0.25% or 0.5%), often with an added opioid (fentanyl or diamorphine); or

- Low dose laevo-bupivacaine solution with or without opioid that will be used for post-operative analgesia (see below).

Post-operative management

- It is now usual practice to use weak local anaesthetic solutions for post-operative epidurals. The use of a synergistic combination of drugs, allows lower concentrations of each to be used, reducing the risk of side effects.
- Common solutions include laevo-bupivacaine 0.1% or 0.125% with fentanyl 2 μg/mL.
- A special infusion pump is used to administer the epidural solution. Modern pumps can be programmed to provide:
  - A background infusion (typically 3–10 mL/h);
  - A patient demand bolus (typically 3–10 mL, with a lock-out period of 10–20 min);
  - Both of the above.
- Infusion and bolus settings are determined by the nature of the operation, the individual anaesthetist's preference and the hospital's protocol.
- Generally, the lumbar epidural space has a greater volume than the thoracic, and so lumbar epidurals require a greater volume of solution.

Post-operative surveillance

- This is very important—nursing staff should document and respond appropriately to the patient's vital signs, pain score, respiratory rate and sedation level.
- Institutional protocols and guidelines often exist and should be readily available.

Obstetric analgesia

- A combination of weak laevo-bupivacaine (0.1% or 0.125%) and fentanyl 2 μg/mL is most commonly used.
- Protocols vary—some units favour infusions, some favour boluses, and some use a combination.
- If conditions are favourable, a 'top-up' bolus of strong local anaesthetic (sometimes with an opioid) can provide adequate anaesthesia for caesarean section.

Complications

Common

- Hypotension is the commonest problem:
  - The mechanism and treatment are the same as for hypotension due to spinal anaesthesia (see Chapter 45);
  - However, hypotension may occur for other reasons and these should be excluded before blaming a working epidural. This is particularly true if the epidural has been in use for several hours.
- Headache occurs in around 1% of epidurals:
  - The cause is the same as with spinals (CSF leakage);
  - Note that the dural puncture may not be evident at the time of siting the epidural;
  - The incidence is reduced with operator experience.
- Failure of block / patchy block:
  - Complete failure usually requires re-siting of the epidural;
  - A patchy block may be improved by altering the patient's position to alter the spread of solution within the epidural space, by using larger volumes of solution, more concentrated solution, or by adding an opioid. If this fails, re-siting may be required (although, a patient may prefer to tolerate some degree of pain, rather than be subjected to a repeat epidural).

Rare

- The catheter may be misplaced:
  - Subarachnoid—resulting in the signs and symptoms of spinal anaesthesia,

> - Epidural insertion is an expert procedure; it is more important that you understand it than gain hands-on experience.
> - Find out your hospital's protocols for post-operative management of epidurals.
> - Aim to see the management of epidurals outside the operating theatre:
>   - Spend some time on an acute pain round, or with the acute pain nurse;
>   - Spend some time with the maternity ward anaesthetist.

    - Intravenously—resulting in signs and symptoms of local anaesthetic toxicity (circumoral paraesthesia, twitching, fitting, progressing to dysrhythmias and cardiac arrest);
    - Misplacement will usually be apparent at the time of insertion or test dose. It is however important to remember that a properly placed catheter can migrate into the sub-arachnoid space or a vessel (although it is rare).
- Haematoma or abscess of the epidural space is an extremely rare consequence of epidural placement.
- Severe or permanent neurological damage has been found prospectively to be about one quarter as common with epidural anaesthesia than with spinal anaesthesia. The risk can be reduced by careful technique.

47

Major peripheral nerve blocks

Martin Herrick

Peripheral nerve blocks provide per-operative anaesthesia and post-operative analgesia for limb surgery. Single-shot injections of local anaesthetic solution may provide analgesia for up to 24 hours if 0.5% solutions of bupivacaine or laevo-bupivacaine are administered. Insertion of a fine catheter close to the nerves permits further boluses or a continuous infusion of local anaesthetic, thus prolonging analgesia. These techniques may also be useful for treating chronic pain states.

Only a brief outline can be presented here. The reader is referred to more detailed accounts *before* attempting any of these blocks.

Nerve stimulation

The majority of peripheral nerves important for anaesthesia are mixed motor and sensory. Direct nerve stimulation, inducing muscle contractions, is now widely encouraged to locate the nerves, minimising the risk of unpleasant paraesthesiae. The important requirements for nerve stimulation include:

- A short square-wave impulse (0.05–0.1 ms). Motor nerves will be stimulated but not sensory nerves, which need a longer pulse width;
- A stimulus frequency of 2 Hz, to minimise the risk of impaling a nerve between impulses;
- An initial current of 1–2 mA;
- The needle to which the stimulator is attached should be the cathode;
- A final current of 0.5 mA producing a muscle twitch suggests that the needle tip is within 1–2 mm of the nerve.

The following criteria are often used to avoid intra-neural injection:

- The muscle twitch is no longer present at a current of 0.2 mA.

- The muscle twitch disappears within 0.5 s after the injection of 0.5 mL of solution.
- The injection of solution is easy without undue pressure.
- Injection is pain-free.

General side-effects of peripheral local anaesthesia

Numbness may be a troublesome sensation for some patients.
Limb paralysis may inhibit normal function (e.g. walking following day-case surgery).

General complications of peripheral local anaesthesia

Accidental limb damage (e.g. burn or pressure sore) may occur in a numb limb.

Systemic toxic reactions may follow if the plasma levels of local anaesthetic become high or if the *rate* of rise is rapid. This may occur with:

- Accidental intravascular injection;
- Absolute overdose;
- Relative overdose—e.g. a 'normal' dose in a frail or debilitated patient;
- Rapid absorption from highly vascular areas—e.g. around intercostal nerves;
- Accumulation during continuous infusions via a catheter.

In practice, intravascular injection is the commonest cause, resulting in symptoms during or immediately after injection. However, after a correctly sited single-shot injection, plasma levels may not peak for up to 45 min. There is no absolute safe dose: the risk of toxicity depends on the site and the rate of injection, as well as the total mass of drug.

None of these nerve blocks should therefore be undertaken without the precautions outlined in previous chapters.

Upper limb

Brachial plexus block

The brachial plexus may be blocked at any point between its origin at the C5–T1 anterior primary nerve roots and the division of the cords into the major terminal nerves in the axilla. The choice of approach will depend on the surgery planned since different brachial blocks preferentially anaesthetise different elements of the plexus. The most commonly used approaches are:

Interscalene approach

Nerves blocked: Anterior primary roots of C4–C6/7.

Indications: Anaesthesia for surgery on the shoulder or upper arm.

Side-effects:

- Ipsilateral phrenic nerve block. This may precipitate respiratory insufficiency in patients with lung disease, especially of the restrictive type.
- Horner's syndrome.

Complications:

- Vertebral artery injection of local anaesthetic. This causes immediate onset of convulsions after a very small dose of drug (e.g. 1 mL bupivacaine 0.5%).
- High spinal anaesthetic, following injection into the subarachnoid space within the vertebral canal or (more likely) into a dural cuff extending lateral to the intervertebral foramen. Respiratory arrest, anaesthesia and cardiovascular depression will rapidly ensue.
- Epidural spread.

Technique: A 50 mm needle is inserted in the groove between the anterior and middle scalene muscles, at the level of the superior thyroid notch, and directed caudally and slightly dorsally and medially, until contractions of the biceps muscle are seen. 30 mL of local anaesthetic solution are then administered.

Diaphragmatic twitch (phrenic nerve stimulation) indicates that the needle is too anterior, while shoulder shrugging (dorsal scapular nerve stimulation) indicates too posterior a position.

Subclavian perivascular/supraclavicular approach

Nerves blocked: The three trunks of the brachial plexus as they cross over the first rib.

Indications:

- Anaesthesia for surgery on the humerus, elbow, fore-arm and hand;
- NOT ideal for surgery on the little finger alone since the inferior trunk, from which the ulnar nerve is derived, is not blocked in 10% of patients.

Side-effects:

- Ipsilateral phrenic nerve block in some patients;
- Horner's syndrome;
- Recurrent laryngeal nerve block, causing temporary hoarseness.

Complications:

- Subclavian artery puncture. This block is therefore unsuitable for patients with abnormal coagulation.

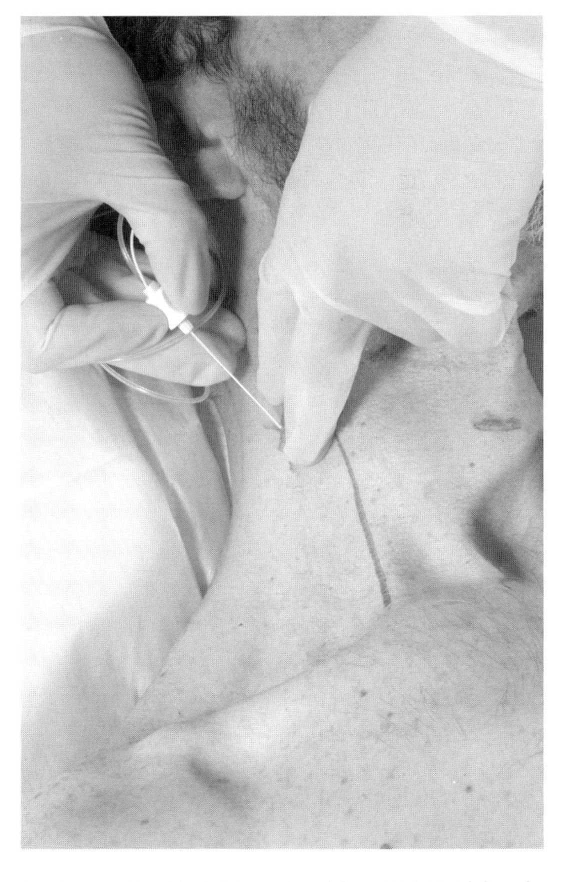

Figure 1. Interscaline block (Reproduced from M.J. Herrick and T.J. Clarke, Upper limb nerve blocks. *Anaesthesia and Intensive Care Medicine*. 2001;2:99 by kind permission of The Medicine Publishing Company).

- Pneumothorax. The incidence of clinically significant pneumothorax is 2–6% for the supraclavicular block and <1% for the Subclavian perivascular block.

Technique: *(Subclavian perivascular)* A 50 mm. needle is inserted at the lowest point of the interscalene groove in the root of the neck,

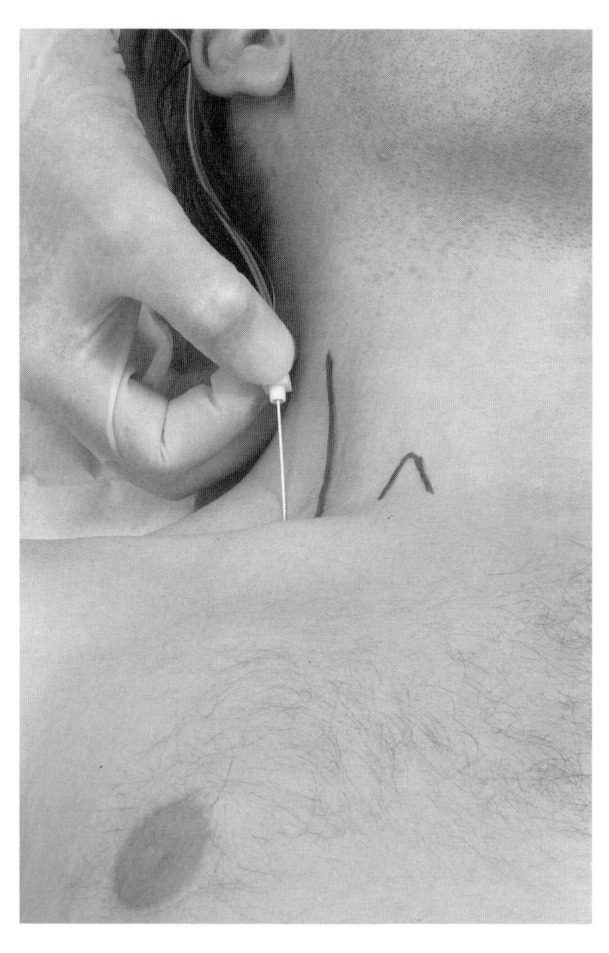

Figure 2. Subclavian perivascular/supraclavicular approach (Reproduced from M.J. Herrick and T.J. Clarke, Upper limb nerve blocks. *Anaesthesia and Intensive Care Medicine.* 2001;2:99 by kind permission of The Medicine Publishing Company).

immediately posterior to the subclavian artery, and directed caudally. It is important that the there is no medial intent, in order to avoid injuring the cupola of the lung. Once flexion or extension of the fingers or wrist has been achieved, 30 mL of local anaesthetic is injected.

If the plexus is not encountered, the needle should insert on the first rib, which acts as a 'backstop'. It should then be redirected either anteriorly or posteriorly.

Axillary approach

Nerves blocked: Cords or major terminal nerves. Single shot injection blocks the median and ulnar nerves more frequently than the radial and musculo-cutaneous nerves. With multiple injections, all four major nerves can be anaesthetised.

Indications:

- Hand and fore-arm surgery, especially if surgery limited to the ulnar side;
- Surgery on the medial side of the elbow.

Complications: There are no specific complications comparable to those associated with more proximal approaches to the brachial plexus.

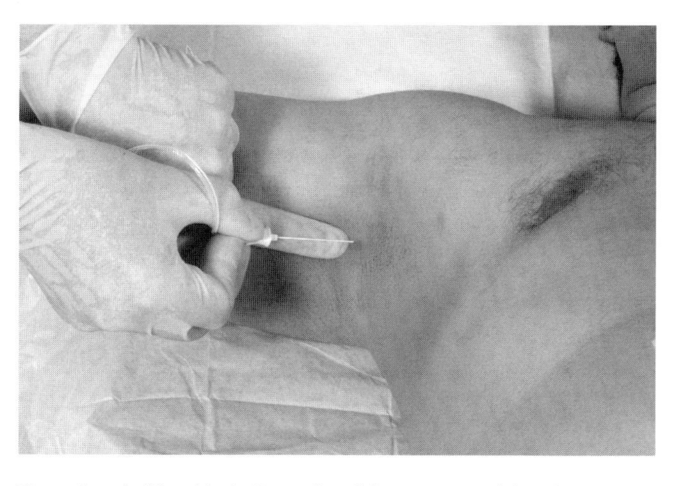

Figure 3. Axillary block (Reproduced from M.J. Herrick and T.J. Clarke, Upper limb nerve blocks. *Anaesthesia and Intensive Care Medicine.* 2001;2:99 by kind permission of The Medicine Publishing Company).

Axillary artery puncture may occur. However, because it is easy to compress the artery, haematoma is unusual even in patients with a coagulopathy.

Technique: With the patients arm abducted to 90° and the elbow flexed, the axillary pulse is palpated high in the axilla. A 25 mm needle is inserted in a cephalad direction at a 45° angle to the skin. The median nerve (thumb, forefinger and long finger flexion) is located above the artery, the ulnar nerve (little and ring finger flexion + thumb adduction) below the artery, and the radial nerve (finger and thumb extension) below and behind the artery. The musculo-cutaneous nerve, important for anaesthetising the radial area of the wrist and hand innervated by the lateral cutaneous nerve of the forearm, lies in the coraco-brachialis muscle, and is identified by inducing biceps contractions. 10 mL of local anaesthetic is injected around each nerve.

Lower limb

It is not possible to anaesthetise the lower limb completely using peripheral nerve blocks, especially for surgery on the hip joint or for surgery requiring a thigh tourniquet. Only spinal or epidural anaesthesia will achieve this.

However, peripheral blocks are very useful adjuncts to anaesthesia, and may provide good post-operative analgesia. All of the following are amenable to the introduction of a catheter for continuous blockade.

Sciatic nerve block combined with femoral nerve or lumbar plexus block provides excellent analgesia following major knee surgery. Additional block of the obturator nerve is rarely required.

Lumbar plexus block

The lumbar plexus, derived from the anterior primary rami of the L1–4 nerve roots, gives rise to the femoral, obturator and lateral femoral cutaneous nerves, which then pass through the psoas muscle. They may be blocked by injection of local anaesthetic into the psoas sheath. This avoids the autonomic side-effects of epidural anaesthesia (hypotension, urinary retention).

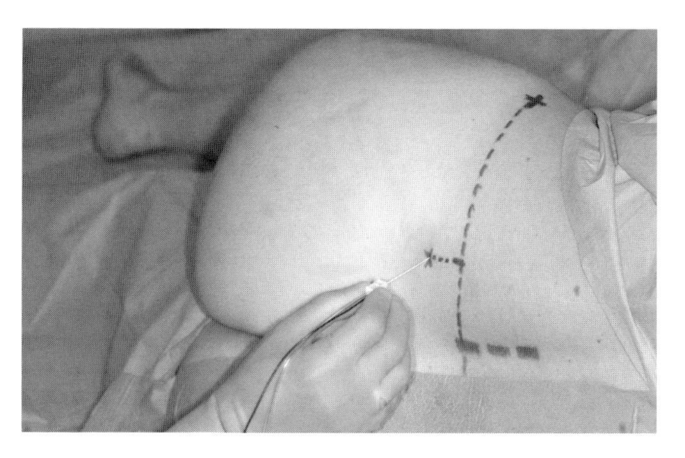

Figure 4. Lumbar plexus block.

Indications: Analgesia following operations on the hip, femur or knee.

Complications:

- Epidural spread
- Intrathecal injection, producing high spinal block.

Technique: With the patient lying on the opposite side and the legs flexed, the spine of L4 is identified on the intercristal line, and a point identified 5 cm lateral and 2 cm caudal to the spine. A 100 mm needle is inserted at this point and directed anteriorly with no medial intent. If the transverse process (of L5) is contacted, the needle is walked off in a cranial direction. When contraction of the quadriceps muscle is noted; 30 mL of local anaesthetic are injected.

Femoral nerve block

The femoral nerve supplies the femur and the anterior part of the knee joint. It also supplies the skin over the anterior surface of the thigh and the antero-medial surface of the knee. Its terminal branch, the saphenous nerve, supplies the skin over the medial aspect of the calf and ankle, and may extend along the medial border of the foot.

The 'three-in-one' block, in which a large volume of local anaesthetic is injected into the sheath around the femoral nerve and encouraged

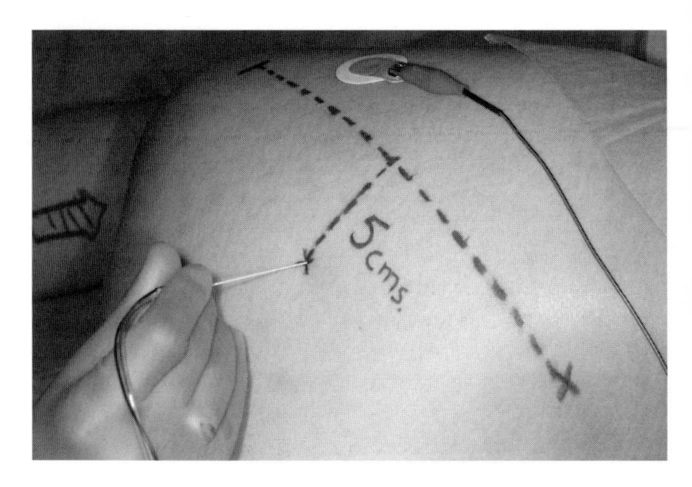

Figure 5. Sciatic nerve block.

to spread proximally, aims to block the femoral, lateral femoral cutaneous and obturator nerves. In practice this goal is rarely achieved.

Indications:

- Analgesia for fractures of the neck or shaft of femur;
- Analgesia for operations on the femur and the knee joint.

Side effects: The nerve supply to the extensors of the knee, notably the quadriceps muscle, is blocked, preventing weight-bearing.

Complications: There are no specific complications.

Technique: The femoral artery is palpated in the groin crease. A 50 mm needle is inserted 2 cm lateral to the artery, angled 45° cephalad, and advanced until quadriceps contraction is obtained, producing a patellar dance. 20 mL of local anaesthetic are then injected.

Sartorius contraction indicates the needle is too medial and superficial.

Sciatic nerve block

The sciatic nerve, which divides into the tibial and common peroneal nerves, supplies the posterior part of the knee joint, the tibia and the foot. It also supplies the skin over the lower leg and foot except for the medial side.

There are many approaches to this nerve, which may be blocked at any point from its emergence below the piriformis muscle down to the popliteal fossa (at which point it has usually divided into its two major components). The classical approach of Labat will be described since it is usually easy to perform, blocks the nerve at its highest point, and incorporates block of the posterior cutaneous nerve of the thigh.

Indications:

- Analgesia for operations on the knee joint (with a femoral nerve block), ankle and foot;
- Controversial in tibial trauma or surgery because the severe pain of compartment syndrome may be masked.

Complications: Prolonged anaesthesia may be associated with pressure sores on the heel.

Technique: The patient lies in the Sim's position, with the dependent leg straight and the leg to be blocked flexed. A line is drawn joining the posterior superior iliac spine and the greater trochanter. At the midpoint of this line, a perpendicular line is drawn 5–6 cm caudally, identifying the needle entry point. This point should lie on a line joining the sacral hiatus and the greater trochanter. A 100 mm needle is introduced at right-angles to the skin and advanced until movement of the foot is observed, either dorsiflexion/eversion (common peroneal component) or plantarflexion/inversion (tibial nerve component), usually at a depth of about 7 cm 20 mL of local anaesthetic are then injected.

Contractions of the gluteal or hamstring muscles suggest that the direction is accurate, but that the needle is still too superficial.

If contractions of the foot are not observed, the needle should be withdrawn and redirected cephalad or caudad along the line of the perpendicular.

Conclusion

None of these blocks are straightforward; and it would be unwise to attempt them without initial supervision from a competent trainer.

Most practitioners learn the skills for lower limb blockade rapidly. However, upper limb blocks may be more difficult to master, especially if the anatomy is not fully understood.

Further reading

1 Brown, DL. *Atlas of regional anaesthesia*, 2nd ed. Philadelphia: Saunders, 1999.
2 Mehrkens, HH. *Peripheral regional anaesthesia*, 2nd ed. B Braun Melsungen AG, 2000.

Section 6

Critical Care Skills

48

Ventilators

Fiona L. Clarke

There are many ways of classifying different types of ventilators, often based on the method of action of the ventilator or the method of operation. Modern ventilators used in the intensive care unit can deliver a wide variety of modes of ventilation, so an understanding of the basic principles of ventilation and an understanding of lung pathophysiology is required to select the appropriate mode for the appropriate condition.

Features of the ideal ventilator

- Simple to use, clean, maintain and repair;
- Robust and possibly portable;
- Integral monitoring systems for airway pressure, tidal volume, respiratory rate, inspiratory and expiratory minute volume and inspired oxygen concentration;
- Disconnection (low airway pressure), high airway pressure, oxygen failure and power failure alarms;
- Versatile so that appropriate tidal volumes, respiratory rates, pressures and inspiratory:expiratory (I:E) ratios and assisted breathing modes can be provided for all age groups;
- Able to supply PEEP and CPAP;
- Able to be used with any gas or vapour mixture, with the ability to entrain air in the event of oxygen supply failure;
- Economical to purchase, clean and use.

Modes of ventilation

Controlled lung ventilation modes are used for patients receiving muscle relaxants or with no intrinsic respiratory effort (e.g. spinal cord injury above C3). If a patient can make some respiratory effort, then sophisticated modern ventilators can use a variety of modes to allow the patient to breathe with greater or lesser assistance from the ventilator.

Controlled ventilation

Fully controlled ventilation is often described as IPPV: Intermittent Positive Pressure Ventilation—which is either volume-controlled or pressure-controlled. Pressure-controlled ventilation is described as BIPAP: biphasic positive airway pressure.

Setting parameters

Ventilators use inspiratory and expiratory pressures and times to achieve a tidal volume and respiratory rate.

To set the parameters on a ventilator, you need to know which variable you can alter on the ventilator. Simple ventilators may only allow you to selected inspiratory time, expiratory time and inspiratory flow rates, e.g. Penlon Nuffield 200 ventilator. Sophisticated ICU ventilators will allow all parameters to be adjusted.

- minute volume ($L\,m^{-1}$) = tidal volume (mL) $\times$ respiratory rate (breaths per minute)
- tidal volume = inspiratory flow rate $\times$ inspiratory time
- rate = 60 s $\times$ (inspiratory time + expiratory time)

so:

$$\text{minute volume} = (\text{inspiratory flow rate} \times \text{inspiratory time}) \times [60\,\text{s} \times (\text{inspiratory time} + \text{expiratory time})]$$

You may need to decide whether it is most important for the patient to receive controlled volumes or controlled pressures. Both excessive volumes and excessive pressures have been shown to damage the delicate lung tissue and increase mortality and morbidity in the critically ill. The appropriate settings will prevent volutrauma due to gas trapping in alveoli, barotrauma due to overdistention of alveoli and atelectrauma or shearing stress due to repeated opening and closing of alveoli.

	Volume-controlled	BIPAP
Control	volume	pressure
Inspiratory flow	constant	decelerating
Inspiratory volume	constant	variable
Inspiratory pressure	variable	constant
Expiration	passive	passive

Intermittent Positive Pressure Ventilation (IPPV)

To use this mode, a tidal volume, the respiratory rate and the upper limits for inspiratory pressure are selected. Current recommendations are for a tidal volume of 5–7 mL/kg, which has decreased from 10–12 mL/kg seen in older textbooks, to minimise volutrauma. The inspiratory pressure will vary depending on the compliance of the patient's lungs and the flow rate, and has an inspiratory peak at the beginning of inspiration, which declines to a plateau. Try not to exceed peak pressures of 35 cm H_2O. This is the simplest mode to choose for the fully ventilated patient, because a set minimum minute volume is delivered, unless the peak inspiratory pressure limits are exceeded.

This is a mode to be used for patients during anaesthesia (those with relatively normal lungs) or when a patient is in a situation where it is more difficult to examine and treat them, e.g. during transfers, or when lung compliance may change very rapidly, e.g. severe asthma or when starting prone ventilation.

Sophisticated ventilators can modify volume controlled ventilation by responding to changes in compliance by altering the inspiratory flow rate to achieve the set tidal volume at the lowest possible inspiratory pressures (e.g. Autoflow).

BIPAP

If you use this mode, you have to select two pressure levels: inspiratory pressure and expiratory pressure (PEEP: positive end expiratory pressure), and the respiratory rate. This mode of ventilation allows the patient to make spontaneous respiratory efforts throughout every phase of the respiratory cycle, unlike IPPV. This may make it more tolerable for a patient able to make respiratory efforts. Inspiratory pressures are generally lower using BIPAP than volume controlled ventilation. The tidal volume is not set, however, and this can vary dramatically as lung compliance changes, with the potential to cause volutrauma. This mode is usually chosen for patients with stiff, non-compliant lungs, e.g. with ARDS (Acute respiratory distress syndrome), and patients where you want to use the minimal amount of sedation possible to allow them to tolerate ventilation. It is possibly easier to wean patients from fully supported ventilation using BIPAP, which can be altered to provide varying levels of pressure support ventilation (see Chapter 34).

Partial ventilation

If a patient can make spontaneous respiratory efforts, then a mode which allows synchronisation of the ventilator breaths with the patient's own efforts should be chosen.

Volume controlled ventilation adjusted to allow patient effort is usually referred to as SIMV: synchronised intermittent mandatory ventilation.

SIMV

When this mode was first developed, it allowed a variable number of pre-set volume breaths to be delivered, and patient effort between these set breaths was detected by either a flow trigger or a pressure trigger. If triggered during a 'trigger window' during expiration, the ventilator would then deliver another pre-set volume breath. This has been modified over time so that the patient breath is now augmented up to a particular pressure or in proportion to the amount of respiratory effort the patient has made (pressure support ventilation or proportional assist ventilation). If a patient is being weaned from full ventilation, it is usual to reduce the set number of breaths so that the patient can make increasing efforts until independence from the ventilator is achieved.

Pressure support

Pressure support ventilation allows a pre-set amount of positive pressure to be delivered when a patient makes a respiratory effort and reaches a certain flow (flow trigger), which assists the patient's own efforts. Expiration is passive, and the respiratory rate and tidal volume will vary depending on the patient's efforts and the impedance of the system. This is used in conjunction with SIMV modes to help wean the patient from ventilation, because a reducing amount of pressure support can be given, as the patient becomes stronger. A minimum amount of pressure support is always needed to overcome the intrinsic resistance of the respiratory system tubing.

PEEP and CPAP

PEEP is defined as artificial maintenance of a pressure above atmospheric at the end of passive exhalation during controlled ventilation.

CPAP is defined as artificial application of a pre-set positive pressure through the inspiratory and expiratory phases of the respiratory cycle in a spontaneously breathing patient (see Chapter 33).

Intrinsic PEEP or auto PEEP refers to the pressure generated when passive exhalation terminates before the lung volume has declined to functional residual capacity (FRC), so that air trapping and hyperinflation of the lung occurs.

PEEP and CPAP are designed to stop alveoli collapsing at the end of expiration and increase FRC above closing capacity, which can improve hypoxia. High levels of PEEP or CPAP may increase the risk of barotrauma, and can reduce cardiac output by increasing intrathoracic pressure. Other effects such as antidiuresis and antinaturesis can be caused, possibly due to effects on renal perfusion, the renin angiotensin system and reduced release of atrial naturetic factor.

Inspiratory:expiratory ratio (I:E ratio)

You should decide whether to use normal I:E ratios (usually 1:2) or to alter them to suit the condition of the patient.

If you have a patient with bronchospasm, you want to allow enough time for expiration to prevent air trapping in the lung, which at worse can cause barotrauma and reduce the cardiac output by increasing intrathoracic pressure.

If you have a patient with hypoxaemia and ARDS you may want to chose inverse ratios (I:E greater than 1:1) to try and hold the lung in inspiration for longer than usual to try and open up collapsed alveoli and give more time for gas diffusion across damaged areas of lung. This is a very uncomfortable mode of ventilation for an awake patient, so generous amounts of sedation should be given, and possible muscle relaxants as well.

Transport ventilators

These usually use O_2 as a driving gas, so when calculating how much oxygen will be required for a transfer you should add (on average) one litre per minute to the patient's minute volume. They generally are less sophisticated than ventilators used in ICU or the operating theatre, so it may not be possible to reproduce the exact ventilator settings during a transfer. This is why you should observe the patient for a suitable period of time when they are connected to the transport ventilator, and ideally confirm acceptable ventilation by checking arterial blood gases before starting the transfer.

49

Conventional tracheostomy

Derek A. Bosman

Tracheostomy is a surgical opening into the trachea, most commonly performed for purposes of ventilation.

This ancient procedure, first performed in 3600 BC, has evolved over the years from a very basic procedure to a sophisticated surgical operation.

For a tracheostomy to be safe and successful it is of paramount importance to adhere to all the principles, especially those pertaining to post-operative tracheostomy care.

Anatomy and Physiology

The larynx is a flexible dynamic organ, which maintains the patency of the airway and is essential for voice production and protecting the airway.

The upper airway is essential for warming, humidifying and purifying ducted air to the larynx. The tracheostomy bypasses the upper airway; therefore post-operative substitution of these functions, by means of humidification and suction is essential.

The trachea extends from directly below the larynx to the bifurcation into the left and right main bronchus.

It has cartilaginous rings, which provide structure and support, and is situated directly in front of the oesophagus. Alongside the larynx and trachea are the carotid artery and jugular vein, as well as cranial and sympathetic nerves. These structures should be identified to avoid injury, especially if there is tracheal displacement and distortion.

Connective tissue, the strap muscles and thyroid gland lie between the skin and trachea.

Indications

- Ventilatory support
- Upper airway obstruction
- Failed Oro-tracheal intubation or inability to intubate
- Pulmonary toilet
- Aspiration
- Laryngeal trauma
- To facilitate head and neck surgery

Preparation

Anaesthesia

Patients are fully consented for the procedure as well as the implications of post-operative care, where long-term tracheostomy is anticipated. General anaesthesia is usually preferred. In un-intubated patients, spontaneous breathing is maintained until the airway has been assessed as suitable for intubation. In these cases it is advisable to have an endoscopy set (with bronchoscopes), prepared together with the surgical tracheostomy set, ready for use at induction of anaesthesia.

In severe upper airway obstruction and critically ill patients, local anaesthesia, using topical lidocaine infiltration is favoured. Conventional tracheostomy is carried out in theatre under sterile conditions.

Tracheostomy tubes

Tracheostomy tubes are produced from various materials ranging from metal through to bio-compatible polyvinyl. There are essentially two groups of tracheostomy tubes for use in conventional tracheostomy as illustrated in Figure 1.

Adult tubes

These are available in cuffed and non-cuffed tubes. A cuffed tube is normally inserted with the initial operation. These tubes are available with inner tubes, which can be removed and cleaned as frequently as necessary without having to remove the outer sleeve, ensuring the tract is maintained.

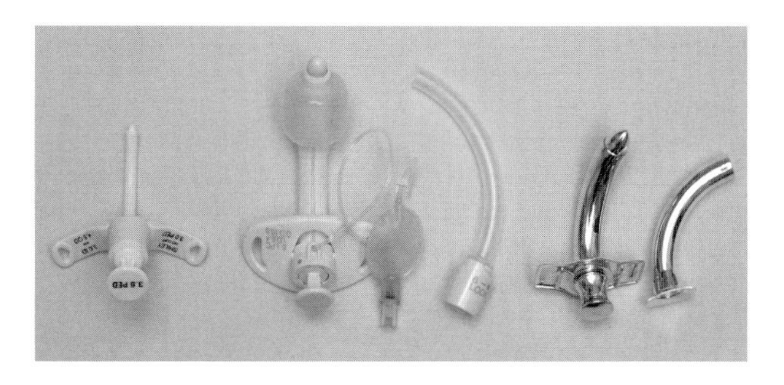

Figure 1. Tracheostomy tubes (Left to right): Paediatric sized tracheostomy tube with introducer; Adult tube with introducer, inflated cuff and inner tube alongside; metal tracheostomy tube with inner tube alongside. (The metal tracheostomy tubes are exclusively used for long-term tracheostomy and are normally not inserted in the acute stage after surgery.)

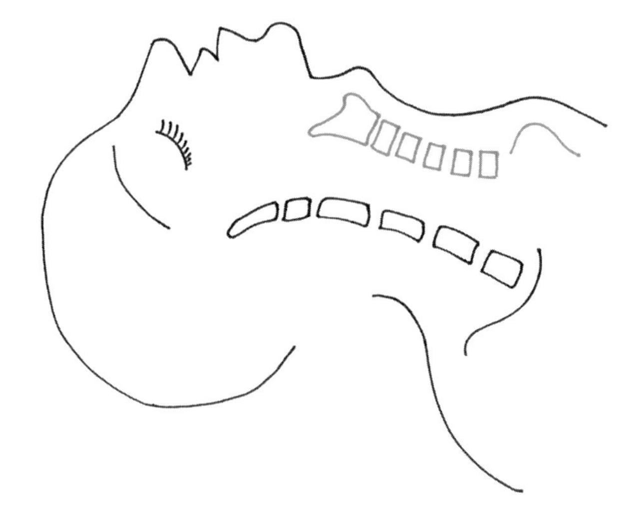

Figure 2. The correct position for tracheostomy with the neck and head extended. Indicated in grey are the thyroid, cricoid and tracheal cartilages and the sternal notch below.

Paediatric tubes

These tubes are non-cuffed and usually do not have an inner tube, as this increases respiratory resistance. All tubes have an introducer to aid insertion, and a collar to secure the tracheostomy using a neck tie.

Technique

Positioning

The head and neck should be fully extended to allow displacement of the trachea to the anterior surface of the neck. Once positioned, the laryngeal cartilages and the trachea are palpated to confirm alignment as well as the position of the cricoid cartilage (above) and sternal notch (below). These positions are marked with a skin marker.

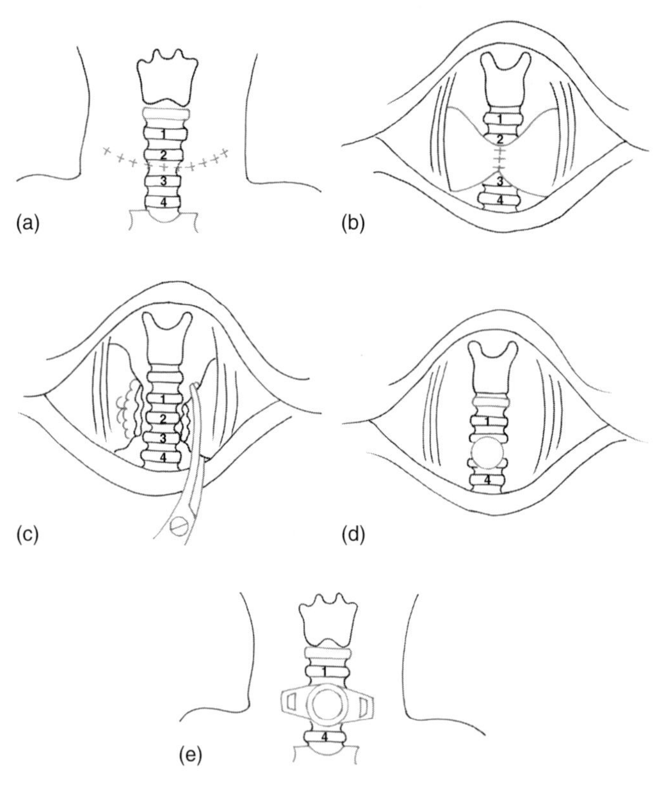

Figure 3. (a) Surface anatomy of the horizontal skin incision, midway between cricoid (above) and sternal notch (below)—indicated in grey. The tracheal rings are numbered 1–4. (b) exposure of the thyroid with strap muscles retracted laterally. (c) division of the thyroid using curved haemostat and ligation. (d) position of fenestration into trachea through the second and third tracheal rings. (e) tracheostomy inserted into correct position.

Skin incision

A horizontal skin incision is used, sited midway between the cricoid and the sternal notch. Once the location of the skin incision is determined it is marked out using a skin marker.

Exposure

The skin is incised with a scalpel. The cervical fascia is opened to reveal the strap muscles. These are separated in the midline, in a vertical plane to reveal the thyroid isthmus.

Division of the thyroid isthmus

The thyroid is clamped with curved haemostats in the midline, divided and ligated.

Tracheal incision

The trachea is opened using a vertical midline incision between the second and fourth tracheal rings. It is normally necessary to incise at least two rings. In adults, where the cartilaginous tracheal rings may be ossified, an elliptical window is excised to improve access.

Intubation

A tracheostomy tube is inserted using a tracheal dilator. Once in place the cuff is inflated (adult tubes only). The introducer is removed, and the tube is connected to the ventilator via a sterile catheter mount. Suction is used to clear the tube and the trachea. Ventilation of both lungs is checked and respiration monitored, certifying normal CO_2 return and saturation. A tracheostomy ribbon is passed through the collar of the tube and firmly secured around the neck. The head and neck is returned into the normal anatomical position, and the patency and position of the tube re-checked.

Post-operative care

Correct and meticulous post-operative care is of essence to achieve a successful outcome. High care or intensive care is advised post-operatively. In addition to standard post-operative monitoring, ensure the following:

- Monitor oxygen saturation;
- Suction and aspiration of secretions;

- Ensure tube patency and position;
- Humidification;
- Chest X-ray to check for pneumothorax and correct tube position;
- Chest physiotherapy;
- Wound care;
- Monitor cuff pressures to prevent stenosis;
- Tracheostomy tube change. (Inner tube may be removed for cleaning as frequently as required to maintain tube patency. The outer tube may only be removed 72 hours post-operatively, after a tract has formed.)

In infants risks are increased and tube obstruction or displacement can rapidly result in cardio-respiratory failure and death.

Complications

- Tube obstruction or displacement;
- Bleeding or haematoma;
- Pneumothorax;
- Surgical emphysema—due to entrapment of air in the tissues;
- Apnoea may occur due to decreased CO_2, reducing the respiratory drive;
- Tracheal erosion;
- Infection;
- Dysphagia—may be caused by over inflated cuff or large tube;
- Cranial nerve injury—may occur when anatomy is distorted;
- Stenosis is a late complication due to trauma caused by the cuff or tube.

> - Always check tube position after changing head and neck posture.
> - If in any doubt as to whether the position of the tube has changed, check immediately by means of fibreoscopy or X-ray.
> - The introducer as well as a spare tube of the same size is left with the patient at all times.
> - The collar of the tracheostomy tube may be sutured to the skin to reduce chances of accidental extubation. Tracheostomy tapes must be firmly secured at all times.

- Close the wound loosely to prevent surgical emphysema and haematoma.
- Always check cuff pressures and deflate if cuff is not required.
- Employing all aspects of post-operative care is absolutely vital.
- Instil saline (2 mL/hr) into the tube to aid suctioning of viscid mucous and prevents crusting.
- Always check the following prior to a tube change or insertion:
  - Correct positioning of the head and neck;
  - Provision of good illumination (preferably a head light);
  - Pre-oxygenation (saturation at 100% prior to change);
  - Suction catheter to aspirate all secretions before and after;
  - The correct tube size and cuff;
  - A tracheal dilator in case the lumen occludes;
- The patient's general condition and respiratory status should be carefully assessed pre-operatively, and should be optimised where possible, to ensure the highest level of safety.
- In critically ill patients the clotting profile should always be checked.

50

Percutaneous dilatational tracheostomy

Stephen Chay

Introduction

Respiratory failure is a common finding in patients admitted to an intensive care unit (ICU). An increasing ability to provide multi-organ support such as renal replacement therapy, cardiovascular support and positive pressure ventilation has led to increasing lengths of ICU stays and days being spent on ventilatory support. Prolonged ventilatory support has resulted in the need for more tracheostomies to be performed.

The Seldinger technique of percutaneous tracheostomy was described in 1957. In 1985, Ciaglia described the percutaneous dilatational tracheostomy (PDT) using sequential curved dilators. There have been further modifications to this technique, including the forceps dilatational technique, the translaryngeal technique and a modification of the original Ciaglia technique using a single tapering dilator marketed as the Ciaglia Blue Rhino (CBR).

Indications

- Upper airway obstruction;
- Airway protection;
- Prolonged ventilatory support;
- Access for tracheal and pulmonary suctioning.

Contraindications

Absolute

- Uncorrected severe coagulopathy;
- Inability to ascertain the position of the tracheal rings;

- Inability to ventilate the lungs should the current airway (usually an oral endotracheal tube) fail during the procedure.

Relative contraindications

- F_iO_2 greater than 50% and positive end-expiratory pressures exceeding 8 cm water;
- Unstable cervical spine injuries;
- Previous neck surgery;
- Presence of blood vessels over the proposed tracheostomy site;
- Head injuries with increased intracranial pressures;
- Previous tracheostomy.

The use of PDT and its long-term complications in children has not been extensively investigated and the technique should not be used in children under 10 years. Currently, PDT cannot be recommended as a standard technique to secure an airway in the emergency setting.

Technique of percutaneous dilatational tracheostomy using the Ciaglia Blue Rhino (CBR) set

- Be familiar with the relevant anatomy (Figures 1 and 2).
- Obtain the appropriate consent or assent in line with local policies.

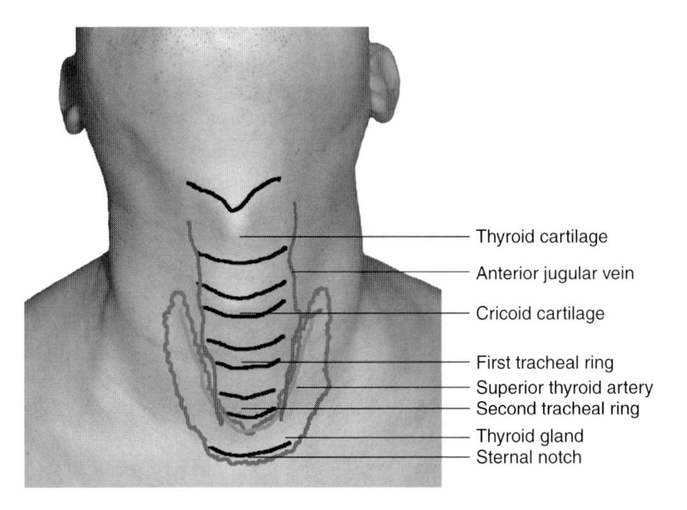

Figure 1. Anatomical landmarks anterior view.

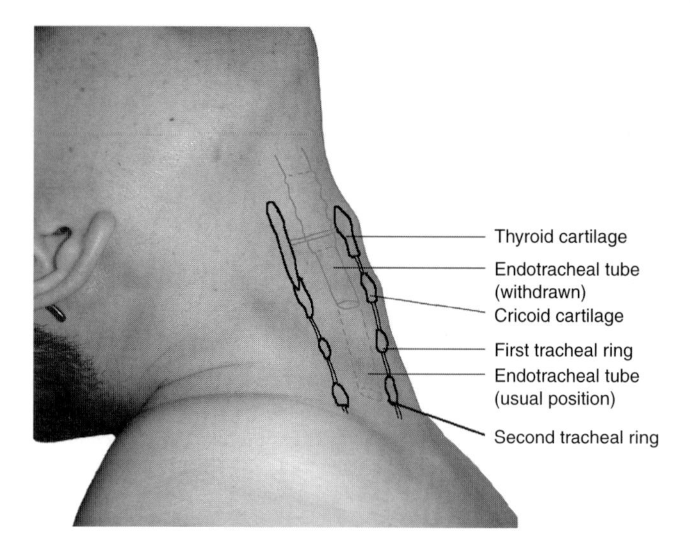

Figure 2. Anatomical landmarks lateral view.

- All resuscitation and other equipment such as extra airways and endotracheal tubes must be available and checked.
- A fibreoptic bronchoscope is highly recommended.
- Full anaesthesia is administered and an appropriate muscle relaxant is given. In critically ill patients, inotropic support may need to be started or increased.
- A translaryngeal endotracheal tube of size 8.0 mm or greater is required for a standard fibreoptic bronchoscope.
- Deflate the cuff of the translaryngeal endotracheal tube under direct vision and withdraw the tube so that the cuff is seen to be between the vocal cords (Figure 2).
- Insert a throat pack under direct vision, ensuring that the endotracheal tube remains in the correct position. This minimises the air leak and stabilises the tube in the correct position for the procedure. If ventilation remains inadequate, inflate the cuff gently to reduce any air leak further.
- Position the patient to achieve the maximum safe neck extension. A sand bag under the shoulders and the use of a head ring may be useful. Elevate the head of the bed by 30 degrees.

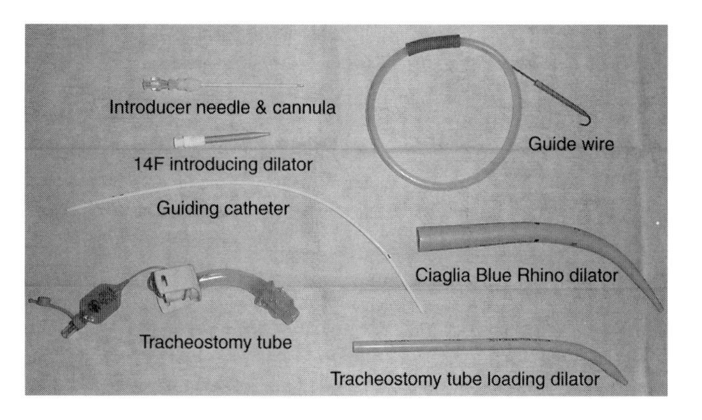

Figure 3. Equipment for PDT.

- Palpate the anterior neck and identify the landmarks. The correct placement of the tracheostomy is between the first and second or the second and third tracheal rings (Figures 1 and 2).
- 5–10 mL of 1% lidocaine with 1:200,000 adrenaline is infiltrated into the site to reduce venous bleeding.
- Prepare and drape the operative site.
- Make a 1.5 cm longitudinal skin incision over the intended insertion site.
- Gently dissect with curved mosquito forceps down to pretracheal fascia. Verify the landmarks with the finger.
- Insert the introducer needle and cannula in the midline into the trachea. The aspiration of air indicates its likely entry into the trachea. If insertion is difficult and the endotracheal tube moves together with the needle, then it is likely that the needle is impaled onto the tube. If uncomplicated, advance the introducer cannula a centimetre and remove the needle. Confirm that there is still easy aspiration of air from the introducer cannula.
- Insert the guide wire into the introducer cannula. This should insert freely until it impinges on a smaller bronchus, when further advancement is not possible. If the guide wire can be freely inserted all the way, then it is possible that the introducer cannula may be in the oesophagus.
- Confirm the position of the guide wire with the fibreoptic bronchoscope. The entry point should be distal to the endotracheal

tube and in the midline of the trachea and the guide wire must be seen going down towards the carina.

- If possible, maintain continuous visualisation of the procedure with the bronchoscope.
- Advance the short 14F introducing dilator over the guide wire to dilate the initial puncture site. The bronchoscopist can provide guidance to prevent over-insertion and possible trauma to the posterior tracheal wall.
- Wet the lubricating coating on the CBR dilator with sterile water, insert it into the guiding catheter ensuring that it is well seated on the safety ridge and advance the whole assembly over the guide wire.
- Dilate gently and slowly—the bronchoscopist can provide guidance to maintain the dilator in a central endotracheal position at all times. It will not be necessary to insert the dilator beyond the black skin level mark.
- Leave the whole assembly in position for 1–2 minutes when the appropriate dilation is reached to allow maximal dilation to occur. Repeated insertions and withdrawals are usually unnecessary and can increase the risk of trauma to the posterior tracheal wall as well as displacement of the guide wire.
- Insert a loading dilator into a lubricated tracheostomy tube.
- Remove the CBR dilator, leaving the guide wire and catheter in place.
- Insert the loading dilator/tracheostomy tube assembly into the guiding catheter, ensuring that the tip of the dilator is seated onto the safety ridge.
- Insert the whole assembly as a single unit into the trachea. The bronchoscopist can again provide guidance.
- Insert the tracheostomy tube to its flange and remove the loading dilator, guiding catheter and guide wire.
- Confirm with the fibreoptic bronchoscope through the translaryngeal endotracheal tube that an adequate length of tracheostomy tube has been inserted. Insert the fibreoptic bronchoscope into the newly inserted tracheostomy tube to confirm that the position is satisfactory, especially with respect to the carina. Any blood or secretions may be quickly cleared before the tracheostomy is attached to the breathing circuit and the cuff inflated appropriately.
- Confirm that ventilation is adequate.
- The translaryngeal endotracheal tube and throat pack are left in place until the tracheostomy tube is safely secured.
- Request a chest radiograph to check for possible complications.

Complications

Early

- Paratracheal insertion;
- Trauma to posterior tracheal wall;
- Pneumothorax;
- Surgical emphysema;
- Aspiration;
- Bleeding;
- Loss of airway and transient hypoxia.

The risk of death has been reported to be less than 1%. Continuous bronchoscopy may reduce some of these complications.

Intermediate

- Para-stomal infection;
- Secondary bleeding;
- Inadvertent displacement of the tracheostomy tube.

The late complications of PDT can be difficult to quantify as the procedure is performed in a group of patients with a high mortality rate. The incidence of symptomatic glottic and subglottic stenosis appears to be comparable to that of surgical tracheostomy, at around 6%.

- Always check tube position after changing head and neck posture.
- If in any doubt as to whether the position of the tube has changed, check immediately by means of fibreoscopy or X-ray.
- The introducer as well as a spare tube of the same size is left with the patient at all times.
- The collar of the tracheostomy tube may be sutured to the skin to reduce chances of accidental extubation. Tracheostomy tapes must be firmly secured at all times.
- Close the wound loosely to prevent surgical emphysema and haematoma.
- Always check cuff pressures and deflate if cuff is not required.
- Employing all aspects of post-operative care is absolutely vital.

- Instil saline (2 mL/h) into the tube to aid suctioning of viscid mucous and prevents crusting.
- Always check the following prior to a tube change or insertion:
  - Correct positioning of the head and neck;
  - Provision of good illumination (preferably a head light);
  - Pre-oxygenation (saturation at 100% prior to change);
  - Suction catheter to aspirate all secretions before and after;
  - The correct tube size and cuff;
  - A tracheal dilator in case the lumen occludes.
- The patient's general condition and respiratory status should be carefully assessed pre-operatively, and should be optimised where possible, to ensure the highest level of safety.
- In critically ill patients the clotting profile should always be checked.

Advantages and disadvantages of the PDT technique

Advantages

- It is a bedside technique;
- Avoids the potentially hazardous transfer of a critically ill patient to the operating theatre;
- May be easily arranged around other procedures such as haemodialysis as it will not be dependent on the availability of surgical and anaesthetic teams and an operating theatre;
- Cheaper than a formal surgical tracheostomy because there is no need for a full operating theatre.

Disadvantages

- Performed by intensivists who may not be surgically trained to deal with unexpected difficulties;
- Lack of operating theatre equipment around the bedside may necessitate an unexpected transfer to the operating theatre in the event of difficulties.

51

Bronchoscopy

Harry Gribbin

Bronchoscopy is the visual examination of the bronchial tree and larynx. There are two techniques: rigid and fibre-optic bronchoscopy. In the past bronchoscopy was largely a diagnostic technique but therapeutic intervention is being increasingly developed.

Bronchial anatomy

Knowledge of bronchial anatomy is required before bronchoscopy can be undertaken. Figure 1 shows the usual anatomy of the bronchial tree with anatomical variants and Figures 2 and 3 the commonest positions for operator and patient.

Common indications for diagnostic bronchoscopy

- Haemoptysis;
- Cough and wheeze of unexplained origin;
- Aspiration of foreign body;
- Tissue diagnosis and extent of lung cancer;
- Pre-operative examination for lung cancer resection;
- Diffuse lung disease for purpose of transbronchial lung biopsy and broncho-alveolar lavage;
- Aetiology of lobar or segmental collapse on chest X-ray;
- Diagnosis of pulmonary infections, particularly TB, when no sputum samples are available.

Rigid bronchoscopy

The adult rigid bronchoscopy (RB) is a hollow tube of approximately 45 cm length and 12–15 mm external diameter. Using intravenous

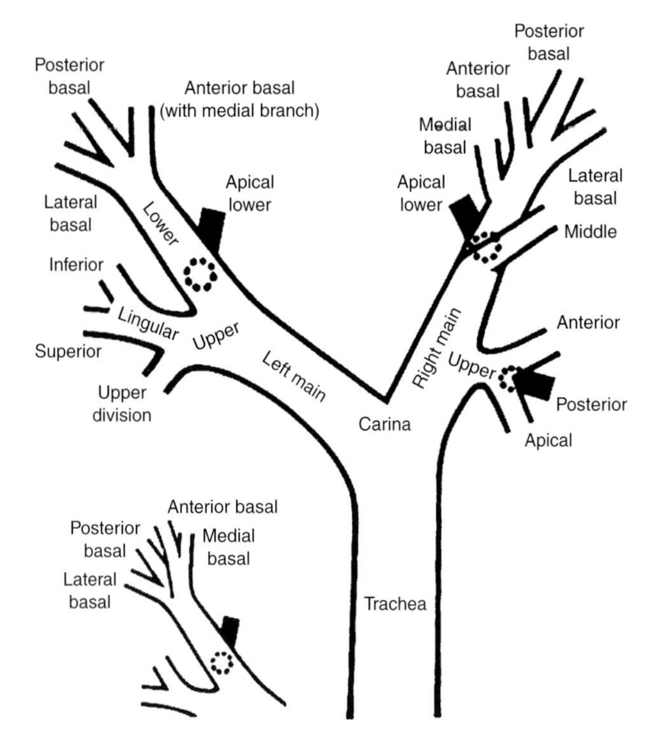

Figure 1. The branching system of the main and lobar bronchi oriented as they would be seen by an operator using a rigid bronchoscope, standing or sitting at the patient's head. For orientation using fibre-optic bronchoscope with the operator facing the patient, the diagram should be rotated through 180°. Solid shading of bronchi indicates a posterior direction.

agents for general anaesthesia and muscle relaxation (e.g. propofol and suxamethonium), with the neck slightly flexed but the head extended, the bronchoscope is passed under direct vision through the vocal cords and into the trachea (Figure 2). Ventilation of the patient is by an oxygen venturi jet into a side arm of the bronchoscope. A variety of straight or side-viewing fibre-optic rigid telescopes are used to inspect the bronchial tree and enable biopsies to be taken.

The great advantage of RB is the ability of the operator to maintain a clear visual field and airway at all times. Secretions and blood can

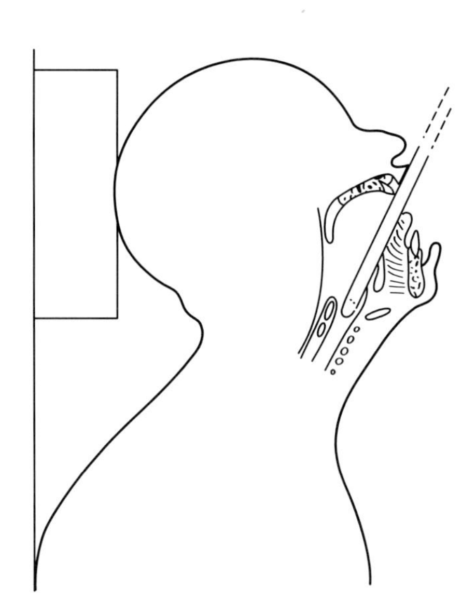

Figure 2. Diagrammatic representation of position of head and neck, and upper airway structures as rigid bronchoscope is introduced into upper trachea. Great care has to be taken to protect the upper incisor teeth from damage. Intubation of the larynx is under direct vision. Best views are obtained with a straight viewing telescope in the lumen of the rigid bronchoscope with the tip just proximal to its distal end.

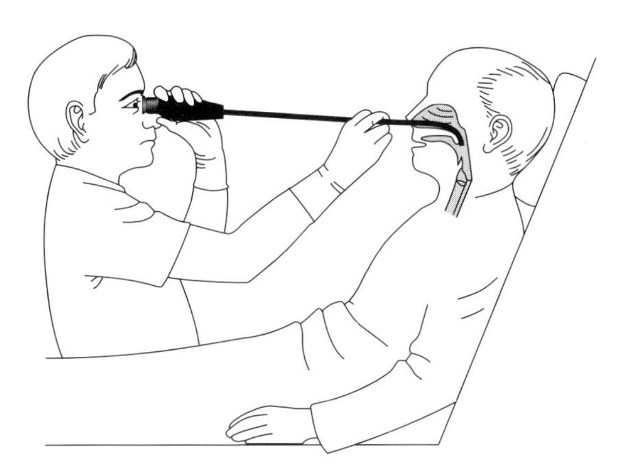

Figure 3. Diagrammatic representation of commonest technique of fibre-optic bronchoscopy.

be removed by aspiration simultaneously as procedures, such as biopsy, are carried out. There is also a tactile element to the examination, which is of value to surgeons in assessing operability of patients with tumours involving the main bronchi. This makes the RB the preferred instrument for operative procedures such as laser photo-resection of endobronchial tumour and stenting of compressed and narrowed bronchi. The main disadvantage is the need for general anaesthesia and the potential risks of this in patients needing bronchoscopy who often have pre-existing cardio-respiratory disease. Trauma to the vocal cords is more common than in fibre-optic bronchoscopy (FB) and post-operative laryngeal spasm and stridor is a problem on occasions for the anaesthetist. The procedure requires operating room facilities and full general anaesthetic monitoring.

Fibre-optic bronchoscopy

The flexible fibre-optic bronchoscope (FOB) has replaced the RB for diagnostic bronchoscopy. Instruments vary in size and external diameter. Adult FOBs are usually about 8 mm in external diameter and contain a single channel of up to 2 mm which is used for suction, instillation of local anaesthesia and flexible instrumentation for biopsy. They can be optical with direct viewing through an eyepiece or, more commonly now, video-linked when the image is transmitted fibre-optically from the distal tip of the FOB to the video screen. The procedure is carried out under conscious sedation with local lidocaine anaesthesia to the nose, vocal cords and bronchial mucosa.

Preparation for FOB

Fasting for 4 hours prior to bronchoscopy is recommended. Patients with diabetes will require glucose–potassium–insulin (GKI) infusions. Written information about the procedure should be given and informed consent obtained. Warfarin anti-coagulation has to be stopped for 72 hours if biopsies are to be taken.

Technique

The commonest technique with the operator facing the patient is to pass the FOB through the nose, negotiating the turbinate bones and identifying first the epiglottis, then the ary-epiglottic folds (false cords) before visualising the true vocal cords. The vocal cords are then entered. The small diameter of the FOB leaves adequate space for normal breathing and ventilation. The FOB allows inspection of the bronchi to sub-segmental level (Figure 1).

Some operators, using the per-nasal route prefer to stand behind the patient and a few prefer to pass the FOB via the mouth using a mouth guard (similar to upper GI endoscopy), but this causes much more gagging. The FOB can also be passed via an endotracheal tube, but care is required in ensuring that the endotracheal tube's internal diameter is sufficient to allow adequate ventilation when the FOB is passed. This is a routine practice in many Intensive Care Units for clearance of bronchial secretions which can be sent for microbiological analysis.

Local anaesthesia

Lidocaine preparations are most widely used. 2% lidocaine gel on the FOB tip gives adequate anaesthesia of the nasal mucosa. A 10% lidocaine nasal spray is also available. 2 mL boluses of 2–4% lidocaine are injected via the FOB suction channel under direct vision on to the vocal cords. Adequate anaesthesia of the vocal cords is the most essential part of the procedure. Further 2 mL boluses of 2% lidocaine are instilled into the trachea and main bronchi. Nebulised 2% lidocaine (4 mL) gives good anaesthesia of the nasal passages, epiglottis and vocal cords but the procedure must be done as soon after nebulisation as possible for maximum anaesthetic effect. Total dose of lidocaine should not exceed 29 mL of 2% solution (or equivalent), or lidocaine toxicity can occur, particularly in those with liver disease.

Sedation

FOB can be performed under local anaesthesia with explanation and reassurance but almost all patients find the procedure more pleasant with sedation. Sedation also reduces coughing and makes it easier for the operator. IV midazolam is the preferred drug. Small incremental doses of 2 mg are used via an indwelling intravenous cannula to induce drowsiness or sleep and provide amnesia of the procedure. The dose required to achieve this in an adult is about 5–6 mg. Flumazenil (250–500 µg), a specific Benzodiazepine antagonist should be available to reverse over-sedation. IV Diazepam (diazemuls) is also safe and has been widely used, the average incremental dose for adults being 7.5–10 mg. Atropine 0.6 mg IM or IV has been used to reduce bronchial secretions but is now thought unnecessary by many

Monitoring during and after fibre-optic bronchoscopy

Pulse oximetry is recommended for all procedures. Supplementary oxygen, given by nasal catheter or face mask, is used to prevent hypoxia, but this is not always possible as many patients undergoing FOB are already hypoxic as a result of chronic lung disease. Two assistants are recommended to help with the procedure and monitor the patient. Patients should be observed for 2 hours after bronchoscopy with oximetry if sedated, and should remain fasting for the same period because of the risk of bronchial aspiration of food through anaesthetised vocal cords.

Procedures undertaken during fibre-optic bronchoscopy

- Visual observation of vocal cords (to identify vocal cord palsy), bronchial mucosa, nature of bronchial secretions, site of bleeding and extent of intra- and extra-luminal tumour to assess operability. Video-assisted bronchoscopy allows a permanent record to be kept;
- Bronchial biopsy;
- Flexible forceps allow bronchial mucosa and intraluminal tumour to be biopsied under direct vision. Five specimens are considered optimal, as the biopsies are necessarily small (1–2 mm);
- Bronchial brushings and washings;
- Small cytology brushes can be used to exfoliate cells for cytological examination. Cytological techniques are also used to examine cells in washings using small aliquots of 5–10 mL of physiological normal saline to ellute the cells, which are then aspirated via the bronchoscope into a trap;
- In the diagnosis of lung cancer, biopsy, cytological brushings and washings are all used. An experienced bronchoscopist should be expected to achieve a definite diagnosis of cancer in 80% of cases with visible tumour;
- Transbronchial biopsy (TBB);
    - Flexible biopsy forceps are passed through the FOB distally into the lung until slight resistance is felt. The forceps are then

opened and the patient asked to breathe out. Lung tissue is forced into the open forceps which are then closed. TBB is useful in the diagnosis of some lung diseases, e.g. sarcoidosis, lymphangitis carcinomatosa and in opportunistic pneumonia. There is a risk of pneumothorax (10%) and significant haemorrhage (2–4%).

- Broncho-alveolar lavage;
  - The cellular content of the alveoli and small bronchi (<2 mm) can be sampled by injecting 30–50 mL of warm normal physiological saline into a sub-segmental bronchus, into which the tip of the FOB is inserted. The fluid is then aspirated through the bronchoscope. Much of the saline is absorbed and repeated lavages have to be made to obtain a satisfactory volume of 30–50 mL for examination. The procedure is safe but causes more hypoxia than bronchoscopy biopsy and fever is common in the day after the procedure (10–30%).
- Insertion of expandable intrabronchial stents for extrinsic bronchial or tracheal compression.

Risk of cross-infection with the FOB

Transmission of infection with mycobacteria and other organisms has been reported with the FOB. Detailed guidance is available on prevention. 2% glutaraldehyde in automated cleaning equipment is recommended with a minimum of 20 minutes immersion between cases. Patients with suspected TB are bronchoscoped at the end of the bronchoscopy list.

52

Intracranial pressure measurement

Kathryn A. Price

Measurement of intracranial pressure (ICP) is rarely seen outside a specialist neurosurgical centre where it has an important role to play in the management of patients with head injuries. Patients requiring having their ICP measured will usually be in a neurosurgical Intensive Care Unit (ICU) or High Dependency Unit (HDU).

It is useful to review some of the underlying physiology in case one is involved in the care of a patient having their ICP measured.

Physiology

The inside of the skull is essentially a bony box. This box contains **brain**, **blood** and **cerebrospinal fluid (CSF)**. The total volume of intracranial contents must remain constant. This is known as the Munro–Kellie Hypothesis and was first described in the early 19th century. This may be expressed as the following equation:

Intracranial Volume = Brain Volume + Blood Volume + CSF Volume

Brain, blood and CSF are all fluids or semi-solids. If any change should occur in any of the principal components there will need to be some compensatory change in the other components if ICP is to remain normal (Figure 1).

Normal ICP in the resting state is approximately 10 mm Hg. When a normal person coughs, sneezes or strains in forced expiration ICP can transiently rise to very high levels (i.e. 40–50 mm Hg). This can be compensated to prevent harm in a patient with normal components of intracranial volume.

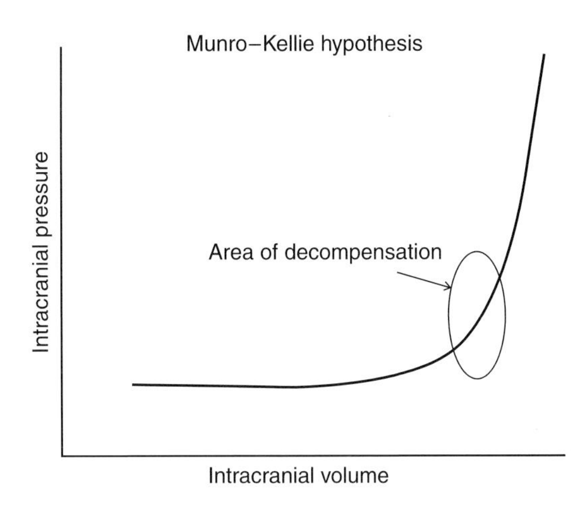

Figure 1. Pressure–volume relationship.

If a patient has cerebral oedema, intracranial haematomata or hydrocephalus, there may be initial compensation by some CSF moving into the spinal canal and some blood may move into the extracranial vasculature. There comes a point when further compensation is impossible and ICP will start to rise dramatically (see Figure 1).

Large ***sustained*** rises in ICP can lead to herniation of the brain internally (the temporal lobe is pushed down through the tentorium incisura) or externally (the cerebellar peduncles are forced through the foramen magnum). Generally, the higher the ICP and the longer raised pressures are maintained, the worse the outcome for the patient.

If a patient has their blood pressure measured invasively via an arterial line, we can relate ICP to mean arterial pressure (MAP) and get a measurement of cerebral perfusion pressure (CPP):

$$\mathbf{CPP = MAP - ICP}$$

In order to maintain adequate cerebral perfusion, the CPP should be kept above 70 mm Hg and the ICP below 20 mm Hg.

CPP gives us an indication of Cerebral Blood Flow (CBF). Normally, CBF is 50 mL/100 g of brain/minute. As cerebral perfusion falls, so does CBF. At around 5 mL/100 g of brain/minute, there is cell death and irreversible damage. By measuring MAP and ICP, it may be possible to maintain CPP and hopefully improve the outcome for the patient.

Indications

Any patient in whom one may predict a high ICP and a compromised cerebral perfusion. This particularly refers to patients where you cannot monitor neurological status clinically, for example any intubated and ventilated patient in ICU where raised ICP may be expected or anticipated i.e.:

Head-injured patients with/without intracranial blood;

Patients with cerebral oedema:

- traumatic
- infective
- metabolic.

ICP pressure measuring devices are usually inserted by neurosurgeons. As patients who require this procedure are usually unable to give consent themselves, assent may be obtained from either next of kin or the responsible physicians.

Contraindications

- This is an invasive procedure and should only be undertaken in units where there is surgical support to treat the complications of insertion.
- Abnormal clotting screen. Coagulation results should be normal before attempting to place an ICP monitor.

Techniques

There are two main methods used for monitoring intracranial pressure.

- **External Ventricular Drainage**
  External ventricular drains (EVD) are inserted to drain CSF where the normal drainage pathways have become ineffective and there is a danger of rising ICP. The EVD may be connected to a closed fluid system which may then be connected to a transducer system allowing ICP to be measured (see Figure 2). The main

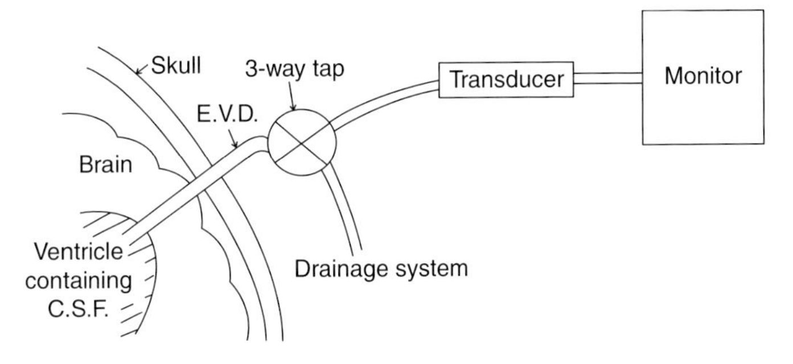

Figure 2. Monitoring equipment for measuring intracranial pressure.

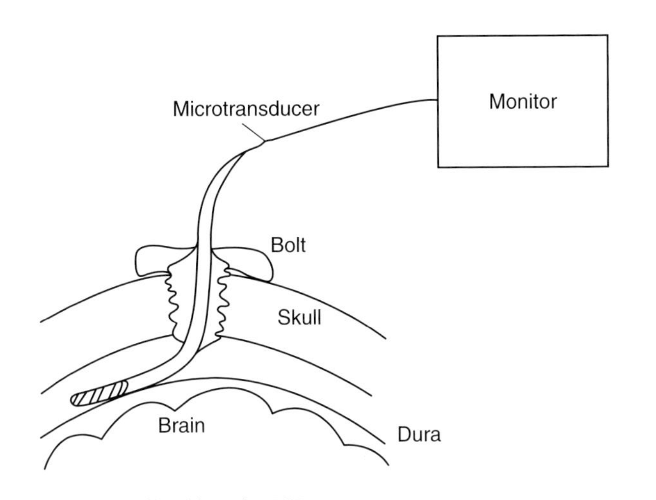

Figure 3. Details of invasive ICP measurements.

advantage of this system is that it may allow ICP to be controlled by draining CSF. The main disadvantage to this system is it is more possible for the patient to acquire an infection. Infection directly into CSF can lead to very serious sequelae for the patient.

- **Extradural microtransducers**
  These are more often used because their accuracy is almost as good as an EVD but there is a much lower rate of infection. In this system, a burr hole is made in the skull vault which allows a bolt to be screwed into position. This bolt allows a catheter containing the microtransducer to be introduced between the

inner table of the skull and the dura mater (see Figures 2 and 3). The microtransducer ***must*** be zeroed ***prior*** to insertion otherwise any measurement of ICP will be inaccurate.

Both of these systems will allow ICP to be measured and, when combined with direct arterial pressure monitoring, CPP may be estimated. If ICP is rising and CPP is falling it may be possible to:

- Give more sedation in case the patient is aware/in pain;
- Give mannitol to try to reduce brain water;
- Raise the MAP by the use of noradrenaline;
- Drain some CSF (if an EVD is used).

All these manoeuvres are aimed at trying to maintain CPP between 65–70 mm Hg and thus prevent further brain damage.

Complications

- May cause bleeding from the formation of the burr hole, which if severe could produce an extradural haematoma and a rise in ICP;
- If microtransducer is inadequately calibrated prior to insertion, measurements of ICP become meaningless;
- May get malposition of microtransducer leading to failure to produce a trace to measure ICP;
- Infection—particularly in the case of external ventricular drainage.

> - Insertion of any ICP measuring device is best done by someone who can adequately manage the possible complications of insertion.
> - Always check the patients' coagulation screen prior to insertion.
> - If inserting a microtransducer, always ensure that it is calibrated prior to insertion.
> - Management of raised ICP and compromised CPP is a joint undertaking between neurosurgeons and intensivists.

Further reading

1 Miller JD. Head injury and brain ischaemia—implications for therapy. *Br J Anaesth.* 1985;45:486.

2 Doppenberg EMR, Bullock R. Clinical neuro-protection trials in severe traumatic brain injury: Lessons from previous studies. *J Neurotrauma*. 1997;14:71–80.
3 Andrews BT, Chiles BW, Olsen WL, et al. The effect of intracerebral haematoma location on the risk of brainstem compression and on clinical outcome. *J Neurosurg*. 1988;69:518–522.
4 Rosner MJ, Rosner SD, Johnson AH. Cerebral perfusion pressure management protocols and clinical results. *J Neurosurg*. 1995;83:949–962.

53

Intravenous feeding lines and total parenteral nutrition

Judith C. Wright

Nutritional support is an essential element of care in both chronically and critically ill patients. In those in whom the gastrointestinal (GI) tract is not functioning normally enteral feeding may not be possible and total parenteral or intravenous feeding becomes necessary.

Total parenteral nutrition (TPN) may be administered via a central or peripheral feeding line, and although the basic insertion techniques are similar to those for other intravenous lines, there are a number of differences.

In patients who are likely to be fed parentally for a short period of time, standard central lines or dedicated peripheral lines can be used. However if TPN is to be continued for longer periods of time, Hickman catheters or peripherally inserted central catheters designed specifically for TPN are the preferred option.

Indications

- GI tract dysfunction where enteral nutrition will not be possible for at least 5–7 days, e.g. Crohns disease/ulcerative colitis;
- Bowel obstruction or surgery where oral/NG feeding cannot be tolerated;
- Pancreatitis (where nasogatric/nasojejunal feeding has failed);
- Chemotherapy/radiation;
- Post bone-marrow transplantation;
- Those with baseline malnutrition are more likely to benefit from TPN. Well nourished patients in whom the duration of starvation is likely to be less than 7 days are unlikely to benefit.

NB: Enteral feeding should always be considered first. In some patients e.g. burns patients, mortality is higher in those fed with TPN compared to those fed enterally.

Contraindications

- Patient refusal;
- Where enteral feeding is possible;
- Coagulopathy (high risk of bleeding from line insertion);
- Infection at insertion site (bacteraemia should be treated prior to line insertion).

Line insertion techniques

- Hickman lines are inserted under radiological guidance by experienced medical personnel. They differ from subclavian lines in that they are buried or tunnelled under the skin.
- Central line insertion is described in the relevant chapter of this book. Lines for feeding should be made from polyurethane. This is important as some central venous lines e.g. dialysis catheters can be dissolved by the intralipid content of TPN. The lumen used for TPN should not be used for any other purpose.

Technique for insertion of Percutaneous Intravenous Central Catheter (PICC) and peripheral feeding lines

- The procedure should be explained to the patient and consent obtained.
- If a PICC is to be inserted ECG monitoring should be used.
- A strict aseptic technique should be used.
- The operator should thoroughly wash hands and arms with antibacterial wash such as chlorhexidine and a sterile gown and gloves should be worn.
- A tourniquet is then applied to the arm above the insertion site.
- The insertion site should be cleaned with betadine or chlorhexidine if the patient is allergic to this.
- Once dry, the area surrounding area should be covered with sterile drapes.

Table 1. A suggested scheme for insertion of a peripherally inserted central catheter and peripheral feeding line.

Peripherally inserted central catheter insertion (Figure 1)	Peripheral feeding line insertion
• An easily palpable antecubital fossa vein should be chosen prior to insertion. • The cannula is inserted into the vein and threaded whilst withdrawing the needle once a 'flashback' of blood is seen. • The tourniquet should now be released. • The needle is with drawn completely and the catheter inserted into the cannula. This should be done reasonably quickly as blood will flow from the cannula once the needle is removed. Watch the ECG whilst inserting the catheter and insert the line far enough to ensure that the tip is within the thoracic cavity. • If an arrhythmia is noticed stop insertion, but if it persists then the line should be withdrawn slightly. • Once the catheter is inserted, the wire from inside it should be removed and a connector fitted to the end. • Using either the wire or a tape measure, estimate how far the catheter needs to be withdrawn to ensure that the tip is placed in a central vein without entering the heart, and withdraw the catheter appropriately (the catheters are marked). • Withdraw the cannula introducer from the skin over the catheter and either peal it off the catheter or click it over the proximal end of the feeding catheter (depending on the type of catheter used). • The catheter should be sutured to the skin following infiltration with local anaesthetic. • A sterile dressing should then be applied. • The catheter can be flushed with a few mL of normal saline but should not be used until correct placement has been confirmed. • A chest radiograph should be obtained to confirm correct placement.	• A suitable vein, in the dorsum of the hand or in the arm should be chosen. • Avoid areas overlying joints as these result in the cannula being bent and are uncomfortable. • The cannula should be inserted into the vein and the needle withdrawn slightly as the cannula is threaded. • The tourniquet is then released. • The needle should be withdrawn and the cap fitted to the end of the cannula. • A sterile dressing should be applied. • The cannula should be flushed with normal saline to ensure patency.

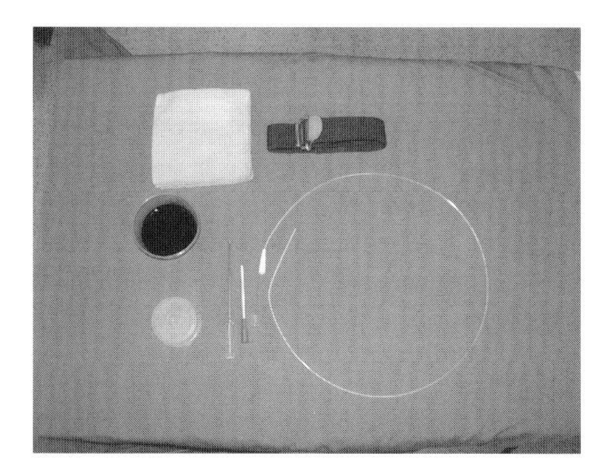

Figure 1. Equipment for insertion of PICC; betadine and swabs, insertion needle with cannula, and the catheter with guidewire which remains in its plastic casing until inserted.

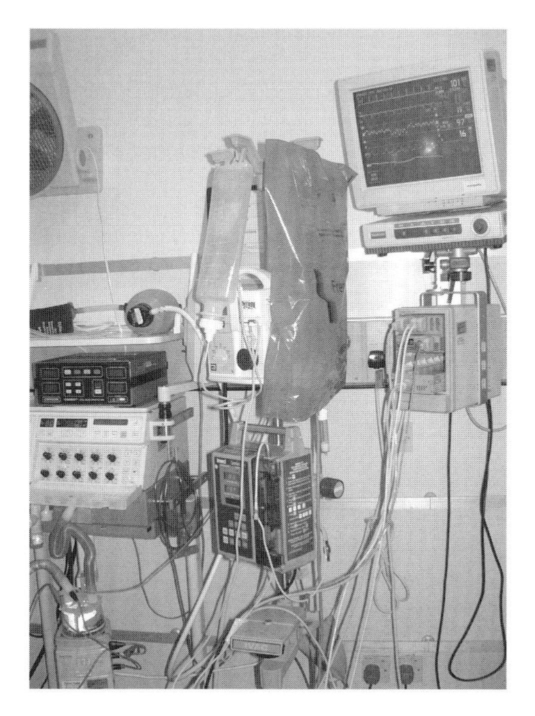

Figure 2. TPN administration in the ICU, notice that enteral feeding has also commenced.

- Local anaesthetic is injected subcutaneously at the site of insertion being careful to aspirate to avoid intravenous injection.

Complications

- Bleeding and bruising at the insertion site;
- Inappropriate placement (PICCs can end up in the internal jugular vein, the right ventricle, even in the hepatic vein);
- Local infection or bacteraemia/septicaemia;
- Arterial puncture—the brachial artery can be easily cannulated inadvertently;
- Thrombophlebitis;
- Catheter blockage;
- Nerve damage.

Care of the lines/Commencement of feeding

The lines should be used solely for TPN. If another line is required for drugs or fluid, a separate cannula should be inserted. Connection of the TPN bag to the feeding line should be performed aseptically, and the insertion site inspected regularly.

Individual feeding requirements are usually calculated by the ward dietician or in many hospitals a nutrition support team. Patients receiving TPN need to be carefully monitored as complications are numerous. In intensive care, patients receiving TPN should also receive glutamine as this reduces infectious morbidity.

Complications of TPN administration include

- Infection;
- Electrolyte imbalance;
- Fatty infiltration of the liver;
- Air embolus;
- Thrombosis;
- Fluid imbalance/pulmonary oedema;
- Hyperglycaemia;
- Respiratory compromise (CO_2 production increases with increased carbohydrate intake);
- Renal dysfunction.

Always

- Consider enteral feeding first;
- Discuss the most appropriate route of access with the nutrition team first;
- Ensure familiarity with the feeding line prior to insertion (there are numerous types);
- Insert feeding lines using an aseptic technique;
- Check insertion site regularly for signs of infection/phlebitis.

Never

- Use feeding lines for any other purpose;
- Use PICCs without first checking correct placement radiographically.

Further reading

1 Sansivero GE. The microcatheter technique for peripherally inserted central catheter placement. *J IV Nurs*. 2000;23:345–351.

2 Godwin ML. The Seldinger method for PICC insertion. *J IV Nurs*. 1989;12:238–243.

3 Galley HF. Critical Care Focus 7—Nutritional Issues *ICS/BMJ Books*, 2001.

4 Duerkson DR, Papineau N, Siemens J, Yaffe C. Peripherally inserted central catheters for parenteral nutrition: a comparison with centrally inserted catheters. *J Parenter Enteral Nutr*. 1999; 23:85–89.

5 Jeejeebhoy KN. Total parenteral nutrition: potion or poison? *Am J Clin Nutr.* 2001;74:160–163.

54

Diagnostic peritoneal lavage

Jonathan R. Easterbrook and Robert Wilson

Introduction

Diagnostic peritoneal lavage (DPL) is a technique that is utilised by surgeons to ascertain the possibility of intraperitoneal bleeding following trauma. It is quick to perform, non-operator dependent and is 98% sensitive.

Indications

In a patient that:

- Has sustained multiple injuries following blunt trauma; and
- Is haemodynamically unstable.

The following circumstances reduce the threshold for performing DPL:

- Reduced conscious level (e.g. head injury, drug or alcohol induced);
- Reduced sensation (e.g. spinal cord injury);
- Vague signs on abdominal examination.

Contraindications

Absolute

- Laparotomy strongly indicated.

Relative

- Previous surgery (adhesions distorting anatomy);
- Morbid obesity, BMI > 35 (difficult access);
- Known liver disease ± clotting disorder.

Materials

- Basic surgical trolley with sterile drapes;
- Betadine;
- 2/0 vicryl suture (for purse-string);
- Non-absorbable suture (for linea alba & skin closure);
- 1% lignocaine with adrenaline;
- 8–10 Fr urethral catheter;
- One litre of warmed isotonic saline/Hartmann's solution;
- Intravenous giving set.

Procedure

- Insert an indwelling urinary catheter to **empty the bladder**.
- Clean and drape abdomen.
- Infiltrate skin, subcutaneous tissue and peritoneum for up to 5 cm in the midline, below the umbilicus with local anaesthetic.
- Make a 3–5 cm infra-umbilical midline incision down to and through the linea alba.
- Grasp peritoneum with two small haemostatic clips, and insert a vicryl purse-string suture around them.
- Insert the catheter through a small incision in the peritoneum (angle the catheter towards the pelvis).
- Tie the purse-string suture.

If blood, bile or bowel contents are aspirated then a laparotomy is indicated and the procedure abandoned.

- Empty 1 litre of solution into peritoneal cavity via giving set and catheter.
- Ensure fluid is dispersed throughout the abdominal cavity by gently shaking and compressing the abdomen.
- Allow fluid to decant back into the bag by placing it on the floor.
- Send the collected fluid for analysis (red cell count and white cell count).

  A laparotomy is indicated if:

  - Red cell count $>$100,000 red cells/mm^3
  - White cell count $>$500 white cells/mm^3

- Remove catheter and tie pursestring suture.
- Close linea alba with interrupted non-absorbable suture.
- Close skin with interrupted non-absorbable suture.

Practical

- An open supraumbilical procedure is recommended in patients who:
  - Are pregnant;
  - Have sustained a pelvic fracture.
- If results unclear, *do not remove* catheter, and repeat lavage in four hours.
- DPL can be performed in haemodynamically stable patients in whom abdominal injury is suspected but ultrasound and CT facilities are not available.
- Strict asepsis must be used.
- Peritoneum may require local anaesthetic infiltration before incision.

Caution

- The following injures cannot be ruled out:
  - Retroperitoneal injuries;
  - Solid visceral subcapsular haematoma/contusion;
  - (e.g. liver, spleen);
  - Hollow organ contusion leading to late perforation.
- Weakly positive results may represent organ contusion not requiring surgery.
- Do not forget to empty the bladder.

Complications

Immediate

- Damage to abdominal structures (e.g. bladder/bowel);
- Bleeding that is difficult to control.

Early

- Wound infection.

Late

- Incisional hernia.

Further reading

1 *Advanced Trauma Life Support® for Doctors, Student Course Manual*. American College of Surgeons Committee on Trauma.
2 Ellis, BW, Paterson-Brown, S, editors. *Hamilton Bailey's emergency surgery*, 13th edition. Arnold Publishers.

55

Haemodialysis and haemofiltration

David Reaich

Introduction

Dialysis and haemofiltration are treatments which are used as a substitute for the solute excretory component of renal function. Patients with end stage renal failure are, on the whole, treated with either regular (thrice weekly) haemodialysis or peritoneal dialysis. Peritoneal dialysis can be used to treat patients with acute renal failure, but is now seldom used. This chapter considers therapies used in acute renal failure and will therefore be limited to discussion of haemodialysis and haemofiltration.

Haemodialysis and haemofiltration are related techniques that can remove water, metabolic waste products and normalise electrolyte balance.

In haemodialysis, the patient's blood is passed through an artificial kidney (the dialyser). The dialyser has a semi-permeable membrane. Blood flows on one side of the membrane, and dialysate on the other side. The dialysate is essentially a sterile, dilute electrolyte solution. The following processes will occur within the dialyser:

- Equilibration of the blood and dialysis fluid electrolyte composition (by *diffusion*).
- Waste products accumulating in blood (e.g. urea) will *diffuse* into the dialysate. Urea will also move with water, increasing its removal (this is referred to as *convective* transport).
- Water will move from plasma into the dialysate because of a hydrostatic pressure gradient induced by the dialysis machine (*ultrafiltration*). This gradient can be varied to remove greater or lesser amounts of fluid.

In haemofiltration, no dialysate is used and therefore metabolites cross the semi-permeable membrane by convection alone. Fluid moves by ultrafiltration, bringing with it solutes by convective transport. Large volumes of fluid can be removed (many litres in 24 hours), which can be replaced by a substitution fluid similar in composition to plasma.

Normal renal function

Normal renal function is necessary for maintenance of fluid and electrolyte balance, excretion of nitrogenous waste, acid-base balance, blood pressure control and appropriate erythropoiesis. The consequences of loss of these homeostatic mechanisms is listed below.

Normal renal function	Acute renal failure
Fluid balance	Fluid overload (generalised oedema, pulmonary oedema, ascites, pleural effusions)
Nitrogen excretion	Nitrogen retention (elevated urea, creatinine, urate)
Potassium homeostasis	Hyperkalaemia
Calcium/phosphate	Hypocalcaemia Hyperphosphataemia Homeostasis
Erythropoiesis	Anaemia (usually multi-factorial in acute renal failure)

Acute renal failure

Acute renal failure (ARF) can be defined as a sudden decline in normal renal function, leading to an increase in serum urea and creatinine concentrations over a period of days or weeks. It is often (but not invariably) associated with oliguria or anuria. There are many potential causes. Many cases are multifactorial, with a number of nephrotoxic insults contributing to the development of ARF. Management involves identification and correction of any reversible causes, and support of the patient until there is a return of renal function.

Indications for acute dialysis

In acute renal failure the commonest indications for the introduction of dialysis are:

- Hyperkalaemia

- Acidosis
- Fluid overload

It may be necessary to initiate **emergency treatment for hyperkalaemia** while making arrangements to commence dialysis. Emergency treatment is indicated if serum potassium is greater than 7 mmol/litre or if there are ECG changes. Treatment consists of:

- 10 mL 10% calcium gluconate IV. This has a stabilising effect on the myocardium but *does not affect serum potassium concentration*.
- 50 mL of 50% dextrose with 10 units soluble insulin, IV over 30 minutes.
  - Potassium moves intracellularly along with the dextrose. *Blood glucose monitoring is mandatory.*
- Calcium resonium 30 g administered as an enema acts as an ion-exchange resin, binding potassium in the G-I tract. It should be washed out after 4–6 hours and can be repeated at that point.

Haemodialysis is also occasionally indicated for the treatment of poisoning. It is efficient at removing water soluble drugs of low molecular weight including salicylate, lithium, ethanol and methanol.

Choice of therapy

Both haemodialysis and haemofiltration can be used in the treatment of acute renal failure. Each has advantages and disadvantages. Both techniques require central venous access and anti-coagulation.

Haemodialysis is rapid and effective at correcting metabolic abnormalities. Specialised equipment, access to appropriately treated water and trained nursing staff are required. Several litres of fluid can be removed during a dialysis session of 4–5 hours. However, in a cardiovascularly unstable patient, such rapid removal of fluid may precipitate hypotension. In patients with chronic renal failure, haemodialysis is usually used thrice weekly, but in a patient with ARF who may be severely catabolic, daily dialysis may be necessary.

Haemofiltration is less efficient than haemodialysis at solute removal and therefore has to be used as a continuous therapy. This, however, leads to its main advantage of allowing slow continuous removal of fluid and solute, thus avoiding rapid fluid shifts and changes in electrolyte concentrations. There are fewer problems with hypotension, meaning that it can be used in patients who are cardiovascularly unstable. As it is continuous it is not usually suitable for patients who are conscious and being mobilised. It is therefore most often used in ventilated patients. The commonest form of haemofiltration currently in use is called Continuous Veno-Venous Haemofiltration (CVVH). In this technique, blood is pumped around a circuit and through a haemofilter. Therefore, as with haemodialysis, special equipment is required. However, it is usually possible for ITU nurses to monitor this equipment while providing all the other aspects of care required by their patient.

Requirements for the therapies

- Central venous access (usually internal jugular or femoral). CVVH requires a double-lumen catheter;
- Anti-coagulation during the procedure. This can be achieved either by heparinisation or use of prostacyclin;
- Appropriate dialysis/filtration equipment;
- Dialysate and appropriately treated water (for haemodialysis); Physiological replacement solution (for haemofiltration);
- Trained nursing staff.

Complications

Complications can be divided into those associated with central venous access (see Chapter 23), those associated with anticoagulation and those associated with the dialysis procedure.

Those commonly associated with the dialysis procedure are:

- Hypotension—in the patient with acute renal failure this is common. Rapid fluid removal contributes, but the patient may well be septic, have cardiac arrhythmias and cardiac dysfunction, all of which increase the likelihood of hypotensive episodes.
- Nausea and vomiting/headache/chest discomfort—these are all common symptoms during dialysis, occurring in up to 10% of routine dialysis treatments. Many episodes of nausea and vomiting are related to hypotension. Obviously these symptoms will not be reported by paralysed ventilated patients!
- Hypothermia—patients on CVVH can drop their body temperature because of the continued exposure of their blood to room

temperature (across the lines and haemofilter). This can be minimised by insulating the lines with tin foil.

- Hypoglycaemia—glucose moves from blood into dialysate. Patients can become hypoglycaemic, particularly if they are on insulin.

Less common but important complications include:

- Dialysis disequilibrium—this consists of systemic and neurologic symptoms occurring during or soon after dialysis. Early manifestations include nausea, vomiting, restlessness and headache but can lead onto seizures and coma. To prevent disequilibrium syndrome, initial dialysis sessions should not aim for excessive urea reduction, with a target reduction of 30% being advised.
- Anaphylaxis—patients can have anaphylactic reactions to the dialyser. Mild cases may present with itch, urticaria, sneezing or watering eyes. However, full blown anaphylaxis can occur. Dialysis should be discontinued and standard treatment for anaphylaxis administered.

- Always exclude reversible causes of acute renal failure.
- Involve a nephrologist in the patient's care.
- Do not use nephrotoxic drugs.
- Look after the arm veins—the patient may not recover renal function and will need good vessels for future vascular access for dialysis.
- Monitor biochemistry before and after dialysis.

Further reading

1 Daugirdas JT, Ing TS. *Handbook of dialysis.* Boston, Little, Brown and Co. 1988.
2 Hoenich NA. The technology and biocompatibility of renal replacement therapy. In: Jamison RL, Wilkinson R, editors. *Nephrology*. London, Chapman and Hill, 1977.

56

Brain stem death testing

Stephen Bonner

Brain death was first described in Paris as late as 1959 and is a product of Intensive Care. Before intensive care, patients with severe brain injury that resulted in coning of the brainstem, inevitably became apnoeic and subsequently asystolic. The advent of artificial ventilation of these patients inevitably resulted in patients whose bodies were resuscitated, but whose brainstems were irrevocably damaged. This produced two distinct new entities. In the persistent vegetative state the brain stem still functions and the patient breathes and is 'awake' but not aware and may survive with artificial feeding for years. In brain stem death the brain stem is dead and even with maximal support from ventilation, inotropes and endocrine replacement, somatic death is inevitable within days. However, whatever the cause of death, cardiac arrest, respiratory arrest or brain stem failure, the common pathway is that of irreversible cessation of brain stem function and this defines death.

In the 1960s and 1970s over 1900 brain dead patients were treated with artificial ventilation and inotropic support, none made any neurological recovery despite continuing all supportive measures until asystole. Brain stem death was accepted as brain death and ratified as a cause of death by the World Medical Association in Sydney in 1968 who declared that "death is when the body as an integrated whole has ceased to function". This statement recognises that brain stem death is the common pathway by which somatic death occurs. Death of the reticular activating system in the brain stem results in inability of the cortex to function, even in the unusual case of residual cortical EEG activity. Usual causes of brain death are damage to the cerebral cortex, e.g. head injury, stroke or global hypoxic damage resulting in increased intra-cerebral pressure forcing the brain stem through the foramen magnum, resulting in death of the brain stem from compression and ischaemia.

The pursuit of brain death as a diagnosis is good medical practice and is completely independent of the potential for organ donation. Guidelines for the diagnosis of brain death in the UK were agreed in 1976 and have recently been confirmed in the UK. Brain death tests are clinical tests of the absence of brain stem function. They are performed by two experienced doctors unconnected with transplant services, one of whom should be a consultant. They should be performed more than six hours after onset of coma, or 24 hours if following cardiac arrest. The legal time of death is the first set of tests. Neither absence of blood flow on cerebral angiography, nor electrical silence on electroencephalography are required for brain death testing in the UK. This is because brain stem death may occur with both the presence of cerebral blood flow and in the presence of residual EEG activity yet the functional integrity of the brain is destroyed and this represents somatic death.

Indications for brain death testing

- Suspected brain death.

Preconditions include

- Apnoeic ventilated ITU patient, fixed pupils, absent brain stem reflexes;
- Known irreversible cause of coma.

Exclusions include

- Markedly abnormal biochemistry, particularly sodium and glucose;
- Significant acid/base disturbance on blood gas analysis;
- Metabolic/endocrine disease such as thyroid disturbance, uraemia, hepatic encephalopathy or Addison's disease;
- Drug intoxication, particularly sedatives in ITU;
- Hypothermia ($<35°$);
- Severe hypotension/hypoxia.

Equipment requirements (Figure 1)

- Endobronchial suction catheter;

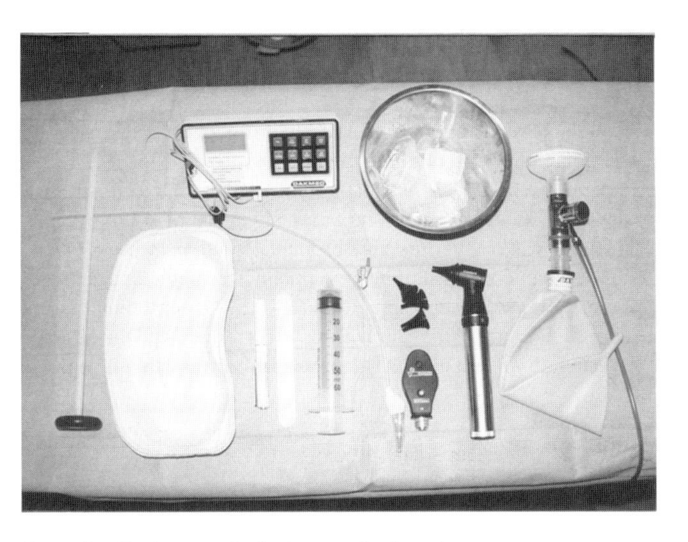

Figure 1. Equipments for brain stem death testing.

- Water's circuit;
- Wooden spatula;
- Otoscope;
- Ice cold water with 50 mL syringe and pipette;
- Bright light (pentorch);
- Cotton wool;
- Nerve stimulator;
- Facilities for instant arterial blood gas monitoring.

Technique

- Pupillary light reflex. A bright light is shone onto each pupil testing both direct and consensual reaction to light (second cranial nerve and parasympathetic outflow).
- Corneal reflex, using light touch of the periphery of the cornea with cotton wool (fifth and seventh cranial nerves).
- Painful stimuli to face, trunk and limbs looking for facial muscle movement (fifth and seventh cranial nerves).
- Oculovestibular reflex. After confirming intact ear drums, ice cold water is slowly injected into each auditory canal using a pipette. Nystagmus will occur if the eighth cranial nerve is intact.

- Orophayngeal reflex ('gag') using the wooden throat spatula touching the posterior pharyngeal wall (ninth and tenth cranial nerves).
- Cough reflex, using carinal stimulation with an endobronchial suction catheter (tenth cranial nerve).
- Apnoea testing. The patient is ventilated with 100% oxygen, then disconnected from ventilation. Oxygen (4–6 L/min) may then be instilled via the endobronchial suction catheter placed down the endotracheal tube to maintain acceptable oxygen saturation. CO_2 will rise at approximately 0.5 kPa per minute during apnoea. Regular blood gas analysis is performed and the absence of respiration with a $PaCO_2 > 6.7$ kPa confirms brain death.

Complications

- Brain death tests may not be positive, in which case they may need to be repeated at a later stage after clinical review of the patient.
- Spinal reflexes may be present particularly during painful stimuli on limb testing.
- Decerebrate posturing during testing indicates some brain stem function.
- Local bleeding can be produced, particularly from the external auditory meatus.
- Perforation of the eardrum is theoretically possible from insertion of the pipette.

- Pupils may be small or irregular, the important fact is that they are fixed.
- Spinal reflexes may be distressing for relatives.
- If the patient desaturates during the apnoea test, consider providing oxygen using a Water's circuit providing positive end expiratory pressure. This has the added advantage of being able to easily see any respiratory movements.
- If patient has pulmonary infection/failure, they may be ventilated at a lower respiratory rate on 100% oxygen to allow the arterial CO_2 to rise so that they have to remain apnoeic for less time to achieve an arterial CO_2 of 6.7 kPa.
- The tests may still be performed in the presence of high spinal injury.

- If the patient has poor premorbid respiratory function, one may allow a higher arterial CO_2 to exclude apnoea.
- Brain death testing on children should be performed by experts in this area, since the tests parameters are slightly different, e.g. a higher arterial PO_2 may be required.

Further reading

1 Mollaret P. Goulon M. Le coma dépassé. *Revue Neurol.* (Paris) 1994;101:3–15.
2 Pallis C. Brain stem death. In: Braakman R, editor. Head Injury. *Handbook of clinical neurology*, Amsterdam, Elsevier, Vol. 13. 1990.
3 Conference of medical Royal Colleges and their faculties in the UK. *BMJ.* 1976;2:1187–1188.
4 *Guidelines on diagnosis of brain death and management of the organ donor*. Intensive Care Society, London, 1999.

Section 7

Specific Advanced Skills

57

Echocardiography—requesting an echocardiogram

Mike J. Stewart

Introduction

Echocardiography is one of the most frequently requested imaging investigations. It is important that clinicians requesting the test and reviewing the report understand the indications, implications and limitations of the technique. This chapter aims to provide a basic understanding of echocardiography, concentrating on transthoracic imaging and introducing transoesophageal echocardiography.

Echocardiographic images are formed by the reflection of ultrasound waves from cardiac structures. There are three main modalities used:

- *Two-dimensional echocardiography* forms a real time image from an array of scan lines arranged in an arc repeating 20–30 times per second;
- *M-mode echocardiography* records just one scan line resulting in increased sensitivity for detecting and timing moving structures. It is commonly used for measuring cardiac dimensions;
- *Doppler echocardiography* examines the frequency shift between transmitted and reflected ultrasound from moving red blood cells to provide information about the direction and velocity of blood flow, according to the Doppler Effect.

A comprehensive echocardiographic study will routinely integrate all three modalities.

Indications for echocardiography

Left ventricular function

An assessment of left ventricular function is the commonest reason for an echo request. Left ventricular systolic dysfunction may be either regional (e.g. ischaemic heart disease) or global (e.g. dilated cardiomyopathy). With global dysfunction, all the walls of the left ventricle are hypokinetic—showing reduced thickening or contraction—and the ventricle may be dilated. Myocardial ischaemia and infarction result in regional wall motion abnormalities where certain walls of the left ventricle may be seen to be akinetic (no thickening) or hypokinetic. Identifying these abnormalities may be helpful in the diagnosis of patients with acute chest pain.

Overall LV function may be assessed in a number of ways. A formal calculation of ejection fraction, made by tracing the endocardial border of the left ventricle at end systole and diastole, is time consuming and requires good image quality. Thus the most widely used method is 'eyeball' assessment. From experience, after imaging the LV in a number of views, the echocardiographer grades the LV systolic function as normal, mildly, moderately or severely impaired.

Hypertrophic cardiomyopathy is characterised by a marked increase in the thickness of the interventricular septum alone ('asymmetric septal hypertrophy'). It may be accompanied by evidence of obstruction to flow out of the left ventricle: systolic anterior motion of the mitral valve, where the anterior leaflet of the mitral valve is 'sucked' against the septum during systole, and increased velocity of flow in the left ventricular outflow tract.

Valvular disease

There are three main aims of an echocardiographic study of a patient with valvular disease (whether previously diagnosed or evaluation of a newly heard murmur):

- Defining the aetiology;
- Quantifying the severity of the valve lesion;
- Assessing the effects on cardiac function.

Quantifying the severity of stenotic valve lesions is made by recording the velocity of blood flow across the valve with Doppler echocardiography (Figure 1). This is directly related to the pressure gradient across the stenosed valve and thus the degree of stenosis. Doppler data can also be used to calculate valve area. In mitral stenosis, the 'pressure half time method' estimates valve area from the slope of the Doppler signal across the mitral valve (Figure 2). For aortic stenosis, the 'continuity equation' is used—this measurement is particularly useful in patients with impaired LV systolic function when low pressure gradients may be seen with severely stenosed valves.

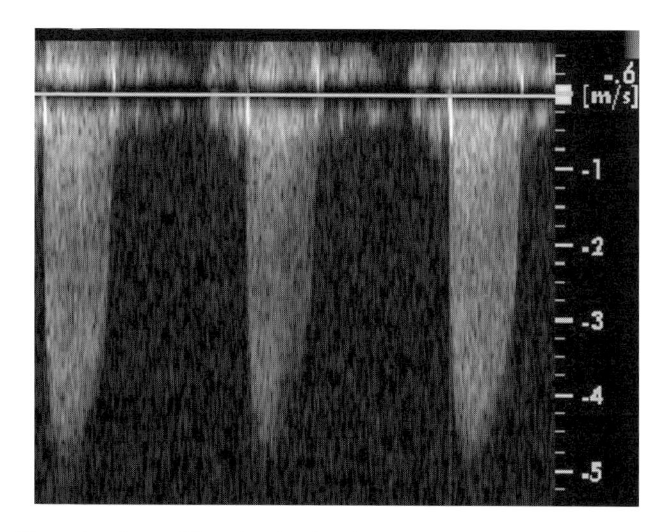

Figure 1. Spectral Doppler: Aortic valve. Note peak velocity 5 m/s, equivalent to peak gradient 100 mm Hg.

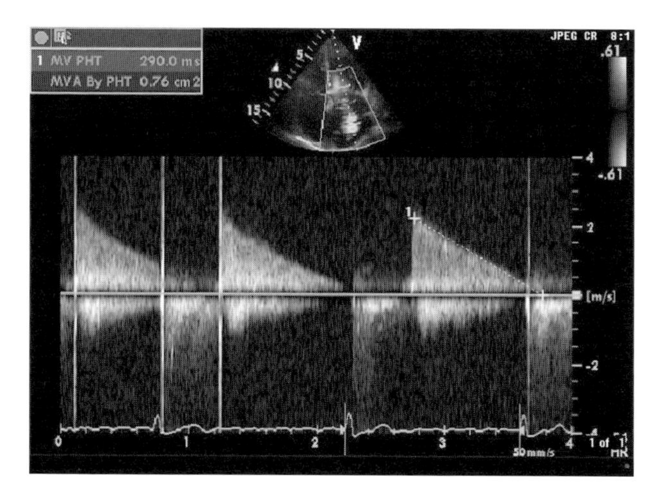

Figure 2. Spectral Doppler: Mitral valve. MV PHT—Mitral valve pressure half time (time taken for pressure to drop by 50% during diastole). MVA by PHT—mitral valve area by pressure half time. This is an estimate of the size of the valve orifice calculated from the pressure drop. 0.76 cm^2 indicates severe mitral stenosis.

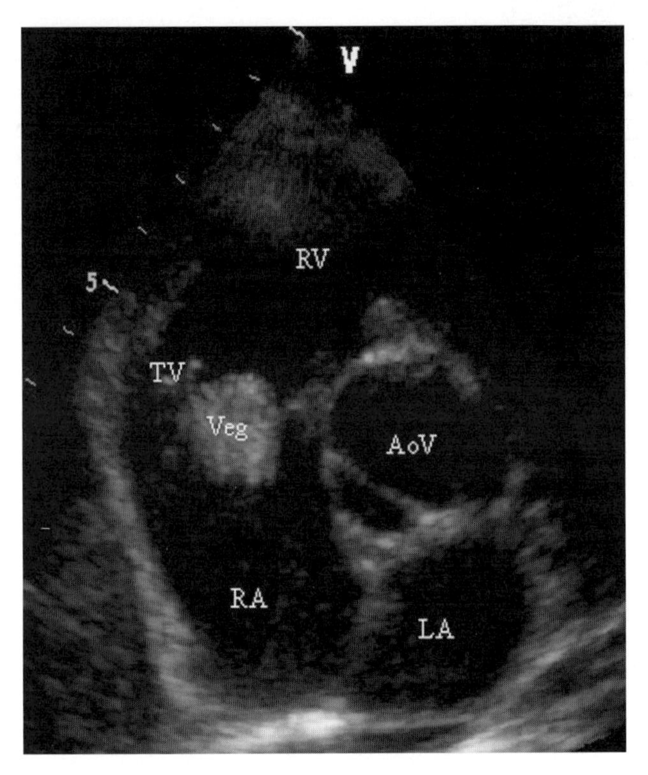

Figure 3. Vegetation on tricuspid valve. Parasternal short axis view, large mass on tricuspid valve leaflet of intravenous drug abuser. AoV—aortic valve; LA—left atrium; RA—right atrium; RV—right ventricle; TV—tricuspid valve.

Aortic and mitral regurgitation are not so straightforward to quantitate. The size of the regurgitant jet on colour flow Doppler provides some indication as to severity. Indirect evidence, particularly left ventricular dilatation, may suggest the regurgitant lesion is significant. Usually, echocardiographers will assess a number of Doppler and 2D parameters to form an overall assessment.

Infective endocarditis

Echocardiographic evidence of endocarditis is one of the keys to the diagnosis of this condition. Vegetations are classically seen as an echogenic mass attached to valvular tissue, moving independently of the valve (Figure 4). Other clues to endocarditis include evidence of valve destruction or abscess formation. The sensitivity of transthoracic echocardiography for detecting vegetations is around 50–60%, thus a 'normal' transthoracic echo certainly does not exclude endocarditis, particularly if the clinical suspicion is high. If there is strong clinical evidence for endocarditis, TransOesophageal Echocardiography (TOE) should be performed if the transthoracic scan is normal or suboptimal quality. TOE is also strongly advised if prosthetic valve endocarditis is suspected, and can be useful in established endocarditis to evaluate for complications.

An echocardiogram is **not** indicated as a screening test in febrile patients if the likelihood of endocarditis is low.

Right heart disease

Increases in afterload to the right ventricle either acutely (pulmonary embolus) or chronically (e.g. chronic obstructive pulmonary disease) may result in a dilated poorly contracting right ventricle. The peak velocity of tricuspid regurgitation (if present) provides an estimation of right ventricular systolic pressure and thus, in the absence of pulmonary stenosis, pulmonary artery systolic pressure.

Intracardiac source of embolus

Echocardiograms are often requested in the investigation of stroke or other embolic events. The usual intracardiac sources of emboli found are:

- Left ventricular (mural) thrombus—usually associated with akinetic or aneurysmal segments post myocardial infarction;
- Vegetation;
- Atrial myxoma.

Atrial thrombus is rarely detected transthoracically. In the absence of clinical or electrocardiographic abnormalities, the yield from a transthoracic echo study is very low indeed. Transoesophageal echo increases the chances of finding an abnormality that may explain the embolic event, detecting aortic atheromatous disease and patent foramen ovale for example.

In younger patients (for example <50 years), in whom stroke is an unusual event, there is a higher likelihood of detecting a rare cause of emboli which may influence further patient management.

Thus most centres advocate investigating this age group with both transthoracic and transoesophageal echo.

Pericardial disease

One of the earliest uses of echocardiography was in the diagnosis of pericardial effusion. This is seen as an echolucent space around the heart. Useful information about the size and location of the effusion can be gained; indeed, pericardiocentesis is often performed under transthoracic echo guidance. Constrictive pericarditis can also be diagnosed with evidence of a thickened pericardium and characteristic pattern of Doppler traces of the mitral and tricuspid valves.

Echocardiography—performing a transthoracic echo

The development of portable ultrasound systems may lead to more widespread use of echocardiography out of the hands of cardiac sonographers and cardiologists. Whilst these may have a useful role in the bedside diagnosis of cardiac disorders, they will not replace formal echocardiographic studies by trained sonographers on full specification machines. However, knowledge of how to acquire basic views on a simple portable system may prove useful.

Anatomy

As transmission of sound waves is attenuated by bone and air, imaging of the heart is limited by the ribs and lungs to small 'windows'. To increase the size of these windows, the subject is usually placed in a left lateral position. Standard views of the heart are obtained that enable examination of all four chambers, cardiac valves and major vessels. Orientation of the echo probe is facilitated by a marker that is displayed on the probe. The parasternal window is found to the left of the sternum in the third to fifth intercostals space. The long axis view is obtained with the marker pointing to the right shoulder. Rotating the probe clockwise through 90° will reveal the parasternal short axis view at mitral valve level. Tilting the probe superiorly and inferiorly will move between a basal view including the aortic valve and right ventricular outflow tract and a left ventricular view. The apical window is located where the apex beat is palpated. The four-chamber view (Figure 4b) is found with the marker directed laterally towards the axilla. Tilting the probe superiorly reveals the aortic valve. Anticlockwise rotation through 60° and 120°

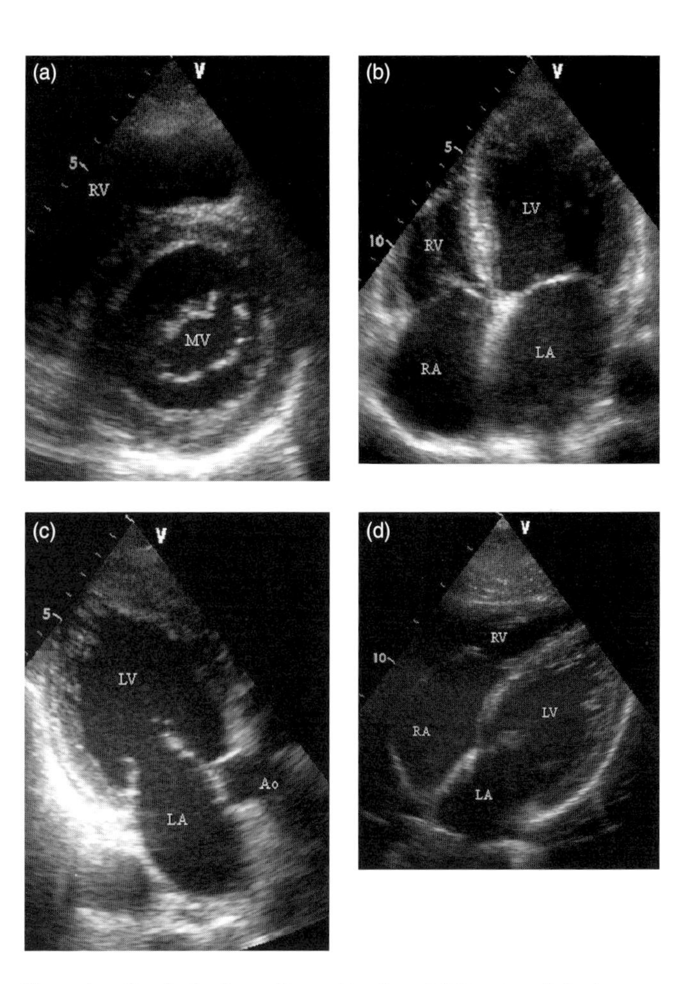

Figure 4. Standard echocardiographic views (a) Parasternal short axis mitral valve level. (b) Apical four-chamber. (c) Apical long axis. (d) Parasternal short axis basal. Ao—aorta; LV—left ventricle; other abbreviations as in Figure 3.

show the apical two-chamber (Figure 4c) and long axis views respectively. The subcostal window (Figure 4d) is found angling upwards from below the xiphisternum with the subject supine. In many patients, not all the standard views can be seen adequately. Obesity, chronic lung disease and chest wall deformities may all reduce image quality on transthoracic scanning.

Trans-oesophageal echocardiography

Anatomy

The close anatomical association of the oesophagus and left atrium provides the basis for the superior image quality of trans-oesophageal echocardiography. A scanner positioned within the oesophagus does not have to contend with rib and lung attenuation and has a direct view into the heart through the left atrium. If the scanner is then directed posteriorly, the descending thoracic aorta is seen. Advancing and withdrawing the probe within the oesophagus can provide imaging of the aorta from arch to diaphragm. If the probe is advanced into the stomach and flexed upwards (transgastric view), the right and left ventricles can be imaged through the diaphragm. TOE is particularly useful for imaging posterior structures (left atrium, mitral valve), which are furthest from a transthoracic probe. Transthoracic evaluation of prosthetic valves, particularly in the mitral position, is hampered by reflection of ultrasound off the prosthetic material resulting in shadowing of the atrial aspect of the valve—the side that TOE shows best. Conversely, the apex of the left ventricle may not be well seen from a TOE, but is usually well seen in an apical transthoracic view. This illustrates the complimentary nature of transthoracic and transoesophageal imaging—the two techniques should be used together.

TOE procedure

The main indications for TOE are listed in Table 1. It should be borne in mind that TOE is an invasive procedure with a risk, albeit small, of

Table 1. Indications for TOE.

Evaluation of prosthetic valve function (particularly mitral)
Endocarditis (diagnosis and monitoring for complications, e.g. abscess formation)
? cardiac source of embolus (in patient <50 years)
Aortic dissection
Assess suitability of mitral valve for
• Repair
• Balloon valvuloplasty
Exclude left atrial thrombus prior to cardioversion (if AF >48 hours and not anticoagulated > three weeks)
Inadequate TTE image quality (particularly on ventilated patient)
Perioperative during cardiac surgery

complications (0.2–0.5%, see Table 2). The transoesophageal echo probe is essentially a gastroscope with a rotatable ultrasound scanning head rather than an optical system. Following preparation of the patient (Table 3), the probe is introduced through a biteguard with the patient in the left lateral position. The procedure takes 10–15 minutes with a further period necessary for recovery from sedation.

Table 2. Complications of TOE.

Relating to sedation	Respiratory depression Hypoxia Aspiration Hypotension
Relating to oesophageal intubation	Dental trauma Oesophageal trauma inc. perforation Aspiration Bronchospasm Arrhythmia

Table 3. TOE procedure.

Ensure no history of dysphagia or oesophageal disease
Nil by mouth for at least four hours
Explain procedure and obtain written consent
Insert intravenous cannula
Remove dentures
Administer oxygen via nasal cannulae
Pulse oximetry throughout procedure
Local anaesthetic spray to oropharynx
Sedation with i.v. midazolam

Essential equipment:
Resuscitation trolley with suction
i.v. flumazenil

How to get the best out of your echo department:

On the request card:
- provide all relevant clinical information;
- be explicit about the question you want answered.

If you're unsure as to whether an echo will help ASK!

- Gain experience of performing scans with the help of an experienced sonographer.
- Become familiar with machine controls.
- Put the patient in left lateral postion to try and optimise windows—other positions worth trying if imaging difficult.
- If one window poor, move to another—it is often better!
- Record what you image.

Further reading

1 Chambers JB. *Clinical echocardiography*. London, BMJ Books, 1995.

2 *A useful introductory text for beginners with many images:* Otto CM. *Textbook of clinical echocardiography*. Philadelphia, WB Saunders, 2000.

58

Neonatal resuscitation

Samir Gupta and Sunil Sinha

Introduction

By adult standards birth is a very hypoxic experience for the fetus. Despite this, babies tolerate it very well. From a study in Sweden, only 1% of babies weighing 2.5 kg or more received mask inflation, and only two required intubation. Whilst there are defined guidelines for attendance at delivery, some other babies unexpectedly require resuscitation. The underlying problem is usually respiratory, which if not managed efficiently may make things worse.

Anatomy

There are certain anatomical differences of importance in babies which have bearing on neonatal resuscitation:

- The relatively large surface area of skin in proportion to weight leads to rapid heat loss in wet infant.
- The airway is likely to be opened in babies, with a neutral neck position.
- The epiglottis is horseshoe shaped and projects posteriorly at 45°.
- The larynx is high and anterior at level of second and third cervical vertebra, and the cricoid ring is the narrowest part of the upper airway.
- The newborn has a deformable cartilaginous rib cage and the ribs are more horizontal in newborn infants.
- Prior to first breath newborn lung is filled with fluid at birth.
- Babies are obligatory nose breathers and rely mainly on diaphragmatic breathing. They also tend to fatigue more easily as they have fewer type 1 muscle fibers.

Physiology

There are numerous physiological adaptations which take place at birth.

- Clamping of cord leads to onset of asphyxia which, with physical stimulation, is a major stimulant of respiration.
- With the first breath, negative pressures of −40 cm to −100 cm water are generated causing alveolar fluid to be enter lymphatic and blood vessels.
- The changes in lung and peripheral resistance, with the resultant change in blood flow cause the closure of the persistent foramen ovale and the duct in the first 72 hours of life.

The sequence of changes (Figure 1) are secondary to the interruption of oxygen supply when baby moves in defined stages from primary to terminal apnea associated with progressive bradycardia. The time taken for the cardiac arrest to occur in absence of resuscitation can be up to

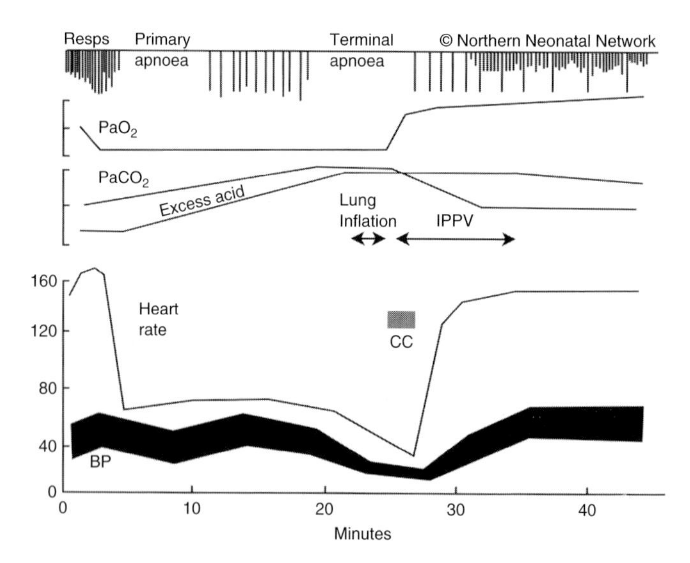

Figure 1. An illustration of the data derived from animal experiments outlining the response of a newborn subjected to hypoxia at birth. (Reproduced with kind permission from Resuscitation at Birth—the Newborn Life Support Provider Course Manual. Resuscitation Council (UK) 2001. Figure drawn by Steven Brindley, 56 Barnwood Avenue, Gloucester, UK.)

20 minutes. The circulation is almost always maintained till all the respiratory activity ceases. Hence, once resuscitation is provided and lungs are inflated, the oxygenated blood can be distributed and recovery usually occurs. During this process blood pressure is initially maintained by vasoconstriction and increased output from the bradycardic heart.

Indications

Although not all neonatal problems can be predicted, the preparation for high-risk deliveries is a key to successful outcome. The list is a guide for the high-risk situations but attendance to any infant requiring support is an emergency.

Preterm delivery	Thick meconium
Hydrops fetalis	Polyhydramnios
GI obstruction	Pulmonary hypoplasia
Diaphragmatic hernia	Acute fetal or maternal hemorrhage
Maternal diabetes	Maternal infection
Oligohydramnios	

Strategy for resuscitation

Preparation

Before the arrival of baby adequate preparation can help in avoiding stress. The key issues are:

- Introduction to family and obstetric staff;
- Review of obstetric notes for information which may help preparation;
- Check the 'resucitaire', oxygen, suction, equipments;
- Do you need help?
- Is transport required?

Resucitation

On delivery if the baby is apnoeic then it is difficult to differentiate between primary and terminal apnoea. A systematic approach usually results in effective resuscitation. The ABC is the rule preceded by drying, during which baby is assessed.

- Dry and cover the baby;
- Assess;

- Airway;
- Breathing;
- Circulation—Chest compressions;
- (Drugs).

Dry and cover the baby
Babies loose heat quickly so every effort should be made to prevent hypothermia. This can usually be done by drying effectively, removing any wet linen and towels and covering the baby with warm dry towel. The availability of resucitaire is beneficial. This is more important for preterm babies and the combination of hypothermia with hypoxia and acidosis can lead to suppression of surfactant production.

Assess
While drying a simultaneous assessment can be made of the infants status of tone and colour followed by heart rate and the effort of breathing.

Airway management
This is the most important part of neonatal resuscitation. This can be divided into two parts:

- Opening the airway;
- Inflating the lungs.

Opening the airway: In an unconscious baby the airway is usually obstructed by collapse of pharynx and falling back of tongue. If the jaw is drawn forward then it would open airway. This can be attempted by (Figure 2) *CHIN LIFT* (holding the head in **neutral position** with chin support) and *JAW THRUST* (move the jaw forward).

Inflating the lungs: The lung inflation can be achieved by using the positive pressure ventilation with a T-piece (Tomb thumb/Neopuff), or bag and mask, using long inspiratory time of about 2–3 seconds and pressures of about 30 cm of water for a term baby. Five such inflations are recommended before further assessment is made.

The adjuncts to airway management are:

- An oro-pharyngeal airway of correct size (hold along the line of lower jaw measuring from the middle of the to the angle of jaw);

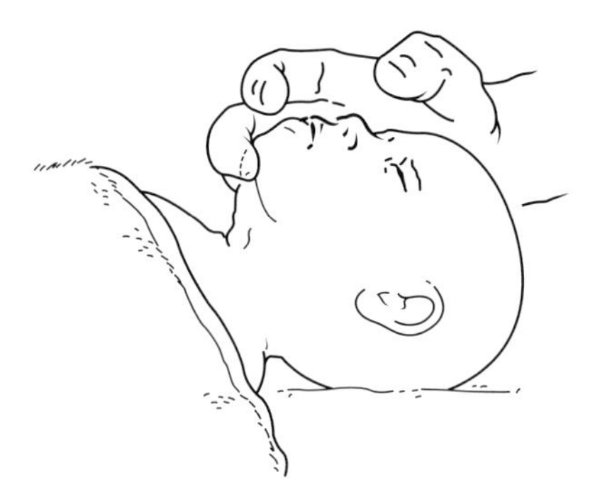

Chin support

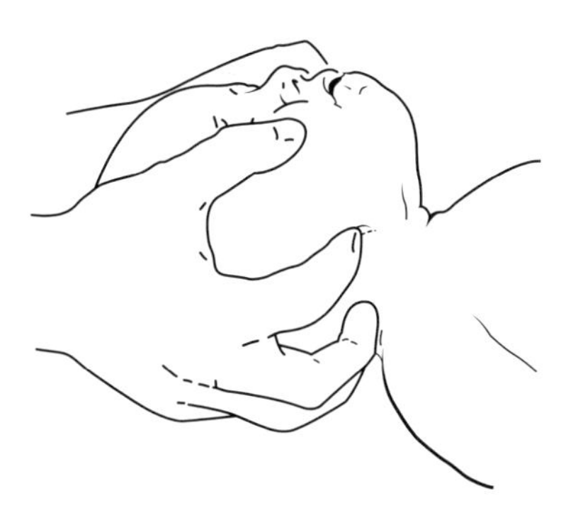

Jaw thrust

Figure 2. Airway opening maneuver. (Reproduced with kind permission from Resuscitation at Birth—the Newborn Life Support Provider Course Manual. Resuscitation Council (UK) 2001. Figure drawn by Steven Brindley, 56 Barnwood Avenue, Gloucester, UK.)

- Choosing the right size of mask (cover the nose and mouth but not chin or orbits);
- Look for the chest movement and if not achieving try with two people (one giving jaw thrust with two hands and other providing ventilation).

The effective use of above techniques will result in success in most situations. Rare exceptions include diaphragmatic hernia, extreme preterm baby, meconium stained flat baby etc. where elective endotracheal intubation with an appropriate size uncuffed tube takes precedence for effective resuscitation.

Circulation

After ensuring that airway is patent and chest is moving, if there is persistent bradycardia, '**CALL FOR HELP**'. The big difference between a neonate and an adult arrest is that the primary event is usually non-cardiac. For effective cardiac compression the sternum needs to be pressed over its lower third using either the 'hand encircling technique' or 'two thumb technique' and pressing about one third the depth towards backbone. The ratio of cardiac compressions to IPPV is 3:1 giving enough time for the filling of heart as there are venous valves at thoracic inlet and the tendency of veins unlike arteries to collapse. The current guidelines recommend 90 compressions and 30 breaths in one minute which are difficult to achieve in 75% cases.

Recheck the heart rate every 30 seconds for the response. A poor response is most likely due to myocardial dysfunction secondary to lactic acidosis, pulse-less electrical activity or exhaustion of myocardial glycogen. At this stage you may resort to drugs.

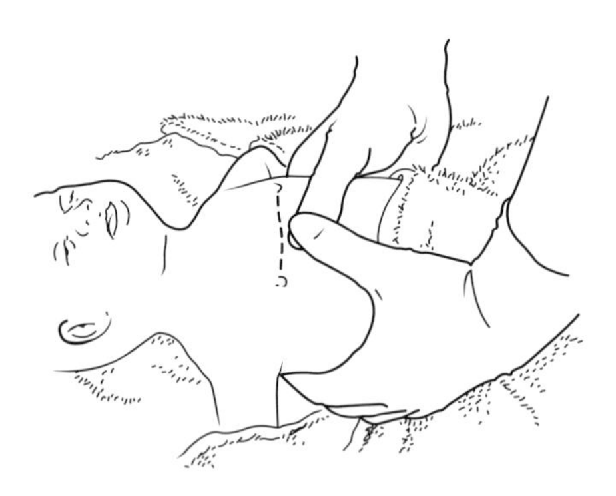

Encircling the whole chest with both hands is the most effective method

Figure 3. Chest compressions. (Reproduced with kind permission from Resuscitation at Birth—the Newborn Life Support Provider Course Manual. Resuscitation Council (UK) 2001. Figure drawn by Steven Brindley, 56 Barnwood Avenue, Gloucester, UK.)

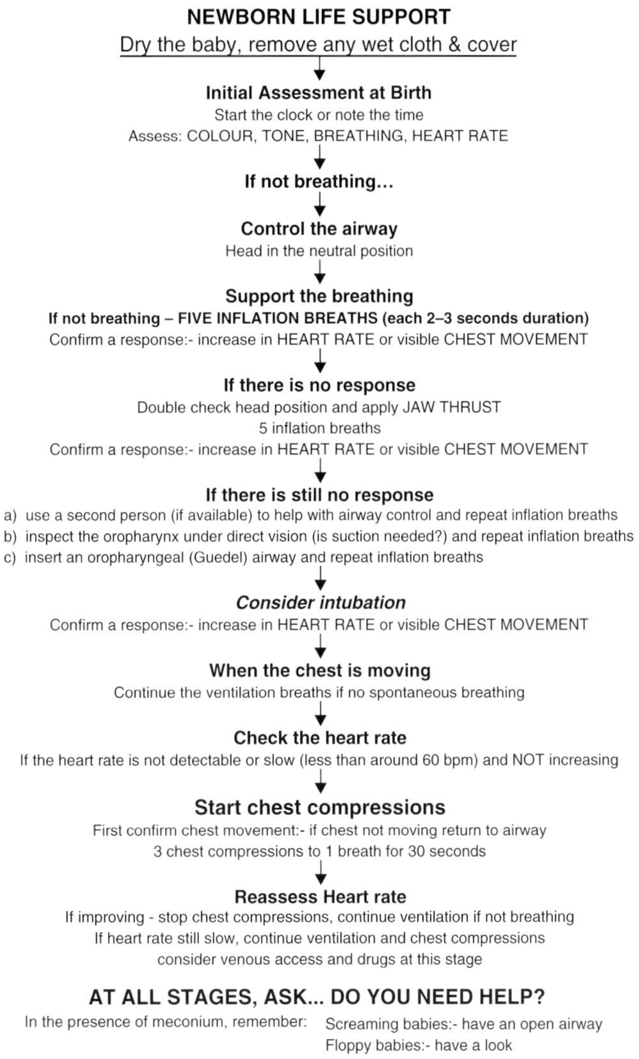

NEWBORN LIFE SUPPORT

Dry the baby, remove any wet cloth & cover

↓

Initial Assessment at Birth

Start the clock or note the time

Assess: COLOUR, TONE, BREATHING, HEART RATE

↓

If not breathing...

↓

Control the airway

Head in the neutral position

↓

Support the breathing

If not breathing – FIVE INFLATION BREATHS (each 2–3 seconds duration)

Confirm a response:- increase in HEART RATE or visible CHEST MOVEMENT

↓

If there is no response

Double check head position and apply JAW THRUST

5 inflation breaths

Confirm a response:- increase in HEART RATE or visible CHEST MOVEMENT

↓

If there is still no response

a) use a second person (if available) to help with airway control and repeat inflation breaths
b) inspect the oropharynx under direct vision (is suction needed?) and repeat inflation breaths
c) insert an oropharyngeal (Guedel) airway and repeat inflation breaths

↓

Consider intubation

Confirm a response:- increase in HEART RATE or visible CHEST MOVEMENT

↓

When the chest is moving

Continue the ventilation breaths if no spontaneous breathing

↓

Check the heart rate

If the heart rate is not detectable or slow (less than around 60 bpm) and NOT increasing

↓

Start chest compressions

First confirm chest movement:- if chest not moving return to airway

3 chest compressions to 1 breath for 30 seconds

↓

Reassess Heart rate

If improving - stop chest compressions, continue ventilation if not breathing

If heart rate still slow, continue ventilation and chest compressions

consider venous access and drugs at this stage

AT ALL STAGES, ASK... DO YOU NEED HELP?

In the presence of meconium, remember: Screaming babies:- have an open airway
Floppy babies:- have a look

Figure 4. Neonatal Resuscitation flow chart (Algorithm). (Reproduced with kind permission from Resuscitation at Birth—the Newborn Life Support Provider Course Manual. Resuscitation Council (UK) 2001. Figure drawn by Steven Brindley, 56 Barnwood Avenue, Gloucester, UK.)

Drugs

They should be given by either an umbilical venous line or an intra-osseous route. Except for adrenaline no other drug can be given by the tracheal route under emergency situations. The peripheral i.v. or direct injection in umbilical cord are ineffective in during cardiac arrest.

The drugs that can be used are:

- Adrenaline: 10 μg per kg (0.1 mL per kg of 1:10,000);
- Sodium bicarbonate: 1–2 mmol/kg (2–4 mL/kg of 4.2%);
- Dextrose: 250 μg/kg (2.5 mL/kg of 10%);
- Volume: 0.9% saline 10 mL/kg.

Complications

The commonest cause of problems is progressing to advanced steps when the primary ones are poorly performed. The long term neuro-developmental effects of ineffective or difficult resuscitation can not be overstressed.

> Ask at every step:
> Do you need help?

Acknowledgements

The figures taken with permission from Northern Neonatal Network & Resuscitation Council UK.

59

Fetal heart rate monitoring in labour

Helen R. Simpson

Physiological basis

Changes in fetal heart rate (FHR) patterns are mediated via the vagus nerve, chemoreceptors and baroreceptors in the aortic arch and carotid bodies. These changes occur in response to change in oxygen, carbon dioxide, hydrogen ion concentration and arterial pressure. The FHR pattern therefore is an indirect measure of fetal acid–base balance, which is a measure of fetal compromise. There are two methods of monitoring the FHR: intermittent auscultation and continuous electronic monitoring.

Structured intermittent auscultation

Intermittent auscultation of the FHR with a Pinard or hand-held Doppler is measured every 15 minutes for one minute after a contraction during the active first stage of labour and after every contraction during the second stage. It is used in low-risk pregnancy. If an abnormality is picked up then continuous monitoring should be commenced.

Continuous intrapartum electronic fetal monitoring (EFM)

In EFM the fetus is monitored continuously and a record of the heart rate and contractions are produced on a strip of paper called a Cardiotocograph or CTG. Figure 1 shows a normal CTG (paper speed 1 cm per hour).

EFM held the promise of preventing fetal morbidity and mortality and fewer law suits but as yet it has failed to live up to these

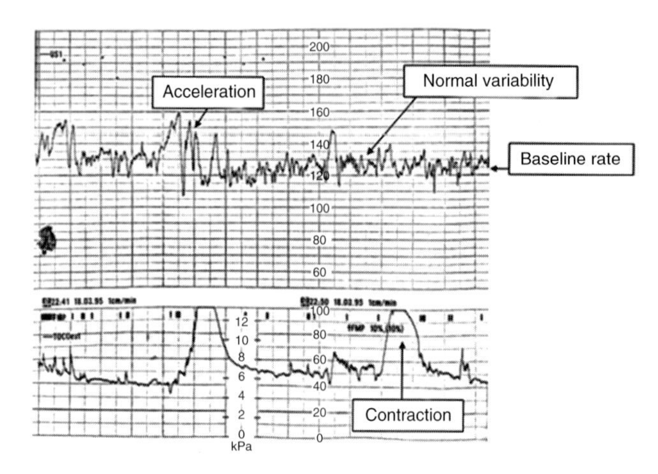

Figure 1. Normal CTG.

Table 1. Suggested indications for EFM.

Labour 1. Induced or augmented labour 2. Epidural, especially after bolus	Suspected fetal compromise in labour: 1. Particulate meconium 2. Suspicious fetal heart rate on auscultation 3. Abnormal FHR on the admission trace 4. Vaginal bleeding in labour
Fetal problems: 1. Multiple pregnancies 2. Intra-uterine growth restriction 3. Preterm labour (<37 weeks) 4. Breech presentation 5. Rhesus isoimmunisation	Maternal medical complications *Common* 1. Hypertension—particularly pre-eclampsia 2. Diabetes *Rare* 3. Cardiac disease 4. Haemoglobinopathy 5. Severe anaemia 6. Hyperthyroidism 7. Collagen disease 8. Renal disease

expectations. EFM used alone increases the Caesarean Section rate by 160%. When used in conjunction with fetal blood sampling (FBS—see later) the rate is increased, but by only 30%. EFM also increases the operative vaginal delivery rate by 30%.

CTGs are often difficult to interpret and inter-observer agreement only occurs 50–60% of the time. Using EFM as a screening test for hypoxia produces a large number of false positives. Thus a 'bad' tracing is not very good at predicting poor outcome, but a 'good' tracing, is predictive of a good outcome. As EFM has been shown to have no benefit in the low-risk population, intermittent auscultation should remain the method of choice. We do need to identify those women who may benefit from monitoring.

Interpretation of fetal heart rate

Risk assessment

Before any CTG can be interpreted the background of the patient should be known, so that risk factors can be identified. It is important to know how much reserve a fetus has. Is this a term, low-risk baby or are there risks present such as growth restriction, or particulate meconium. Is labour progressing well or is there associated failure to progress. Is an assisted vaginal delivery possible?

Contractions

Contractions should be described as the number in a 10-minute period of time. Unless an in-utero pressure catheter is being used the duration and strength of contractions cannot be determined. Is there evidence of hyperstimulation (>5:10)? It is impossible to interpret decelerations without a satisfactory contraction trace.

Baseline rate

The normal range is 110–160 bpm.

Both bradycardia and tachycardia can be a sign of fetal hypoxia.

Bradycardia

Mild bradycardia is defined as a rate of 100–110 bpm. When not associated with other abnormalities, it does not indicate hypoxia. It is associated with post-dates infants and occipito-posterior position. Rates less than 100 bpm may be seen in fetuses with congenital heart disease or myocardial conduction defects associated with collagen vascular disease in the mother. Prolonged bradycardia either alone or associated with other abnormalities is often a terminal event and may indicate severe hypoxia.

Tachycardia

Fetal movement, maternal anxiety or fever, maternal dehydration or ketosis and beta-adrenergic agents may cause tachycardia without hypoxia. Variability will be normal and the tachycardia is usually less than 180 bpm. Fetal immaturity, thyrotoxicosis and anaemia may also cause a mild tachycardia. A gradually increasing baseline accompanied by decreased variability and/or decelerations frequently indicates fetal hypoxia. Persistent tachycardia greater than 180 bpm, especially if maternal fever is present, suggests chorioamnioitis. A FHR greater than 200 bpm is frequently due to fetal arrhythmia or other congenital abnormalities.

Variability

The FHR normally exhibits short-term variability with an average change of 10–15 bpm about the baseline rate. (The trace will appear to have a jagged appearance rather than a straight line.) This variability is linked to the fetal central nervous system and reflects fetal cerebral activity. It is therefore a vital clue in determining the overall fetal condition. Its presence is correlated with a good outcome.

Sleep cycles of 20–40 minutes or longer may cause a normal decrease in FHR variability. Medications, including analgesics, anaesthetics, barbiturates, tranquillisers, atropine and magnesium sulphate may also induce quiet periods in the FHR pattern without fetal compromise. Steroid administration to induce fetal lung maturation also reduces variability. Loss of variability, especially when accompanied by late decelerations or variable decelerations increases the possibility of fetal acidosis if it remains uncorrected.

Accelerations

These are increases in the FHR of 15 bpm, lasting for 15 seconds or more, often associated with fetal movement or stimulation. Their absence does not necessarily indicate fetal compromise, but does indicate the need for further evaluation. The presence of accelerations is reassuring.

Decelerations

These are decreases in the FHR below the base line. There are three types.

Early decelerations

Transient decreases in FHR, occurring with and **mirroring the uterine contraction**, are termed early decelerations. They should not usually fall more than 60 beats from the baseline. They are nearly always benign if no other abnormalities of FHR are noted and probably indicate 'head compression'. To accurately distinguish early decelerations from late decelerations, uterine contractions MUST be adequately monitored.

Late decelerations

Transient decreases in FHR begin **after the onset** of the uterine contractions, as shown in Figure 2. Their nadir occurs later than the peak of the contraction. If uncorrected, repetitive late decelerations are frequently associated with fetal hypoxia. When associated with decreased variability or other FHR abnormalities, there is an increased likelihood of significant fetal compromise and immediate evaluation and intervention are indicated. Subtle, shallow late decelerations are extremely significant, they are easily missed but can be detected by holding a straight edge along the baseline.

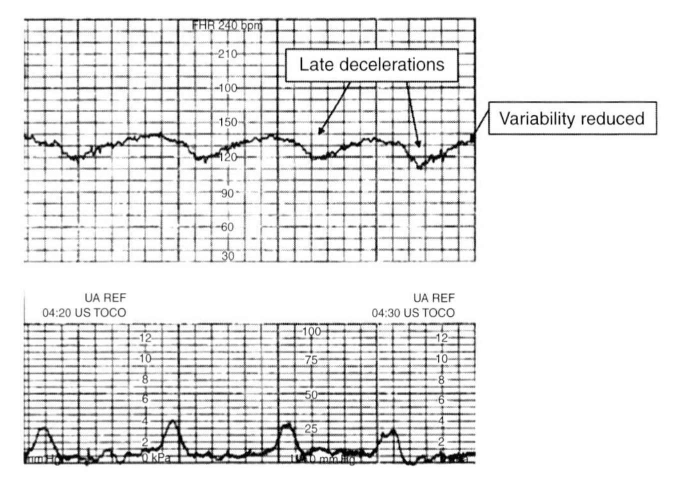

Figure 2. Late decelerations.

Variable decelerations
Variable decelerations have variable shape and relationship to the contraction. Cord compression is the most common mechanism. They are extremely common, occurring in 50–80% of labours in the second stage. Most are benign. Characteristics that indicate benign variable decelerations include rapid descent and recovery, good baseline variability and accelerations at the onset and at the end of the contraction (the classic or 'M' shape). Ominous signs include late onset (in relation to contractions), slow recovery, decreased variability, baseline tachycardia, loss of accelerations or shoulders if previously present and increased severity of the variable decelerations.

To determine severity of a deceleration, consider depth, frequency and duration. A single deceleration is meaningless and may be triggered by an immediate preceding event such as vaginal examination or a change in position or vomiting.

Assessment and plan of management

Having assessed the FHR trace and defined risk, an assessment of the situation and management plan should be made. The FHR trace can be classified as 'reassuring', 'suspicious' or 'pathological'. If the FHR trace is reassuring then the question should be asked whether monitoring is continuous or by intermittent auscultation. A suspicious or pathological FHR trace may require:

- Close observation and reassessment;
- Assessment by fetal blood sampling;
- Immediate delivery.

Abnormalities in FHR traces can be related to specific events, e.g. vaginal examination. If the fetus was not previously compromised, recovery will usually occur with discontinuation of the inciting event or agent. Factors known to cause hypoxia should be sought and corrected.

Fetal blood sampling

Ideally EFM should not be used without the facility to measure fetal blood pH. This reduces the number of unnecessary caesarean sections. A small sample of blood is taken from the fetal scalp. In the first stage of labour, during which a mild acidosis normally occurs, the mean fetal scalp blood pH is 7.33. A pH greater than 7.25 is therefore considered to be normal. pH values between 7.20 and 7.25 reflect a borderline or 'low normal' situation. A pH below 7.2 is 2 SD below the mean and is regarded as abnormal and requires delivery. When the FHR pattern is ominous only 50–65% of the new-borns are depressed as judged by the Apgar score, i.e. a 35–50% false positive prediction. The false prediction by scalp blood pH <7.20 is only 10–20%. A single sample, no matter how reassuring, means nothing if a FHR tracing remains non-reassuring. It is necessary to repeat the sample in 1/2–1 hour if the FHR tracing does not improve.

Antepartum fetal monitoring

Many of the principles of FHR trace interpretation discussed above can be related to antepartum fetal monitoring. Biophysical profiles (fetal breathing, amniotic fluid volume, fetal tone, fetal movements and FHR trace) and Doppler studies of the umbilical artery can be used to help gauge fetal well being but are beyond the scope of this chapter to discuss in detail.

Conclusion

Electronic monitoring of the fetus must be initiated with an understanding of the physiological basis. Changes need to be interpreted in the light of the clinical background, the overall pattern, the stage of labour, and in conjunction with fetal scalp sampling (when appropriate) if outcome is to be improved without increasing the operative delivery rate.

Section 8

Emergencies

60

Hypovolaemia

L. Jeyaraj and Gerard Danjoux

Definition

Hypovolaemia is defined as a reduced circulating blood volume. It may be further classified as absolute hypovolaemia and relative hypovolaemia.

- *Absolute hypovolaemia*—total circulatory blood volume is reduced resulting in an inadequate cardiac output to meet the metabolic demands of the tissues.
- *Relative hypovolaemia*—this arises secondary to increased vascular capacitance (vasodilatation) resulting in less blood available for circulation despite an unchanged blood volume. Examples of this are sepsis and spinal anaesthesia.

The cardinal feature of hypovolaemia is inadequate tissue perfusion resulting in tissue hypoxia and anaerobic metabolism. In the rest of this chapter, the discussion that follows pertains to ***absolute hypovolaemia***.

Physiology

In the average adult, water accounts for 60% of body weight (BW). This water is distributed into the intra- and extracellular body compartments as outlined in Figure 1. Essentially one third of total body water (TBW) is extracellular and two thirds intracellular. TBW (as a percentage of body weight) and its distribution into intra- and extracellular compartments can also be affected by age and gender.

The main ions in extracellular fluid (ECF) are sodium and chloride with potassium and phosphate being predominant in intracellular fluid (ICF). In order to maintain body homeostasis water is able to move freely between all compartments. The intracellular compartment is relatively impermeable to sodium, restricting it predominantly to ECF. Four simple rules help tie this physiology to fluid resuscitation in the clinical setting:

- Hypovolaemia refers to fluid loss from the intravascular compartment.
- The intravascular compartment comprises one third of the ECF, and only one tenth of TBW.
- Infused intravascular sodium remains in the ECF. Water infused with the sodium will also remain in the ECF.
- Infused intravascular solutions without sodium, e.g. dextrose, will distribute into TBW.

Examples

- One litre of infused sodium chloride distributes into 14 litres (ECF volume) and only one third of this (333 mL) remains in the intravascular compartment. Therefore one litre of blood loss from the intravascular space must be replaced by three litres of sodium chloride i.e. three times the volume lost (3:1 rule).

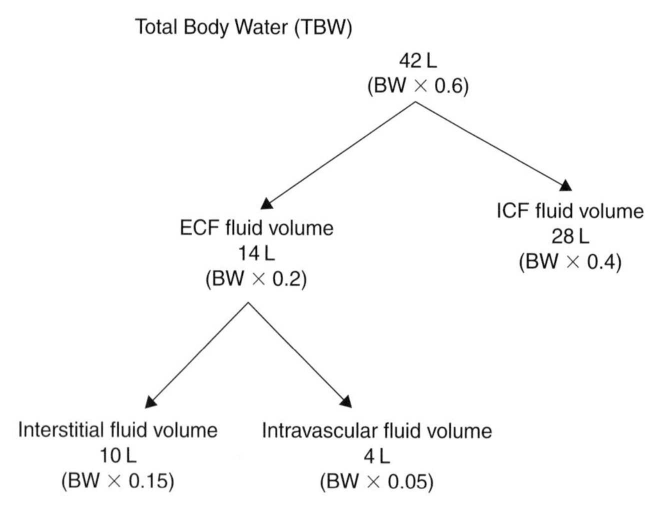

Figure 1. Distribution of ICF and ECF in a 70 kg adult. (For differing body weights the compositions are calculated as shown in parentheses.) ECF = extracellular fluid; ICF = intracellular fluid; BW = body weight.

- One litre of infused dextrose distributes into 42 litres (ICF volume) with only one tenth (100 mL) remaining in the intravascular compartment. Here one litre of blood loss from the intravascular space must be replaced by 10 litres of dextrose i.e. ten times the volume lost.

Clearly from these examples it is appropriate to treat hypovolaemia secondary to intravascular fluid loss with sodium chloride (or other sodium-containing solutions, e.g. Hartmanns solution) but not dextrose containing solutions. This concept is taken to its clinical application in the 'management' part of this article.

Causes of hypovolaemia

Loss of blood (haemorrhagic shock)

- Trauma;
- Gastrointestinal tract bleeding;
- Iatrogenic e.g. surgery

Loss of plasma

- Burns

Loss of fluid and electrolytes

- Bowel obstruction;
- Vomiting and diarrhoea;
- Hyperosmolar states, e.g. diabetic ketoacidosis;
- Pancreatitis.

Pathophysiology

It is useful to consider the effects of haemorrhage because they illustrate the features of a major form of hypovolaemic shock and the multiple compensatory reactions that come into play to defend ECF volume. Generally there are immediate, early and late compensatory mechanisms which are outlined below:

- ***Immediate* (Mainly autonomic)**—When blood volume is reduced and venous return is decreased, the arterial baroreceptors are stretched to a lesser degree and sympathetic output is increased. This causes a decrease in pulse pressure, reflex tachycardia and vasoconstriction. The vasoconstriction is generalised sparing only the vessels of the brain and the heart.

- ***Early* (Neurohumeral)**—Up to 12 hours. The rennin–angiotensin system, aldosterone and antidiuretic hormone all play active roles. ECF volume is restored by retention of sodium and water by the kidneys and an increase in thirst. There is also a generalised arteriolar vasoconstriction to increase systemic vascular resistance and maintain systemic blood pressure.
- ***Late* (endocrine)**—After a moderate haemorrhage, the circulating blood volume is restored within 12–72 hours. Erythropoietin appears in the circulation and reticulocyte count increases. The red cell mass is restored in 4–8 weeks.

Clinical signs and symptoms

Hypovolaemic shock is also called '**cold shock**'. It is characterised by hypotension, a rapid low-volume pulse, cold pale clammy skin, intense thirst, rapid respiration and restlessness or alternatively stupor. The degree to which symptoms and signs exist depends upon the degree of hypovolaemia. This can be classified as mild, moderate and severe and the clinical signs/symptoms are outlined in Table 1.

Management

Management of hypovolaemia should follow the ABC approach. Airway and breathing problems should be identified and treated first and all patients should receive supplementary high flow oxygen (>15 L/min via a face mask and reservoir system). This is followed by assessment of the degree of hypovolaemia.

Table 1. Degrees of hypovolaemia and clinical signs/symptoms.

	Mild	Moderate	Severe
Blood loss (mL)	750	750–1500	>1500
Blood loss (% blood volume)	<15%	15–30%	>30%
Pulse rate	<100	>100	>120
Blood pressure	Normal	Normal	Decreased
Pulse pressure	Normal	Decreased	Decreased
Urine output (mL/hr)	>30	20–30	5–15
Respiratory rate	14–20	20–30	30–40
Mental state	Slightly anxious	Mildly anxious	Confused, lethargic

General management

Direct pressure can be applied to control obvious external bleeding points. Internal bleeding should be sought during the primary survey to identify concealed haemorrhage within the chest, abdomen or pelvis. At the same time treatment of hypovolaemia should occur.

Initial circulatory resuscitation should commence by placing two, short, wide-bore (14 or 16G) peripheral cannulae (antecubital fossa often preferable). Blood should be sent for baseline haematological and biochemical tests and a crossmatch ordered. An initial fluid challenge of one to two litres of warmed sodium containing crystalloid should be started and given over 30 minutes. Further fluid management should be based on continual re-evaluation of the patients' clinical status, urine output, and response to the initial fluid challenge. All patients should receive a urinary catheter (aim to maintain urine output >0.5 mL/kg/hour) and nasogastric tube (to reduce likelihood of aspiration).

Failure to respond to the initial fluid challenge suggests ongoing concealed blood loss especially in cases of multiple trauma. Immediate surgical referral and operative intervention may then be required to enable bleeding to be stopped and intravascular volume to be replaced.

Specific fluid therapy

Initial fluid therapy should be instigated with crystalloid solutions (avoid dextrose containing solutions). Colloid solutions and blood may be required depending on the degree of hypovolaemia and estimated blood loss:

- $<15\%$ circulatory volume—crystalloid resuscitation (remember 3:1 rule);
- 15–30% circulatory volume—crystalloid $+/-$ colloid resuscitation;
- $>30\%$ circulatory volume—blood transfusion will be indicated.

Fully cross-matched blood is preferable if time permits. If blood is required more urgently then type specific or 'O rhesus negative' blood (universal donor blood) should be requested.

Controversy exists regarding the use of **colloids *vs.* crystalloids** as replacement therapy. Proponents of colloids argue that by maintaining plasma oncotic pressure, colloids are more effective in restoring normal intravascular volume and cardiac output. Colloid solutions are far more expensive than crystalloids, but they more effectively restore intravascular volume. Crystalloid proponents on the other hand maintain that the crystalloid solutions are equally as effective when given in sufficient amounts. Crystalloid solutions are readily available and inexpensive.

Further points regarding fluid resuscitation:

- Warm all fluids to prevent hypothermia and coagulopathic states;
- Use rapid infusion device (e.g. Level I® blood warmer) if high very flow rates are required;
- Frequent re-evaluation of clinical signs (Table 1) should guide fluid therapy;
- Massive transfusions can result in coagulopathic states. Blood products, e.g. FFP, platelets may be required in addition to blood.

Continuing management

All patients with significant hypovolaemia should ultimately be managed in a critical care environment (high dependency or intensive care unit) irrespective of the need for surgical intervention. Central venous or pulmonary artery pressures may need to be measured in some circumstances to guide on-going fluid therapy especially in refractory patients or those sustaining multiple trauma. Inotropic or vasopressor therapy may also be needed in the critical care environment.

Conclusion

Hypovolaemia is the cause of shock in most trauma patients. Management should initially be aimed at ABC resuscitation. The goal of therapy is prompt restoration of organ perfusion with oxygen and aggressive fluid therapy. Hypovolaemia refractory to aggressive fluid therapy may warrant the need for early surgical intervention.

- Initial resuscitation begins with ABC.
- Use short, wide-bore cannulae in peripheral veins.
- Avoid dextrose containing crystalloids.
- Warm all resuscitation fluids.
- Continually re-evaluate signs and symptoms.

- Refractory hypovolaemia requires early surgical intervention.
- Large transfusions may require other blood products to avoid coagulopathies.

Relevant Physics

Fluid flow through a tube follows certain physical principles (Poiseuille's law):

(a) Flow rate (Q) is proportional to (radius)^4; (b) Q is inversely proportional to tube length; (c) Q is directly proportional to the pressure gradient across the tube ($P_1 - P_2$).

Therefore high flow rates are best achieved via short, wide-bore cannulae with a high driving pressure.

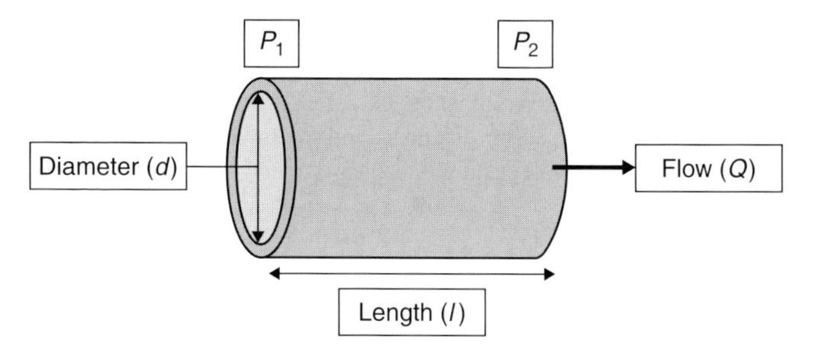

Figure 2. Factors affecting flow through a tube. P_1 = upstream pressure; P_2 = down stream pressure; radius = $d/2$.

61

Acute asthma

Harry Gribbin

Acute asthma is a common emergency but its diagnosis is not always easy. Worsening wheeze, shortness of breath, chest tightness and cough are the commonest symptoms but in adults the same symptoms occur in other common respiratory disorders, e.g. chronic obstructive pulmonary disease (COPD). A clear past history of asthma is the best guide. COPD is unlikely in the younger patient. Many patients with asthma now carry emergency plans which include details of their therapy and peak expiratory flow (PEF) and confirm the diagnosis. Previous acute attacks with restoration of normal activities point to asthma. Chronic symptoms in a smoker with persistent respiratory disability are more likely in COPD, although can occur in chronic asthma. In the emergency room, however, there are occasions when the physician may be uncertain of the specific diagnosis and treatment has to be started based on available history and clinical assessment.

The acute asthma attack

Asthma is a chronic inflammatory disorder of the airways. The factors which precipitate the complex cascade of mediator release and inflammatory cell infiltration of the bronchial mucosa, and cause the acute attack, are often obscure. Mast cell IgE antibody–inhaled antigen reactions are the likely initiators, although many other factors may be involved. In most patients, symptoms deteriorate over days or hours. In a minority, the acute episode can come on very rapidly, within minutes. A reduction in airways calibre is caused by a combination of bronchial smooth muscle contraction, bronchial mucosal oedema and increased amounts of mucus in the bronchial lumen, which contains desquamated bronchial epithelium. Increasing resistance to airflow into and out of the lung causes increases in work of breathing, recruitment of accessory muscles of breathing (sternomastoid and abdominal) and a progressive rise in the end expiratory lung volume. Patients become anxious, tired, with tachypnoea, expiratory wheeze and hyperinflation.

Measurement of airways obstruction

Measurement of the degree of airways obstruction is the best objective guide to the severity of an asthma attack. PEF and forced expiratory volume in one second (FEV1) can be used but PEF is easier. The value recorded has to be compared to the predicted value for the patient (Figure 1). Many patients with chronic asthma, however, do not have normal PEF when well and the PEF during an acute attack should be related to the patient's recent 'best' PEF. If this is not known, comparison with the predicted normal value is advised.

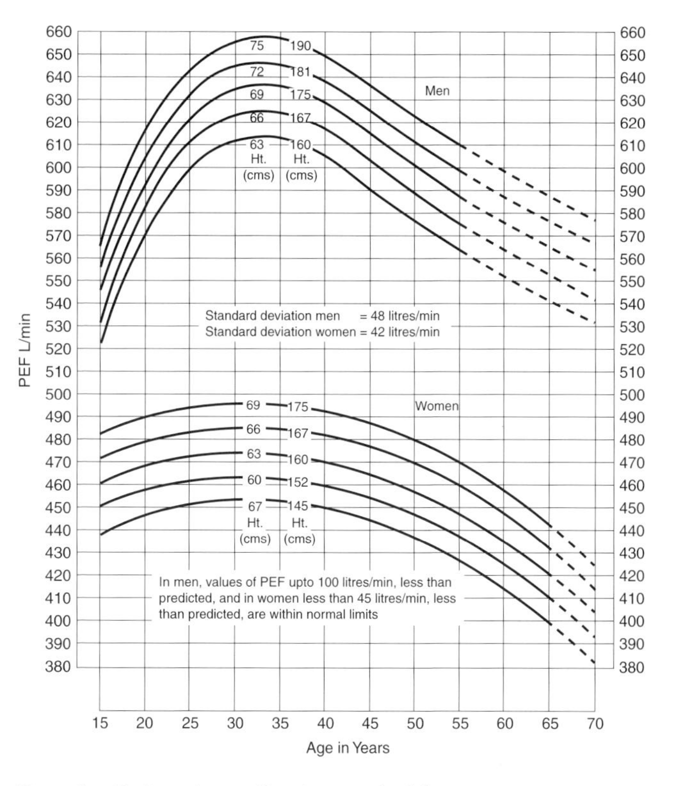

Figure 1. Peak expiratory flow in normal adults.

The chest X-ray in acute asthma

Apart from showing signs of hyperinflation, the chest X-ray is usually normal in acute severe asthma. Chest X-ray should be obtained in all patients whose symptoms do not improve or who have life-threatening asthma, to rule out the presence of acute and sometimes tension pneumothorax.

Assessment of severity of acute asthma attack

Acute severe asthma

One or more of the following:

- PEF 33–50% recent best or predicted;
- Respiratory rate $>$25/minute;
- Heart rate $>$110 bpm;
- Inability to complete sentences in one breath.

Life-threatening asthma

One or more of the following:

- PEF $<$33% recent best or predicted
- PaO_2 $<$8 kPa or SaO_2 less than 92%
- Dysrhythmia
- $PaCO_2$ $<$6.0 kPa
- 'Silent' or quiet breath sounds
- Exhaustion and failing respiratory effort

Bradycardia
Hypotension
Confusion
Coma
Cyanosis

Near-fatal asthma

Any one of the indicators of acute severe or life-threatening asthma with:

- $PaCO_2$ $>$6.0 kPa indicating requirement for Intermittent Positive Pressure Ventilation.

Management of acute asthma

Oxygen therapy

High fractional concentrations of inspired oxygen (e.g. Hudson-type mask with an oxygen flow rate of 6–8 litres/minute) should be given to all patients with acute severe asthma, with the aim of achieving normal oxygen saturation. Unlike exacerbations of COPD, a rise in arterial PCO_2 is an indicator of worsening asthma and not oxygen-induced depression of ventilation.

Beta-agonist bronchodilators

The beta-agonist bronchodilators, salbutamol and terbutaline, given by oxygen-driven nebulisers, are the most useful drugs in the immediate management of the acute attack. In acute severe asthma give:

- Salbutamol 5 mg or terbutaline 5 mg every 15–30 minutes until patient improves; or
- Continuous nebulised salbutamol 5–10 mg/hour. This requires specialised nebuliser equipment.

Steroid therapy

Inhaled beta-agonists relieve the symptoms of acute asthma but steroids are required to shorten the duration of the attack by switching off, at the cellular level, the inflammatory mechanisms responsible. They act over a longer period than beta-agonists and it takes several hours and sometimes days before the acute episode is relieved. Oral steroids are as effective as the intravenous route, providing the patient can swallow and is not vomiting.

In acute severe asthma give:

- Intravenous hydrocortisone 100 mg six-hourly; or
- Prednisolone 40–50 mg daily.

Prednisolone 40–50 mg daily should be continued for at least five days or longer until recovery, as indicated by peak flow readings and symptoms returning to their normal level.

Other drugs used in acute severe asthma

The following drugs are used either singly or in combination in patients who do not improve on nebulised beta-agonists and steroids:

- Ipratropium bromide
  - 0.5 mg 4–6 hourly by oxygen-driven nebuliser.
- Intravenous aminophylline
  - Loading dose: 5 mg/kg by slow IV infusion over 20 minutes;
  - A loading dose should not be given in patients already taking oral aminophylline;
  - Maintenance infusion: 0.5 mg/kg/hour;

  - Side effects of palpitation, cardiac arrhythmia, nausea and vomiting can occur. Hypotension is a rare but frightening complication. Monitoring of aminophylline blood levels is recommended to avoid exceeding therapeutic range (10–20 mg/litres).
- Intravenous magnesium sulphate
  - Magnesium sulphate (1.2–2 g) by IV infusion over 20 minutes.

Discharge from hospital

There is no single clinical or physiological measure of fitness for discharge. Morning PEF greater than 75% of best or predicted values and diurnal variation in peak flow of less than 25% are reasonable guides when used with clinical signs and discussion. The patient's GP should be informed of the discharge within 24 hours, and wherever possible the patient seen by the GP within two working days.

Asthma maintenance therapy

It is important at the time of discharge to check that the patient understands the nature of regular asthma therapy and has an adequate supply. Inhaler technique requires checking. Changing to an alternative device can help some patients.

All patients should have:

- A beta-agonist inhaler for as-required use for relief of symptoms;
- An inhaled steroid. In patients not already on an inhaled steroid, start beclomethasone dipropionate by metered dose aerosol or dry powder inhaler 200 μg bd;
- A standard stepwise approach to asthma therapy is recommended, according to current guidelines;
- Following admission to hospital with acute severe asthma, all patients should be given a simple self-management plan with instructions to start oral steroid therapy in the event of worsening asthma and peak flow values falling below a given threshold, usually set at about 50% of the predicted normal or best recent values. Patients should be provided with an emergency supply of prednisolone at the time of their discharge from hospital.

Acknowledgements

The version of Nunn and Gregg's graph of peak flow values in the normal population appears in the *current British Guideline on the Management of Asthma* (*BMJ*. 1989;298:1068–1070).

62

Anaphylaxis

Jacqui Gedney

Definition

Anaphylaxis is a severe, potentially life-threatening systemic allergic reaction. It presents as either respiratory difficulties or hypotension and collapse.

Mechanism

An anaphylactic reaction is a severe type 1 immediate hypersensitivity reaction. It occurs on re-exposure to an allergen to which the individual has become sensitised. Previous exposure has resulted in the production of specific IgE antibodies to the allergen and these antibodies are bound to IgE on mast cells and basophils. On re-exposure the allergen binds to the IgE leading to mast cell activation and release of mediators stored within granules in the cell. These mediators include histamine, serotonin, eosinophil chemotactic agent, and neutrophil chemotactic agent. There is also increased arachidonic acid production from the cell membrane leading to the production of prostaglandins, thromboxanes and leukotrienes.

These mediators produce increased capillary permeability, mucosal oedema, smooth muscle contraction and vasodilatation.

Triggers

The commonest triggers are foods (peanuts, other nuts, fish, shell fish, eggs) and insect bites. In hospital common causes include drugs (antibiotics, intravenous anaesthetic agents, aspirin, contract media) and latex allergy.

Anaphylactoid reactions

An anaphylactoid reaction is also caused by the activation of mast cells, but does not involve IgE antibodies. The clinical picture and immediate management of anaphylactic and anaphylactoid reactions are identical. Triggers include opiates, exercise, aspirin, complement activation.

Incidence

Accident and emergency department data suggest an incidence of 1 in 10,000 population/year. In hospital the incidence rises to 1 in 3000. The mortality is between 3 and 4.3%. It is more common in women than men (3:1) and the incidence appears to be increasing.

Presentation

The commonest presentations are cardiovascular collapse (88%), erythema (45%) and bronchospasm (36%). Other symptoms include pruritus, urticaria, rhinitis, conjunctivitis, angio-oedema, generalised oedema, nausea, abdominal pain, diarrhoea, vomiting, laryngeal oedema, and a sense of impending doom. The skin may look flushed or pale.

Respiratory problems result from severe upper airway oedema or bronchospasm. Hypotension and collapse result from massive fluid shifts from the intravascular to the extra-vascular space due to increased capillary leak combined with vasodilatation.

The presentation varies with the trigger. Ingested allergens usually cause lip and laryngeal oedema. Intravenous drugs and insect stings produce predominantly cardiovascular effects.

Symptoms usually occur within minutes of exposure but may be delayed by several hours. Improvement also usually occurs very quickly, but symptoms may last up to 24 hours and can rarely be biphasic with a deterioration occurring 1–8 hours after the initial symptoms.

Differential diagnosis

Differential diagnoses include panic attacks, vaso-vagal episodes, cardiac arrhythmias, myocardial ischaemia, food aspiration, pulmonary embolus, seizures.

Management

First line of management

- Airway
- Oxygen
- Circulation

Also consider

- Epinephrine
- Intravenous fluid
- Antihistamine
- Hydrocortisone
- Inotropes
- Bicarbonate
- Bronchodilators

The immediate management guidelines from Resuscitation Council (UK) are given in Figures 1 and 2.

A history is required as soon as situation permits to provide information of all possible triggers.

Any drug, which could be a trigger, should be stopped immediately.

The airway must be maintained. This may be difficult because of laryngeal oedema and early intubation should be considered because the airway may continue to get worse.

Oxygen (100%) should be given, either by face mask with reservoir bag in the spontaneously breathing patient or by Ambu-bag in the patient needing mechanical ventilation.

Circulation—monitor the circulation closely. Cardiac arrhythmias and arrest can occur due to severe hypotension.

If the patient is hypotensive, lying the patient down with feet elevated will improve systemic blood pressure. If respiratory symptoms predominate the patient may prefer to sit up.

In the event of cardio-respiratory arrest, the airway may be difficult because of oedema and the patient should be intubated and

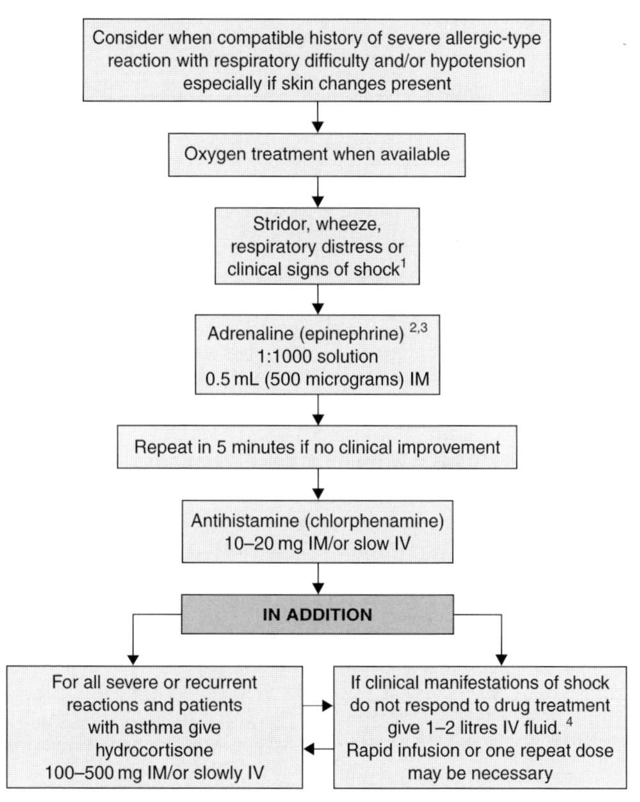

1. An inhaled $beta_2$-agonist such as salbutamol may be used as an adjunctive measure if bronchospasm is severe and does not respond rapidly to other treatment.
2. If profound shock judged **immediately** life threatening give CPR/ALS if necessary Consider **slow** IV adrenaline (epinephrine) 1:10,000 solution. This is **hazardous** and is recommended only for an experienced practitioner who can also obtain IV access without delay. Note the different strength of adrenaline (epinephrine) that may be required for IV use.
3. If adults are treated with an Epipen, the 300 micrograms will usually be sufficient. A second dose may be required. Half doses of adrenaline (epinephrine) may be safer for patients on amitriptyline, imipramine, or beta blocker.
4. A crystalloid may be safer than a colloid.

Figure 1. Anaphylactic reactions: Treatment algorithm for adults by first medical responders. Reproduced with kind permission from Resuscitation Council (UK).

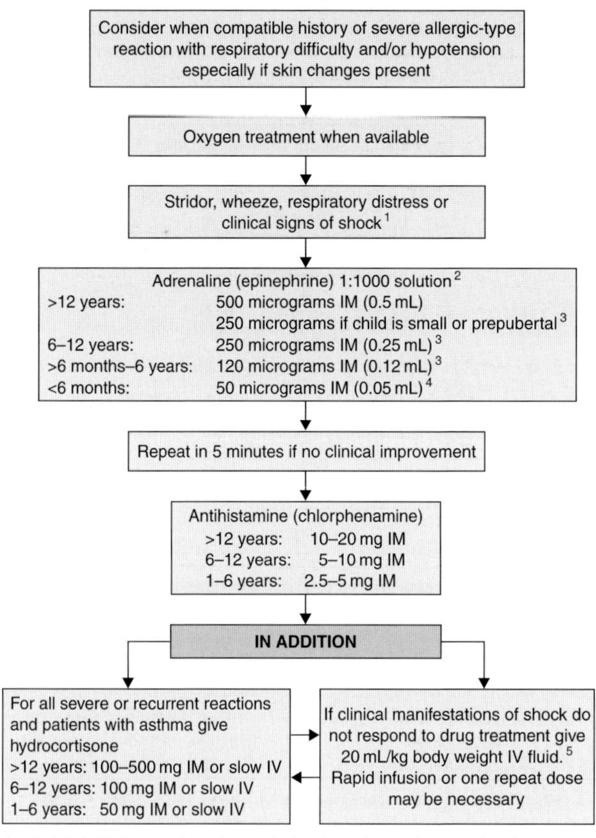

1. An inhaled beta$_2$-agonist such as salbutamol may be used as an adjunctive measure if bronchospasm is severe and does not respond rapidly to other treatment.
2. If profound shock judged **immediately** life threatening give CPR/ALS if necessary. Consider **slow** intravenous (IV) adrenaline (epinephrine) 1:10,000 solution. This is **hazardous** and is recommended only for an experienced practitioner who can also obtain IV access without delay. Note the different strength of adrenaline (epinephrine) that may be required for IV use.
3. For children who have been prescribed Epipen, 150 micrograms can be given instead of 120 micrograms, and 300 micrograms can be given instead of 250 micrograms of 500 micrograms.
4. Absolute accuracy of the small dose is not essential.
5. A crystalloid may be safer than a colloid.

Figure 2. Anaphylactic reactions: Treatment algorithm for children by first medical reponders. Reproduced with kind permission from Resuscitation Council (UK).

ventilated. The rhythm is often PEA or asystole. CPR is often prolonged. These patients are usually young people with healthy hearts and should make a good recovery provided the circulation is restored. Rapid volume expansion and high doses of adrenaline are required (see below). Transcutaneous pacing may be required.

Adrenaline (epinephrine) is the most important drug in the treatment of anaphylaxis. A dose of 0.5 mg to 1 mg (0.5–1.0 mL of 1:1000) adrenaline should be given intramuscularly as soon as possible to all patients with respiratory difficulties or hypotension. This may be repeated every ten minutes until improvement occurs.

The α-agonist effects of adrenaline cause vasoconstriction, increasing blood pressure and reducing angio-oedema and urticaria. The β-agonist actions of adrenaline reduce bronchoconstriction, produce positive inotropic and chronotropic effects and increase cyclic AMP which reduces mediator release.

Intravenous adrenaline may be used in severe cases with cardiovascular collapse in the hospital setting. A solution of 1 in 10,000 should be used and must be given slowly in aliquots of 50–100 μg. Cardiac monitoring is essential when intravenous adrenaline is given. Intravenous adrenaline can result in arrhythmias, severe hypertension, myocardial infarction and intracerebral haemorrhage. Cardiac complications with intramuscular adrenaline are rare, but can also occur.

Beta-blockers may increase the severity of anaphylactic reactions and antagonise the effects of adrenaline. Patients on beta blockers can fail to respond to adrenaline. In these patients, glucagon may be helpful. This agent is short acting and a dose of 1–2 mg every 5 minutes is required.

Patients receiving tricyclic antidepressants and monoamine oxidase inhibitors should receive half the dose of adrenaline.

Fluids—Patients need large volumes of fluids to compensate for the intravascular leak and vasodilation, usually between 2–4 litres of crystalloid. The use of crystalloids may be safer than colloids.

Antihistamine—Chlorpheniramine 10–20 mg should be given by slow intravenous infusion or intramuscular injection to antagonise the histamine response.

Hydrocortisone 100–300 mg should be given intravenously. The benefit of steroids does not occur until 4–6 hours after administration, however biphasic anaphylactic reactions with a late worsening of symptoms at 1–8 hours have been described. The use of hydrocortisone reduces this late stage response.

Inotropes—Catecholamine infusions may be needed to increase the blood pressure, adrenaline (4–8 $\mu g\,min^{-1}$) or noradrenaline (4–8 $\mu g\,min^{-1}$).

Bicarbonate—If the patient is acidotic, bicarbonate 0.5–1.0 $mmol\,kg^{-1}$ (equivalent to 0.5–1.0 mL of an 8.4% solution of sodium bicarbonate) may be required.

Bronchodilators should be given if there is persistent bronchospasm.

Observation for late effects should continue for 8–24 hours.

Investigations

Blood samples should be taken for mast cell tryptase. Tryptase is the principle protein of mast cell granules. It is an indicator of mast cell activation and is raised in both anaphylactic and anaphylactoid reactions. The basal tryptase level is 0.8–1.5 $ng\,mL^{-1}$. Levels of greater than 20 $ng\,mL^{-1}$ may be seen after anaphylactic reactions. The half life of tryptase is approximately 2.5 hours. Levels peak one hour after the onset of the reaction. Therefore approximately one hour after the beginning of the reaction 10 mL venous blood should be taken in a plain or EDTA bottle (check with your local lab). Plasma or serum may be stored at −20°C. A negative result does not completely exclude anaphylaxis.

Follow-up

After resuscitation it is essential to take a detailed history to determine all possible triggers. This is best done early to avoid missing possible triggers. The patient should be referred to an allergist for further investigation. All adverse drug reactions should be reported to the Committee of Safety of Medicines on a yellow card.

Patients should receive a written record of the reaction and be encouraged to carry a hazard card or Medic-alert bracelet. The general practitioner must also be informed.

Further reading

1 *Resuscitation Council (UK) Guidelines—The Emergency Medical Treatment of Anaphylactic Reactions for First Medical Responders and for Community Nurses*. Revised 2002; available at www.resus.org.uk
2 *Suspected Anaphylactic Reactions Associated with Anaesthesia*, revised edition 1995. London, The Association of Anaesthetists of Great Britain and Ireland. The British Society for Allergy and Clinical Immunology. Available at www.aagbi.org
3 Ewan PW. AC of allergies: Anaphylaxis. *Br J Anaesth.* 1998;316: 1442–1445.

63

Epilepsy

Peter Newman and Maureen Pearce

Epilepsy affects at least 1 in 150 of the population and will impinge in many ways during hospital treatments, whether these be emergency epilepsy admissions or for other purposes.

Epilepsy classification

Seizures are graded as partial or generalised.

- Partial (focal or localised onset) seizures such as a focal motor event or an olfactory disturbance are called ‘simple’ if there is no loss of awareness, or ‘complex’ if this occurs.
- Simple or complex partial seizures may become secondarily generalised.
- Other patients have primary generalised seizures, common examples of which are absence attacks seen in children or tonic-clonic attacks at any age.

Some drugs are more effective in some seizure types than in others, so it is important to classify seizures in all patients, and it is unacceptable to just state that someone has epilepsy.

When to start treatment

After a single seizure treatment is usually withheld unless a second attack occurs (50% risk). Exceptions are where there is an underlying condition such as a tumour or encephalitis when recurrence risk is high.

- Most patients are offered treatment if a second fit arises within an interval of weeks or months of the first.

- Consider the alternative causes of a 'seizure'—syncope, functional, cardiac—before starting therapy.
- If in doubt, wait.

When to stop treatment

After two or three years on treatment free of seizures there is a 60–70% chance that remission will continue even if the antiepileptic drug (AED) is withdrawn.

- Patients should be counselled about drug withdrawal and if proceeding, this should be cautious and gradual over 4 to 6 months.

Which treatment to use

The choice of AED is based on the seizure type, side effect profile, age and sex of the patient. For example, sodium valproate would be avoided in young women because it is teratogenic, but in other circumstances may be the drug of choice.

- The selected AED is introduced gradually, usually over 2–4 weeks to minimise adverse effects, but individual product advice should be consulted.
- Routine monitoring of drug levels is unnecessary and should be restricted to patients who are on high doses, who have side effects, or in whom poor compliance is suspected.
- Aim for an average dose, but be prepared to go higher if seizure control is not achieved, or to drop the level if dose related side effects develop.

Most patients respond to a single drug. If unsuccessful it should be withdrawn and an alternative substituted. About 10% of patients benefit from treatment with two drugs, or rarely with three, but these will be under specialist care.

For treating generalised tonic–clonic seizures use:

- Sodium valproate (Epilim) except in women who may become pregnant;
- Lamotrigine (Lamictal) is first choice in young women;
- Carbamazepine (Tegretol) is a reasonable alternative to valproate in most cases;

- Levetiracetam (Keppra), lamotrigine or topiramate (Topamax) are second line alternatives.

In childhood absence seizures use:
- Sodium valproate or ethosuximide (Zarontin).

For partial seizures the recommended anti-epileptic drugs are:
- Carbamazepine or valproate as first line;
- Phenytoin (Epanutin) as a second line, or possibly first choice in the elderly;
- Levetiracetam, topiramate, gabapentin (Neurontin) or lamotrigine as alternative second line.

Specialist advice should be sought before using unfamiliar drugs
Phenobarbitone is not generally used because of a relatively high level of side effects, but it is a very effective anticonvulsant and its cheapness makes it together with phenytoin one of the first choice drugs in developing countries.

Adverse effect of anti-epileptic drugs

All anti-epileptic drugs act on neurotransmitter pathways or brain cell ion channels. Central nervous system side effects are therefore common.

- Drowsiness, dizziness, double vision, sedation, memory or concentration impairment, unsteadiness, fatigue, headache and insomnia may be alleviated if the AED dose is reduced, but if persistent will require switching to an alternative drug.
- Systemic effects such as rash, hepatitic reaction or blood dyscrasia usually lead to urgent withdrawal and substitution.
- Drug interactions are common, especially with the AEDs which are liver enzyme inducers (particularly carbamazepine and phenytoin), but complex interactions are also seen when valproate is used with other drugs. Note that lamotrigine levels are lowered by concomitant carbamazepine or phenytoin, but raised by valproate, so smaller lamotrigine doses and slower increments are used when added to valproate.

Emergency anti-epileptic drugs loading

It is sometimes necessary to rapidly load a patient with an anti-epileptic drug, for example before a neurosurgical procedure or when a head injury is followed by seizures. Phenytoin or its pro-drug fosphenytoin are used. The advantages of the latter are speed of safe administration and, because of water solubility, reduced liability to cause thrombophlebitis. Each requires blood pressure and ECG monitoring.

- Phenytoin is injected or infused intravenously at a rate not exceeding 50 mg/minute to a loading dose of 15 mg/kg. Further increments of 100 mg each 6–8 hours maintains a therapeutic level which can be monitored in the plasma. Intravenous phenytoin should be flushed with physiological saline.
- Fosphenytoin can be infused more rapidly and is given as phenytoin equivalent (PE) at a rate of 100–150 PE/minute and a dose of 10–15 PE/kg.

Status epilepticus

- This is defined as prolonged or repetitive seizures without recovery in between, persisting for more than 30 minutes.
- It is thankfully now uncommon because of improved epilepsy treatments but it is a medical emergency and seizures must be rapidly controlled if irreversible brain damage is to be avoided.
- **Involvement of a senior clinician is mandatory in treating status epilepticus.**

The principals of treatment also apply to the more common problem of serial seizures. Clinicians should be aware of the existence of partial seizure status as well as the better known condition in which tonic–clonic seizures predominate.

- Note also that in some cases of apparent status epilepticus, the seizures are psychogenic, mimicking true status and providing a pitfall for the unwary.
- Patients in status epilepticus should usually be treated on the intensive care unit but initial measures are taken before transfer.
- Airway safety and oxygen administration are the first essentials.
- Blood gases and routine metabolic tests are assessed.
- Fifty mL of 50% glucose are given intravenously, as well as in adults in whom alcoholism is possible, 250 mg of thiamine.
- Oximetry, blood pressure, ECG and neurological status are carefully monitored.
- Hypoxia, acidosis, hypotension and cardiac irregularities may need to be corrected.

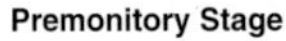

Premonitory Stage
Diazepam 10 mg IV (given over 2–5 min) or rectally,
repeated once 15 min later if status continues to threaten
or Lorazepam 4 mg IV bolus
↓
If seizures continue or status develops

↓

Stage of early status
Lorazepam 4 mg IV bolus (if not given earlier)

If status continues after 30 minutes

Stage of established status
Phenobarbital IV infusion of 10 mg/kg at a rate of 100 mg/min
(i.e. about 700 mg in an average adult over 7 min)
or
Phenytoin IV infusion of 15 mg/kg at a rate of 50 mg/min
(i.e. about 1000 mg PE in an average adult over 20 min)
or
Fasphenytoin IV infusion of 15 mg PE/kg at a rate of 100 mg PE/min
(i.e. about 1000 mg PE in an average adult over 10 min)

If status continues over 30–60 min

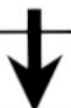

Stage of refractory status
General anaesthesia with either.
Propofol 2 mg/kg IV bolus, repeated if necessary,
and then followed by a continuous infusion of 5–10 mg/kg/h
initially, reducing to 1–3 mg/kg/h.
When status have been controlled for 72 h,
the drug dosage should be slowly tapered over 12 h
or
Thiopental: 100–250 mg IV bolus given over 20 s, with further 50 mg
boluses every 2–3 min until seizures are controlled, followed
by a continuous IV infusion to maintain a burst
suppression pattern on
The EEG (usually 3–5 mg/kg/h).
Thiopental should be slowly withdrawn 12 h after the last seizure

Figure 1. Emergency treatment of status epilepticus. (Reproduced with kind permission from S. Shorvon (2000) *Handbook of Epilepsy Treatment*. Blackwell Science Ltd.)

- In resistant cases or where there is an underlying structural lesion, raised intracranial pressure should be controlled by intravenous dexamethasone, mannitol or neurosurgery.
- Do not forget to maintain levels of the routine AED regime.

In treating a patient in status epilepticus, *time is of the essence*. The above measures are dealt with while at the same time the emergency drug treatment is instigated, according to the principles in the Figure.

- The staged process is time capped and leads to anaesthesia with propofol or thiopental on the ICU if initial measures fail to resolve the seizures.
- Early involvement of anaesthesia colleagues is therefore vital.
- Electroencephalographic monitoring becomes important in ICU management.

The high morbidity and significant mortality of status epilepticus can be substantially improved by attention to the above principles in which urgent, focussed and timed treatment is given by well trained clinicians.

64

The management of near-drowning

Jason Easby

Introduction

Drowning is defined as death due to asphyxia following submersion in a fluid; usually water. Near-drowning therefore implies survival (however temporary). Drowning accounts for up to 1000 deaths a year in the UK, and is the third most common cause of accidental death in children (after road traffic accidents and burns).

The majority of all drowning victims are aged less than 20 years, and as much as 50% are less than four years of age. The incidence of near-drowning is unknown. Risk factors include: inadequate responsible supervision, alcohol, recreational drugs, suicide, trauma, epilepsy and myocardial infarction. Therefore the potential for an underlying cause must be sought on presentation, and cervical spine injury must be considered in every diving accident.

Pathophysiology

Wet drowning is associated with aspiration of fluid into the lungs and accounts for up to 85% of cases. Dry drowning occurs in 15%, and is found when no fluid is aspirated, possibly due to reflex laryngospasm and apnoea, or by the absorption of fluid into the bloodstream before the onset of cardiac arrest secondary to hypoxia. Drowning is dissimilar to the immersion syndrome, in which sudden immersion into cold water causes an intense sympathetic response with increased vasomotor tone and bradycardia. Death occurs secondary to myocardial ischaemia and cardiac arrest.

The difference between fresh and saltwater drowning has been over-emphasized, and does not change the initial management. The volume of fluid aspirated is usually insufficient to produce the major electrolyte disturbance and fluid overload that has been sought in the past.

Hypoxia is the final common pathway resulting in death. The principal mechanisms leading to hypoxia include: a reduction in pulmonary compliance due to the inactivation and dilution of lung surfactant, intrapulmonary shunting due to lung atelectasis and pulmonary oedema, and alveolar obstruction due to the aspiration of fluid, debris and vomit.

Clinical presentation

The clinical picture encompasses a broad spectrum of illness. Most present awake and alert, and probably have not sustained a significant hypoxic injury. Others will have significant hypoxia, and may have suffered a cardiac arrest at some point. Care must be taken for patients presenting in the mid spectrum. Delayed respiratory failure, due to pulmonary oedema has been reported in previously normal patients up to 72 hours after the initial event. This 'secondary drowning' warrants admission for all near drowning victims, as up to 15% of patients who are conscious on arrival may die from respiratory failure.

Management

At the scene

- Safety of the rescuer is of prime importance.
- Help should be sought at the earliest opportunity, and the victim transported to hospital.
- In-water resuscitation should not delay the landing of the casualty.
- The duration of hypoxia is critical to outcome, and requires immediate relief. The ABC of emergency management must be emphasized. Vital signs should be assessed and basic life support initiated when appropriate.
- The potential for cervical spine injury should be considered and appropriate immobilization techniques employed.
- If spontaneously breathing returns, management in the recovery position, to reduce the risk of aspiration is appropriate. (Care is needed if cervical spine injury suspected.)

- No attempt should be made to remove water from the lungs; this increases the incidence of aspiration. The Heimlich manoeuvre is no longer recommended. If vomit or debris is present in the upper airway this can be removed by a finger sweep.
- Hypothermia is common. Therefore the victim should be kept as dry and warm as possible.

In hospital

- Near-drowning is an emergency; and victims who appear normal on admission can deteriorate rapidly.
- Many patients arrive hypoxic, acidotic and hypothermic.
- A rapid detailed assessment is required. Advanced Trauma Life Support algorithms are useful, following the primary and secondary survey approach.
- Resuscitation should be continued and if cardiac arrest is present, Advanced Cardiac Life Support algorithms should be followed.
- All patients should receive 100% oxygen, and endotracheal intubation should be performed early if required.
- A nasogastric tube should be passed once the airway is protected, to empty the stomach contents and reduce the incidence of aspiration.
- The application of PEEP to ventilated patients or facial CPAP to those spontaneously breathing may prove valuable in correcting hypoxaemia.
- Suggested indications for mechanical ventilation include:
  - Inability to maintain PaO_2 >100 mm Hg in 40% O_2;
  - An AaO_2 gradient >150 mm Hg;
  - Borderline ventilation/oxygenation with associated brain injury;
  - Glasgow coma score <8;
  - Inability to maintain a patent, protected airway.
- Haemodynamic support maybe required including the use of warmed intravenous fluids and the use of inotropes.
- Hypothermia should be prevented and corrected by passive and active means. This may include; warm air blowers, peritoneal lavage or cardiopulmonary bypass. A low core body temperature (<30ºC) adversely affects resuscitation and predisposes to spontaneous refractory ventricular fibrillation, coagulopathy and altered drug metabolism.
- As a general rule it is recommended that resuscitation should not be discontinued until core temperature is at least 32ºC or cannot be raised despite active measures. This may prove to be difficult.

- A secondary survey should be performed and the patient examined fully, to exclude injury or predisposing cause.
- Early neurological assessment is vital, as these parameters are closely linked to ultimate outcome.
- Prophylactic antibiotics and anticonvulsants have been used empirically, but have not been shown to improve outcome. Corticosteroids are of no benefit.

Investigations

- Routine non-invasive monitoring should be applied including; pulse oximetry, ECG and NIBP;
- Core temperature measurement; usually by an oesophageal or low reading rectal thermometer;
- Arterial blood gases;
- Baseline laboratory investigations; FBC, U&E, blood glucose, cardiac enzymes, LFTs and clotting screen;
- Chest X-ray. Radiological findings are variable and correlate poorly with clinical findings;
- Hourly urine output (low threshold for urine catheter);
- Invasive monitoring may be required, including; arterial blood pressure analysis, central venous access, or a pulmonary artery catheter;
- Drug screen for overdose of paracetamol, alcohol, aspirin, etc.

Definitive care

- Patients should be admitted to a HDU/ITU environment for further monitoring and care. The potential for secondary drowning must not be forgotten.
- The development of Acute Respiratory Distress Syndrome (ARDS) may occur early or late in the disease process. Pulmonary oedema and intrapulmonary shunting result in further hypoxaemia and hypercarbia necessitating advanced respiratory care.
- Hypoxia results in a multisystem insult, and the incidence of multiple organ failure (MOF) may be increased by bowel ischaemia and the translocation of bacteria. Gastrointestinal bleeding may arise. Cerebral oedema is common and is associated with an elevation in intracranial pressure, and this may be exacerbated by the

Table 1. Favourable prognostic indicators.

Children >3 years

- Evidence of spontaneous respiratory effort
- Females
- Water temperature <10°C
- Duration of submersion <5 minutes
- No aspiration
- Start of effective basic life support within 10 minutes
- Spontaneous cardiac output on arrival in the hospital
- Minimum blood pH >7.1
- Blood glucose <11.2 mmol litre^{-1}
- Glasgow Coma Score >6. No coma on admission
- Pupillary response present

onset of ARDS. Acute renal failure is less common in the early stage but maybe precipitated by rhabdomyolysis. The development of MOF may also be delayed, as sepsis ensues, commonly secondary to aspiration pneumonia.

- Electrolyte derangement is not uncommon, and requires appropriate therapy. Frequently encountered abnormalities include hypo- and hypernatraemia, hypo- and hyperkalaemia, hypocalcaemia, hyperglycaemia and hyperosmolality.

Outcome

- The duration of submersion and hypoxia are the critical factors determining outcome.
- 70% of children survive a near-downing episode if effective basic life support is provided at the scene. Survival falls to 40% without on scene resuscitation.
- Of these survivors around 70% will make a good recovery (Table 1), 25% will have a mild neurological deficit. The remainder will be severely disabled or remain in a persistent vegetative state.
- The onset of hypothermia is crucial to survival. Reports exist of children submerged in icy cold-water surviving prolonged resuscitation attempts. In this instance, hypothermia develops rapidly and provides cerebral protection from hypoxaemia. If hypothermia develops at a later stage, due to heat loss by evaporation, it is not protective.

65

Hypothermia

Diane Monkhouse

Definition

Hypothermia is defined as a core temperature of less than 35ºC. Three degrees of severity are recognised:

- Mild (32–35ºC)
- Moderate (30–32ºC)
- Severe (<30ºC)

Classification

- Therapeutic hypothermia—temperature is deliberately lowered as part of a therapeutic strategy (for example, circulatory arrest during cardiac surgery).
- Accidental hypothermia
  - Primary—associated with extreme cold exposure in an individual with normal thermoregulation (for example, cold water immersion);
  - Secondary—associated with abnormal thermogenesis (for example, hypothyroidism).

Aetiology

- Decreased heat production;
- Increased heat loss;
- Underlying disease process.

Hypothermia is more common in extremes of age, where poor thermoregulation increases susceptibility to cold. In young adults, the most common cause is environmental exposure confounded by immobility and/or impaired conscious level.

Pathophysiology

- **Cardiovascular**—With mild to moderate hypothermia, there is an initial increase in cardiac output due to sympathetic activity. However, as core temperature decreases, heart rate, blood pressure and cardiac output all fall resulting in decreased tissue perfusion. ECG changes include sinus bradycardia, prolongation of PR, QRS and QT intervals and generalised T wave inversion. Below 33°C, J waves may appear. They are extra deflections at the QRS–ST junction and are pathognomonic of hypothermia. Supraventricular dysrythmias, most commonly atrial fibrillation, occur below 30°C while refractory ventricular fibrillation is common at temperatures below 28°C. If cooling is rapid, VF can occur at higher temperatures. VF can be precipitated by stimulation such as endotracheal intubation or central venous catheter insertion. Below 20°C, asystole occurs.
- **Respiratory**—After an initial reflex stimulation of respiration, there is a progressive reduction in respiratory rate and tidal volume until spontaneous ventilation ceases at 24°C. Hypoxia results from impaired hypoxic pulmonary vasoconstriction, diminished gas transfer and a reduction in oxygen availability at tissue level (the oxygen-dissociation curve is moved to the left). Loss of consciousness and impaired cough reflex increase the risk of aspiration.
- **Gastrointestinal**—Gastroparesis and ileus occur below 34°C.

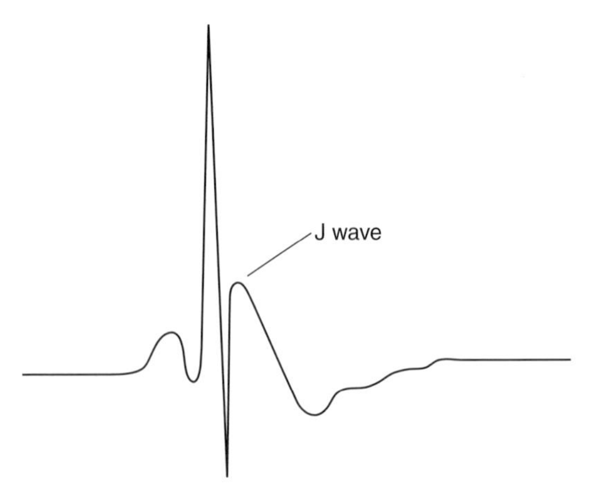

Figure 1. ECG changes showing 'J wave'.

- **Metabolic**—The shivering phase occurs between 30 and 35ºC. This compensatory mechanism stimulates energy production by breakdown of glycogen stores. When the temperature falls below 30ºC, the non-shivering phase commences. At this stage, thermoregulation starts to fail, metabolism slows dramatically and organ dysfunction ensues. The metabolic rate decreases by 6% for every degree Celsius reduction in body temperature. Reduction in oxygen consumption, however, conveys some degree of protection from hypoxia. Severe mixed metabolic and respiratory acidosis due to tissue hypoperfusion and hypoventilation is common. Insulin resistance and impaired peripheral glucose utilisation lead to hyperglycaemia. However, hypoglycaemia may ensue due to glycogen depletion in prolonged hypothermic states. Hepatic enzymatic activity is depressed.
- **Renal**—Initial peripheral vasoconstriction causes a cold diuresis. This is followed by a reduction in renal blood flow and glomerular filtration rate secondary to reduced cardiac output and increased vascular tone.
- **Neurological**—There is generalised cerebral depression culminating in loss of consciousness and papillary dilatation at 30ºC. Both cerebral blood flow and cerebral metabolic rate decrease in a linear fashion. The EEG is isoelectric below 20ºC.

Diagnosis

- Relies upon a high index of clinical suspicion and accurate temperature measurement using a low-reading thermometer;
- Sites for monitoring core temperature include tympanic membrane, nasopharynx, distal oesophagus, pulmonary artery and rectum;
- Death cannot be confirmed until core temperature has been corrected to 35ºC.

Investigations

- Urea and electrolytes, full blood count and coagulation screen;
- Blood glucose;
- Arterial blood gas (correct for temperature);
- ECG (check for dysrhythmias and prolongation of PQRST complex);

- Amylase (high levels do not necessarily imply pancreatitis);
- Toxicology screen including blood alcohol level;
- Thyroid function tests to exclude hypothyroidism;
- CXR to exclude aspiration and LVF.

Management

The basic principles include:

- ***Reduction of further heat loss***—Patient should be placed in a warm environment and have wet clothes removed. Gentle handling is imperative to minimise the risk of precipitating VF. **Do not elevate cold limbs!**
- ***Restoration and maintenance of cardio-respiratory stability*** using the ABC approach. Patients with GCS <8 or in respiratory failure should be intubated and ventilated with warmed, humidified oxygen. Insertion of a central venous catheter may precipitate dysrhythmias but is often technically easier than peripheral access in a profoundly vasoconstricted patient. It can also be used to guide (warmed) fluid resuscitation and deliver vasoactive drugs. Arrhythmogenic vasopresssors should be avoided. Tachydysrhythmias usually resolve with re-warming and are characteristically resistant to chemical and electrical cardioversion. Temporary pacing may be required for refractory bradycardia. In event of cardiac arrest, advanced life support should be continued until core temperature reaches 35ºC. When core temperature is <28ºC, cardiac massage may precipitate VF and is therefore best avoided even if pulses are absent.
- ***Re-warming*** is the mainstay of treatment. Passive external re-warming is achieved by wrapping the patient in blankets and is adequate for mild hypothermia where core temperature increase is typically 0.5ºC per hour. Hot air blankets are an ideal way of providing active external warming and should be used for mild to moderate hypothermia. Peripheral vasodilatation may cause hypotension and a further drop in temperature. Active core re-warming methods allow rapid temperature correction but are invasive. They include airway re-warming; gastric, rectal, pleural or peritoneal lavage; haemodialysis using a blood warmer and cardiopulmonary bypass. These methods are reserved for the management of refractory cardiac dysrhythmias in the severely hypothermic.

- ***Treatment of the underlying condition***—The cause may be obvious but other conditions such as drug and/or alcohol intoxication, hypoglycaemia, CVA, hypothyroidism or hypopituitarism should be excluded.
- ***Prevention of complications*** requires careful monitoring and early intervention, particularly with regard to infection.

Prognosis

- Mortality varies from 20 to 85% depending on the age, significant co-morbidity, severity of hypothermia and lag-phase to treatment.

Always

- Use a low-reading thermometer to measure core temperature;
- Look for and treat the underlying cause;
- Remove wet clothing prior to re-warming;
- Handle the patient with care to minimise the risk of precipitating VF;
- Avoid arrhythmogenic vasopressors;
- Avoid cardiac massage in patients with core temperature <28°C;
- Watch for after drop and hypotension on re-warming.

Never

- Confirm death until core temperature reaches 35°C.

66

Overdose

Samit Mitra and Gaynor Creaby

Introduction

Overdose is a common presentation to the Emergency Department and causes significant morbidity and mortality. The pattern of overdose is continually changing as newer drugs are developed and abused. Overdoses are either accidental (usually children) or intentional to cause self-harm. Even if the substance ingested does not require active medical treatment, any patient having taken a deliberate overdose should be observed until a full and thorough psychiatric assessment is made. It is vital to act in a timely manner as many overdoses can deteriorate quickly. This usually means simultaneous history taking, examination and emergency treatment.

It is important to consider your own safety together with that of your team's, as patients can be agitated, aggressive or carrying dangerous objects (e.g. syringes and needles).

These patients can present in many ways and overdose needs to be considered in all unconscious, convulsing or confused patients and those where the diagnosis is not immediately obvious. Pre-hospital personnel, family or the patient themselves may have useful information about medications, possible amounts taken and overdose timing. It is also important to note that overdose patients may give inaccurate histories in particular in relation to the substances taken and also the timing of the ingestion.

It is good practice to utilise poison centres and also information databases for detailed specific information on individual overdoses and poisoning. This is especially relevant with regard to combined overdoses.

General priorities

Although it may be tempting to reach for specific antidotes when an overdose patient arrives, it is essential that all patients are assessed from an Airway, Breathing and Circulation point of view. It is important to consider the possibility of co-existent injury, underlying medical conditions and the patient's usual medications.

- You need a good reason not to use Toxbase or the Poisons centre.
- The overdose patient gives a notoriously inaccurate history.
- Take paracetamol and salicylate levels unless strong reason not to.
- The nasopharyngeal airway is often better tolerated than an oropharyngeal airway.
- If a patient can tolerate an oropharyngeal airway call an anaesthetist.
- Pulmonary oedema can be caused by several drugs.
- Take early glucose levels, urea and electrolytes and blood gases.
- Gastric lavage rarely needed and not to punish patient.
- Inducing vomiting rarely needed.
- Charcoal may need to be repeated.
- Beware aware of sustained release drugs.
- Don't discharge patient without full psychiatric assessment.
- Antidotes themselves can cause problems—be prepared.
- X-ray of the abdomen may show iron, iodide, enteric-coated tablets.

Airway

Any drug that can reduce conscious level (opiates, benzodiazepines) or that can cause vomiting (paracetamol, iron) can cause airway compromise. This is often compounded by ingestion of alcohol.

All patients need a clear airway, and this can be obtained by simple airway manoeuvres, or by airway adjuncts. Any overdose patient that can tolerate a Guedel airway should be assessed by an experienced anaesthetist for consideration of airway protection by endotracheal intubation.

Great care must be taken if a Guedel airway is inserted as this may induce vomiting. A nasopharyngeal airway is helpful and is often better tolerated. High-flow oxygen is essential initially in patients with airway, breathing or haemodynamic compromise. However, in cases of paraquat poisoning, supplemental oxygen may actually worsen outcome. Hyperbaric oxygen can be used for carbon monoxide poisoning.

Breathing

Overdose can cause respiratory depression (ethanol, barbiturates, opiates, benzodiazepines) and so ventilation must be supported when required. Adequacy of ventilation must be assessed clinically and also by use of oxygen saturation and blood gas monitoring. Several medications taken in excess can cause an increased respiratory rate (theophylline, cyanide, salicylates, methanol, ethanol and ethylene glycol).

Circulation

Many overdoses cause tachycardia (tricyclic antidepressants, bronchodilators, amphetamines, cocaine), any many cause bradycardia (beta blockers, insecticides, digoxin). Hypotension may be associated with sedatives, narcotics, antihypertensives, theophylline, tricyclic antidepressants, iron, phenothiazines, and phenytoin. General measures in the management would include a fluid challenge (providing there is no pulmonary oedema) and the appropriate antidote if indicated (e.g. glucagon in beta-blocker overdose). Occasionally inotropic support may be required. However, concurrent trauma, hypothermia and infection must be considered and excluded. Hypertension may be associated with cocaine, ecstacy, amphetamines.

ECG manifestations of overdose

Prolonged QT interval	Ethylene glycol
	Tricyclic antidepressants
	Class 1 anti-arrhythmics
Prolonged QRS interval	Phenothiazines
	Tricyclic antidepressants
	Class 1 anti-arrhythmics
Atrioventricular block	Beta-Blockers
	Calcium channel antagonists

	Digoxin
	Tricyclic antidepressants
Ventricular tachyarrythmias	Amphetamines
	Cocaine
	Digoxin
	Theophylline
	Tricyclic antidepressants
	Class 1 anti-arrhythmics

Disability and pupils

Overdoses can cause a fall in conscious level (opiates), and can cause severe agitation (Ectasy). Some can cause marked fluctuations in conscious level (Gamma hydroxybutyric acid—GHB). Pinpoint pupils are commonly seen with opiates and in rare cases, organophosphate and phenothiazine overdose. Dilated pupils are commonly seen with amphetamines, carbamazepine, cocaine, atropine and tricyclic antidepressants. Convulsions may be caused by carbamazepine, organophosphates, phenothiazines, and tricyclic antidepressants.

Exposure

Hypothermia can be due to exposure or the drug itself (sedatives or alcohol) and should be managed according to standard guidelines. Hyperthermia can be seen in ecstasy, amphetamines, cocaine, phenothiazine and salicylates. For dangerous core temperatures (above 41°C) the patient needs to be rapidly cooled with immersion in cool water, fanning and treatment of seizures as these may be the underlying cause. Dantrolene can be considered after discussion with the poisons centre. Cyanosis occurs as a result of hypoxaemia and can be mimicked in cases of methaemoglobinaemia and also by ergotamine. Flushed red skin can be seen with carbon monoxide (rare and late), cyanide (rare), and anticholinergics (hot, red and dry). Barbiturates can cause skin rashes (bullae).

Gastric lavage

This procedure was previously widely used until several years ago. It is now clear that routine gastric lavage is no longer appropriate and in fact can cause significant morbidity (aspiration, oesophageal perforation, local trauma and electrolyte disturbance) and even death. There is also no clear evidence that gastric lavage favourably affects outcome. Gastric lavage however may be considered if the overdose was taken within one hour, and a potentially fatal amount of substance has been ingested. It must not be performed after ingestion of corrosives or hydrocarbons. Delayed gastric emptying occurs with anti-cholinergics, opiates, salicylates, iron and gastric lavage may be appropriate after one hour after discussion with a poison centre.

If the technique is to be performed then the following should be used as a guide:

- Lavage may compromise the airway. Therefore, if the GCS is reduced or a fall is anticipated, the airway needs to be protected by endotracheal intubation. This usually means that an anaesthetist needs to be present.
- Monitoring must include a minimum of ECG monitoring, oxygen saturation and non-invasive blood pressure.
- Full resuscitation facilities must be available.
- If the patient is awake a full explanation should be given and verbal consent taken.
- Use a large bore gastric tube by the oral or nasal route.
- The patient should be lying on their left side with head down on a tiltable trolley.
- Aspirate first prior to fluid lavage and check acidity of aspirate by litmus paper.
- Instill 200 mL water or normal saline into stomach.
- Aspirate fluid back—send for toxicology if required.
- Repeat lavage until aspirate is clear.

Emesis

Previously ipecacuanha was widely used to induce vomiting. It is now seldom used as no clear benefit has been shown and there is risk of increased morbidity.

Charcoal

This may be effective up to one hour post ingestion to decrease drug absorption. Charcoal is not effective in ingestion of the following substances; cyanide, ethanol, ethylene glycol, iron, lithium, methanol, petroleum products, strong acids and strong alkalis.

Haemodialysis

Potentially useful for lithium, methanol, salicylates, anti-freeze, phenobarbitone.

Haemoperfusion

Potentially useful for theophylline, paraquat.

Investigations

Full blood count, urea/electrolytes, clotting screen and blood gases can be of value initially and offer clues to the diagnosis. ECG should be considered if there is a clinical indication or an overdose is taken that can abnormal cardiac rhythm. With certain overdoses measuring blood levels can aid in management (e.g. antifreeze, carboxyhaemoglobin, digoxin, iron, lithium, methanol, paracetemol, salicylate, theophylline and valproate). However, it is essential to be sure of the timing of the overdose to the drawing of blood.

X-rays may be useful for iron, chloral hydrate, heavy metals and condoms containing illicit drugs.

Monitoring

All overdoses require initial monitoring of cardiac rhythm, pulse oximetry and blood pressure.

Antidotes

- **Opiates:** Naloxone 0.4–2 mg intravenously reverses opiate overdoses. Naloxone 0.8 mg intramuscularly should be given at the same time as intravenous naloxone wears off quickly. An infusion of naloxone may be required.
- **Benzodiazepines:** The reversal agent flumazenil should not be used in mixed overdoses and can precipitate seizures.

Table 1. Treatment of specific overdose.

Drug	Treatment
Anti-freeze	Ethanol, fomepizole
Benzodiazepines	Flumazenil (not if any possibility of mixed overdose)
Beta blockers	Glucagon
Calcium blockers	Calcium chloride/gluconate
Cyanide	Sodium nitrite/thiosulphate, amyl nitrate, dicobalt edetate
Digoxin	Digibind
Isoniazid	Pyridoxine
Methanol	Ethanol
Opioids	Naloxone
Paracetemol	N-acetylcysteine, methionine
Warfarin	Vitamin K, fresh frozen plasma
Organophosphates	Atropine, pralidoxime
Hydrofluoric acid	Calcium gluconate
Iron	Desferrioxamine
Tricyclics	Sodium bicarbonates

- **Paracetemol:** Remember that a level before four hours is meaningless. N-acetylcysteine before four hours has no benefit—wait for a level. Large overdose (>12 g in adults) after seven hours start N-acetylcysteine after level taken. Don't forget to ask about enzyme inducers, malnourished, excessive alcohol—high risk line on treatment graph. Methionine (oral) can be used instead of N-acetylcysteine.
- **Tricyclic antidepressants:** If patient unwell (cardiovascularly) give sodium bicarbonate to alkalinise.
- **Ecstasy:** Need supportive care—rehydation, rate and temperature control and prevention of renal failure.
- **Cocaine** can cause ECG changes of acute myocardial infarct or ischaemia

Further reading and help

1 National Poison Information Centre (United Kingdom) 0870-600-6266

2 TOXBASE Website: www.spib.axl.co.uk

67

Stridor

Mike Tremlett

Introduction

Listening in a quiet room, the breathing of a normal subject at rest is inaudible at more than a foot away from the mouth. Breathing becomes 'noisy' (audible) when airflow in the proximal (upper) airways (pharynx, larynx or trachea) is turbulent. This occurs in one of two circumstances:

(a) High rates of air flow (e.g.: exercise);
(b) Narrowing of these upper airways.

Stridor is noisy breathing, with sound occurring predominantly on inspiration. It is easily audible without the need for a stethoscope. It tends to be relatively high pitched, and differs from snoring in that the patient is not asleep. Stridor is different from wheeze in a number of ways. Wheeze occurs during exhalation rather than inspiration. When audible, wheeze is due to vibration of the larger intra-thoracic (lower) airways as they narrow on breathing almost to the point of closure.

The presence of stridor in a subject at rest indicates partial obstruction of the upper airways, and always requires urgent assessment and management.

Aetiology

Upper airway obstruction may occasionally exist without stridor, but only when airway obstruction is complete or almost complete, and therefore airflow is minimal. The two usually go together. The age of the patient and speed of onset of symptoms and signs give important clues to the possible underlying cause (Tables 1 and 2).

Table 1. Common causes of upper airway obstruction in adults.

Sudden onset: (Minutes to hours)	Gradual onset: (Days to weeks)
Anaphylaxis	Pharyngeal tumours
Toxic gas inhalation	Vocal cord palsies
Acute epiglottitis	Laryngeal tumours and polyps
Inhaled foreign body	Crico-arytenoid rheumatoid arthritis
	Thyroid enlargement
	Post tracheostomy granulomas
	Tracheal tumours
	Paratracheal compression by lymph nodes (e.g. tuberculosis)
	Post intubation strictures

Table 2. Common causes of upper airway obstruction in children.

Sudden onset: (Minutes to hours)	Gradual onset: (Days to weeks)
Laryngotracheobronchitis (Croup)	Laryngomalacia
Acute epiglottitis	Tracheomalacia
Bacterial tracheitis	Sub-glottic stenosis
Foreign body aspiration	Vascular ring
Anaphylaxis	Micrognathia
Post intubation oedema	Down's syndrome
Retropharyngeal abscess	Mucopolysacharidoses
Diphtheria	Laryngeal papillomatosis
Acute tonsillitis	

Assessment

The presence of stridor is a medical emergency. Successful management requires the ability to rapidly assess the severity of the upper airway obstruction present. The presence of stridor in a child is especially important. Small changes in size of an initially small larynx or trachea markedly increase the resistance of the tube to airflow. If the resistance of the upper airways is considerably raised, then either the negative intra-thoracic pressure needed to cause inspiration or the duration of inspiration itself, will need to increase to keep the amount of air going into and out of the lungs (alveolar ventilation) unchanged. The energy required to breath, that is to contract the diaphragm and intercostals muscles to move the chest wall on inspiration and thus expand the elastic lung tissue and overcome the heat expended resisting expiration must increase. This is the 'work of breathing'. If this cannot increase adequately to maintain alveolar ventilation, then alveolar ventilation falls and respiratory failure is present. Assessment should only take a matter of minutes, with much of the examination being undertaken simultaneously with obtaining the key points in the history. The key questions to answer are:

(a) How much **effort** is being expended to breathe? (= how much **work** is being done to breathe?)
(b) What is the **efficacy** of the breathing? (= for all the work of breathing taking place, how much alveolar ventilation is actually occurring?)
(c) Is respiration **effective?** (= is the combination of ventilation and blood flow around the circulation adequate to deliver enough oxygen to important end organs, such as the brain?).

All three questions can be answered predominately by simple clinical examination, without the need for complex investigation. Each will be considered in turn. The answers will indicate the general management required.

(a) EFFORT of breathing

Sitting on the bed, watching a subject breath over one minute will tell you how much effort is being expended to breath. The **respiratory rate** is the first important assessment. A faster than normal rate indicates increased work being undertaken, but more worrying a slow rate with shallow breaths may suggest exhaustion.

Children have a thin and compliant chest wall. **Recession** (the in-drawing of tissue between the ribs on inspiration), is a common sign of increased work of breathing in all conditions causing breathing difficulty. Recession of the sternum indicates significant upper airways obstruction.

The **use of accessory muscles** (contraction of the sternocleidomastoid muscles on inspiration) also indicates increased work of breathing.

(b) EFFICACY of breathing

Again sit on the bed and look at the breathing. Watch the amount of **chest expansion** on inspiration, and also abdominal excursion.

With severe upper airways obstruction, a see-saw type ventilatory pattern may be seen, with the chest sucking in on inspiration and the abdomen bulging out, and the opposite on expiration.

Auscultation of the chest with a stethoscope for **breath sounds** will also give some idea of the amount of air movement occurring in and out of the lungs. The loudness of the stridor does NOT signify the degree of upper airways obstruction present. Very little air movement may cause quite quiet stridor, so beware!

(c) EFFECTIVENESS of respiration

Simple observation will give clues as to the effectiveness of respiration. An altered **level of consciousness** may reflect inadequate oxygen delivery to the brain. The stress of hypoxia stimulates catecholamine release (adrenaline/noradrenaline), producing vasoconstriction and pallor (altered **skin colour**). The presence of central cyanosis (blue discolouration of the lips) indicates at least 5 g of deoxygenated haemoglobin in the blood. It is a very late sign of sign of acute respiratory failure, and if present suggests a patient close to completely stopping breathing (respiratory arrest). **Pulse oximetry** rapidly gives an excellent estimate of the effectiveness of respiration.

The patient with stridor may thus present a range of clinical pictures. At one extreme, the patient may have relatively quiet stridor. The subject may be a child with a slow, laboured respiratory rate. Marked recession may be present. The subject is sitting with arms providing support allowing more effective use of accessory muscles. Auscultation of the chest may elicit minimal air movement. Exhaustion is clearly present, with pulse oximetry readings of less than 90% despite high flow facial oxygen. This child clearly demonstrates features of severe respiratory failure due to upper airways obstruction, and subsequent management will be very different from the other clinical extreme.

Alternatively, the subject may have very load stridor, a relatively normal respiratory rate with minimal recession or use of accessory muscles. If the subject is a child it may even be playing contentedly. Auscultation may reveal good airflow with saturations at normal levels breathing room air. The majority of patients lie between these extremes and management will depend on where they lie on the continuum and whether they improve or not on initial definitive care. There is no substitute for experience. Do not be reticent in requesting senior help when faced with a subject with stridor.

Management

All patients presenting with stridor should receive high flow oxygen via a facemask with a reservoir while initial clinical assessment is made.

Management will then vary according to the age of the patient, and whether respiratory failure is felt to be absent, pending or present.

(a) Adults

If respiratory failure is pending or present, multiple investigations are neither appropriate nor safe. The history and clinical assessment may suggest the level of likely obstruction, e.g: hoarseness suggests a lesion at laryngeal level. The quick use of a nasal-endoscope will allow rapid examination of pharynx and larynx, and demonstrate the level and severity of the obstruction.

Inexpert use of a fibreoptic scope and biopsy of any obstructing tumour, may cause to bleeding or oedema. The obstruction may rapidly worsen and death follows. With gross obstruction at or above the larynx, an immediate threat to life or impending respiratory failure, where a non-infective cause of obstruction is present, the formation of a tracheostomy by an Ear, Nose and Throat surgeon under local anaesthetic may be the safest first option. If obstruction is due to advanced laryngeal malignancy, debulking of the tumour to enlarge the airway is often possible with the use of a laser.

Infective causes, such as acute epiglottis may be fatal in adults as well as children, and a short history of symptoms, high fever, significant pain with drooling of saliva suggests the diagnosis. Early involvement of an anaesthetist to potentially intubate the patient ('secure the airway') and intravenous antibiotics are required.

In cases of sub-glottic obstruction or where respiratory failure is not present or pending, assessment of the upper airway with both fibreoptic and rigid scopes (under general anaesthesia) may be appropriate. The cause of the obstruction is often readily identifiable from the history and examination, and definitive treatment may then be started.

Patients should not be sent for radiological investigations (neck or chest X-rays or more complex imaging) unless absolutely no risk of significant obstruction of the airway is present.

(b) Children

Children are different. Initial clinical assessment will identify present or pending respiratory failure and those without (Table 3).

All infants and children with evidence of actual or pending respiratory failure should not be upset in any way. No attempts to view the airway should be undertaken. They should be allowed to stay sitting up and not laid flat. Cannulation probably should be avoided. Senior paediatric, anaesthetic and ENT staff must be called rapidly to help. High flow oxygen should be given by mask if tolerated. Where an infective cause of the obstruction at laryngeal level is suspected, administration of nebulised epinephrine (5 mg [5 mL of 1:1000] in oxygen) may bring about short-term improvement, giving time for senior help to arrive. The child will need to be intubated under controlled circumstances. Anaesthesia will need to be induced in theatre or similar environment, with spontaneous respiration maintained. The distance from ward to theatre should be short, and transfer undertaken with full resuscitative equipment including facilities to perform and oxygenate the child via cricothyroid puncture should complete obstruction occur. **No patient should be transferred between hospital sites unless or until a safe airway has been secured.** Only when the level, cause of the obstruction, its severity established by direct vision, and an endotracheal tube placed, will controlled ventilation be started. The presence of a senior ENT

Table 3. Extremes of clinical presentation of stridor in small children.

Stridor	Loud	Quiet
Respiratory rate	Fast	Slow
Recession	Mild intercostal	Severe intercostals and sternal
Breath sounds	Good	Markedly reduced
Heart rate	Mildly raised	Significant tachycardia or bradycardia
Skin colour	Normal	Pale
Mental status	Alert	Agitated or drowsy
Assessment	Child at present compensating for upper airway obstruction	Severe respiratory failure secondary to upper airway obstruction; respiratory arrest likely
Management	Give definitive treatment according to probable underlying cause; reassess regularly	'Secure' the airway; subsequently, control the breathing

Surgeon in theatre able to perform emergency tracheostomy if complete obstruction of the airway occurs is valuable.

In children coping well with a degree of airway obstruction, definitive treatment reflecting the likely diagnosis should be started. In those children who deteriorate, where stridor has been present from birth or where a foreign body is suspected, examination of the airway under anaesthesia may be required on an emergency or planned basis. Definitive care for specific conditions is as follows:

- Croup—There is good evidence that steroids modify the natural history. Administer either dexamethasone 0.15 mg/kg intravenously or budesonide 1 mg inhaled as a nebuliser. Few require endotracheal intubation.
- Epiglottis—Less common in UK since routine *Haemophilus influenzae* type B vaccination. Endotracheal tube placement commonly required. Blood cultures and intravenous cefotaxime or ceftriaxone.
- Bacterial tracheitis—Frequently life threatening requiring intubation. Possible infective organisms include *Staphylococcus aureus*, *Haemophilus influenzae* B or *Streptococcus*. Commence intravenous cefotaxime and flucloxacillin.
- Foreign body—See Foreign body chapter
- Anaphylaxis—See Anaphylaxis chapter.

Close observation with regular reassessment should occur frequently to ensure improvement is occurring.

- Stridor is an emergency requiring urgent assessment and management.
- Bedside clinical examination forms the basis of successful and safe patient care.
- Assessment of breathing should be under the following headings:
  - Effort of breathing (respiratory rate, recession, accessory muscle use);
  - Efficacy of breathing (chest expansion, auscultation);
  - Effectiveness of breathing (skin colour, pulse rate, pulse oximetry).
- Assessment of severity of airway obstruction and management takes precedence over establishing a diagnosis.

- Children present a particular risk due to the small size initially of their upper airway.
- Patients with stridor should receive high flow oxygen whilst assessment is undertaken.
- All patients require senior involvement at or soon after presentation.
- Do not upset any children with significant airway obstruction.
- Where respiratory failure is pending or present, intubation in theatre under general anaesthesia (undertaken by senior staff) is required.
- Frequent reassessment of clinical condition is required.

Further reading

1 Anon. The child with breathing difficulties. In: Mackway-Jones K, Molyneux E, Phillips B, Wieteska S, editors. *Advanced paediatric life support—the practical approach*. London BMJ Publishers, 2001;79–97.

2 Empey DW. Upper airway obstruction. In: Brewis RAL, Corrin B, Geddes DM, Gibson GJ, editors. *Respiratory medicine*. London. W.B. Saunders, 1995;1015–1020.

3 Browning GG. *Updated ENT*. London, Heinemann, 1994; 139–145.

68

The immediate management of head injuries

Roger Strachan

Introduction

Head injuries are extremely common. Every year, they account for about one million attendances to A & E departments, of which 150,000 are admitted to hospital. Severe head injuries requiring neurosurgical care account for 7,500 patients, of which approximately 50% die, 10% remain significantly disabled, and 40% retain some independence.

Head injuries are generally divided into minor, moderate or severe. This classification is largely based on their Glasgow coma scale (GCS, Chapter 7) on admission. Minor injuries are GCS 14 or 15, moderate GCS 9 to 13, and severe GCS 8 or less (in coma). Minor head injuries are those where there has been no or only a brief period of loss on consciousness, with return to normal function and no clinical or radiological evidence of skull fracture. Moderate head injuries will be more significant, with evidence of skull fracture, dural tear and brain injury. Severe injuries are patients in coma, often with other associated injuries, and it is this group that this article will concentrate on.

Anatomy and physiology

There are two basic mechanisms that lead to head and brain injury.

Direct trauma to the skull

This causes:

- Local injury, with bruising, swelling, or skull fracture;
- Intracranial injury with dural tear, brain laceration, or brain contusion;

- Arterial or venous injury within the cranial cavity causing haematomas to collect (extradural, subdural or intracerebral);
- Cranial base fractures leading to cranial nerve palsies (e.g. facial weakness, deafness, anosmia).

Acceleration/Deceleration injuries

These occur particularly in road traffic accidents, but also when the rapidly moving head is brought to an abrupt halt in certain falls. Rotational forces are particularly dangerous, because the density of bone, dura, and grey and white matter in the brain are all different, and if the head is twisted or spun rapidly the angular momentum of each will be different, leading to shearing forces between adjacent layers or tissues. This leads to diffuse axonal injury within the brain, or laceration of veins causing subdural and intracerebral haemorrhages. In this group, patients can often suffer severe brain injury without any evidence at all of local trauma to the head.

The primary insult that occurs to the brain at the time of the injury is often thought to be irreversible, but some aspects of neuronal injury may still be potentially reversible within the first several hours of the injury if appropriate treatment is established.

The main purpose of good early management is to prevent secondary insults. The brain may be only 2% of the total body weight, but requires 15% of the resting cardiac output, and 25% of the total inspired oxygen. These insults maybe:

- ***Hypoxia.*** Obstruction of the airway, impaired respiratory function, shock and impaired cardiac function will all contribute to reduced oxygen delivery to the brain.
- ***Ischaemia.*** Shock, reduced blood volume, and reduced cardiac output will lead to impaired cerebral perfusion, even where blood oxygenation appears adequate. Cerebral perfusion pressure (CPP) is linked to intracranial pressure and blood pressure by the simplified formula CPP = MABP − CP (Cerebral perfusion pressure = Mean arterial blood pressure − Intracranial pressure).
- ***Raised intracranial pressure.*** The skull vault is a tight box. Any additional increase in its contents will lead to a rise in intracranial pressure. This might happen as a result of a mass lesion (e.g. haematoma), increased cerebral blood volume (hyperaemic state), brain swelling (cerebral oedema) or a rise in CSF volume if obstructive hydrocephalus contributes.

- ***Seizures.*** During an epileptic seizure, the cerebral metabolic rate can rise as much as seven times, with an associated higher oxygen requirement. Even if oxygen delivery is only marginally impaired, further neuronal damage will occur.

All these factors are interlinked. For instance, a rise in intracranial pressure will reduce brain perfusion, causing further tissue hypoxia, leading to further injury, swelling, and increasing pressure. Moreover, neuronal damage causes massive increases in tissue neurotransmitter levels, such as glutamate, which can cause further neuronal damage. A variety of other metabolites, such as lactic acid, nitrites and oxygen radicals, damage cells and their ability to utilise oxygen. The final common pathway for all these insults will be lack of oxygen to drive the energy-producing pathways within the neurons, and without energy, the cells cannot continue to function or repair themselves. If oxygen depletion is significant enough for long enough, neuronal death is inevitable.

Immediate management

The initial management of head injuries must begin where the patient is found after the injury, and is directed at reducing the potential for secondary brain damage.

Airway, Breathing and Circulation (ABC)

- ***Airway.*** Comatose patients cannot maintain their airway. Obstruction may occur from the tongue in a supine position, or blood, vomit, teeth or other foreign material in the oropharynx. Associated facial injuries may contribute to airways obstruction.
- ***Breathing.*** Chest injuries and the head injury itself (brain stem injury or compression) may impair respiration and reduce blood oxygenation.
- ***Circulation.*** Other injuries, particularly fractures of the pelvis or long bones and abdominal injuries, may lead to hypotension from hypovolaemia, thus impairing brain perfusion. Rarely, direct chest injuries may impair cardiac function (e.g. pericardial tamponade from haemopericardium).

Head injury

- ***External examination.*** Swelling, bruising, lacerations to skin, compound fracture, brain haematoma, and CSF rhinorrhea or otorrhoea are all indications of head trauma, indicating the site and possible extent of the injury.

- ***Cranial nerve signs.*** Pupillary size, asymmetry and reactivity should be assessed. A dilated fixed pupil on one side with a contralateral hemiparesis will usually indicate a mass lesion causing compression of the brain on the side of the dilated pupil. This is likely to require urgent CT scanning and neurosurgical intervention. If the dilated pupil is on the same side as the direct head trauma, it may represent an expanding extradural haematoma. If the dilated pupil is on the opposite side, this represents a contra coup injury, usually indicating a contralateral subdural haematoma or intracerebral contusions, with associated swelling and compression of the opposite hemisphere. (Caution—significant midline shift of the brain structures may cause compression of the opposite cerebral peduncle against the edge of the tentorium leading to an ipsilateral (same side) hemiparesis.)
- ***Neurological examination.*** In a patient who is still responding to stimuli, assessment of limb movements looking for lateralising signs and appropriate recording of the Glasgow coma scale is important (see Chapter 7).

In deeply unconscious patients, it is helpful if (prior to intubation and/or sedation/paralysis of the patient) the anaesthetist makes a quick assessment of cough and gag reflexes and also a corneal (blink) reflex (trigeminal nerve), as this gives some indication of intact or absent brain stem function.

Where there is little or no evidence of external head trauma, yet the patient remains deeply comatose after resuscitation and is exhibiting abnormal limb movements, particular after high-speed road accidents, this indicates a severe diffuse axonal injury to deep brain structures. It is unlikely that such patients can be assisted by immediate neurosurgical intervention. Appropriate resuscitation is still the mainstay of treatment in these patients.

Thus, the immediate management of head injuries includes:

- Control of the airway, by intubation and mechanical ventilation if necessary;
- Oxygen therapy, and arterial blood gas analysis;
- Restoration of circulating blood volume, using fluid, colloid and blood infusion. Adequate venous access is required (at least two large intravenous cannulae);
- Cervical spine examination and imaging;

Table 1. Risk of an operable intracranial haematoma in head injured patients* (PTA = Posttraumatic amnesia).

GCS	Risk	Other features	Risk
15	1:3615	None	1:31,300
		PTA	1:6700
		Skull fracture	1:81
		Skull fracture + PTA	1:29
9–14	1:51	No fracture	1:180
		Skull fracture	1:5
3–8	1:7	No fracture	1:27
		Skull fracture	1:4

* From Guidelines for the Initial Management of Head Injuries. Recommendations from the Society of British Neurological Surgeons. *Br J Neurosurg*. 1998;12:349–352.

- Assessment and treatment of other life-threatening injuries;
- Temporary immobilisation of limb fractures;
- Treatment of suspected internal injuries;
- Treatment of suspected raised intracranial pressure. Give mannitol 20% 0.5–1.0 g/kg, usually about 200 mL for an average 70 kg adult, intravenously over 20 minutes. Consider *temporary* hyperventilation—the cerebral vessels are reactive to blood CO_2 levels and will vasoconstrict if the arterial CO_2 pressure is reduced. This reduces cerebral blood volume;
- Imaging of the patient. Cervical spine. Chest, pelvis and long bones where appropriate. CT scanning—brain and cervical spine (if required, particularly C1/2 and C6/7). If the patient cannot be scanned quickly in the hospital at which he presents, consider transfer to the neurosurgical unit instead. Table 1 illustrates the risk of an operable haematoma in patients with head injuries.

Further reading

1 Gentleman D, Dearden M, Midgley S, Maclean D. Guidelines for resuscitation and transfer of patients with serious head injury. *BMJ*. 1993;307:547–552.

2 Bartlett J, Kett-White R, Mendelow AD, Miller JD, Pickard J, Teasdale G. Guidelines for the initial management of head injuries. Recommendations from the Society of British Neurological Surgeons. *Br J Neurosurg*. 1998;12:349–352.

3 Flannery T, Buxton N. Modern management of head injuries. *J R Coll Surg Edinb*. 2001;46:150–153.
4 *Recommendations for the Transfer of Patients with Acute Head Injuries to Neurosurgical Units*. London, The Association of Anaesthetists of Great Britain and Ireland, 1996.
5 *Report of the Working Party on the Management of Patients with Head Injuries*. The Royal College of Surgeons of England, 1999.

69

Adult cardio-respiratory resuscitation

Carol Tennant

Introduction

Following cardiac arrest effective basic life support (BLS) within the first 3–4 minutes may increase the chance of patient survival. The manner in which the initial stages are managed may determine success or failure. The role of the healthcare professional can be summarised as an assessor, manager and coordinator of the initial situation.

BLS is the maintenance of the airway and support of breathing and circulation by performing rescue breathing and external chest compressions. By definition this implies the use of no equipment. Within a healthcare setting this should not be the case. One of the priorities in this emergency situation is the delivery of high flow oxygen to ventilate a patient who is not breathing. Therefore, all patient areas should be equipped with basic airway equipment and have immediate access to a supply of oxygen. This can then be referred to as BLS with airway adjuncts.

Respiratory arrest

Can occur for a number of reasons, for example foreign body obstruction, disease process such as epiglottitis, drug overdoses, near drowning, electrocution and cerebrovascular accident (CVA), additionally respiratory arrest may be secondary to a decreased conscious level. When primary respiratory arrest occurs, the heart and lungs can continue to oxygenate the blood for several minutes, and oxygen will continue to circulate to the brain and other vital organs. Such patients initially demonstrate signs of circulation. When respiratory arrest occurs or spontaneous respirations are inadequate, establishment of a patent airway and ventilation can be lifesaving.

Cardiac arrest

Circulation ceases and vital organs are deprived of oxygen. Ineffective 'gasping' breathing efforts (agonal respirations) may occur early in cardiac arrest and should not be confused with effective respiration. Cardiac arrest can be accompanied by the following cardiac rhythms; ventricular fibrillation (VF), pulseless ventricular tachycardia (VT), asystole and pulseless electrical activity (PEA).

Resuscitation should be carried out in an unresponsive patient where there is an absence of breathing and/or circulation.

Technique

Universal precautions

Healthcare providers should ensure the use of universal precautions by the use of gloves as protection during any resuscitation attempt. Special care must be taken with any sharps; a sharps container must be immediately available.

Safety

On discovering or being called to a collapsed patient, the first consideration is safety, firstly for yourself and those around you. Having determined there are no immediate dangers and the scene is safe; shout for help, pull the emergency buzzer in the room (if available) assess responsiveness, stimulate the patient, and speak loudly to the patient: 'Are you alright?'

- ***If there is a response***: Leave the patient in the position in which you find them (provided they are not in further danger), shout for help and check their condition, get help if needed, reassess at regular intervals.
- ***If there is no response***: Shout for help if you have not already done so. It can be assumed that the patient is unconscious and may be unable to maintain their airway. Patients can, and very often do, suffer cardiac arrest in difficult locations such as the toilet, bathroom or places with limited space in which to work. There may be a need to position the patient in order to carry on with your assessment.

Manual handling and lifting

When a patient collapses (in their haste) staff members may be side-tracked from using safe manual handling and lifting techniques. Once positioned (supine) the patient should now be quickly assessed using the structured **ABC** (airway, breathing, circulation) approach.

- **(A) Open the airway.** There are two methods of achieving an open airway, first the head tilt/chin lift manoeuvre and second, in the case of any suspected trauma or injury to the neck a jaw thrust. To carry out a head tilt/chin lift place one hand on the patients forehead and apply pressure to tilt the head back, simultaneously placing your fingers under the bony part of the jaw and lifting the chin. To carry out a jaw thrust manoeuvre place your fingers at the angle of the jaw and life upwards and forwards ensuring the neck does not move.
- **(B) Check for breathing.** Whilst keeping the airway open assess for breathing by looking for any effective chest movement, listen for sounds of breathing and feel for airflow for no more than 10 seconds. Simultaneously check for signs of a circulation, although this may prove difficult whilst attempting to maintain an open airway.
    - ***If the patient is breathing normally*:** The recovery position can be used to prevent airway obstruction from the tongue, mucous or vomit. Continually observe for adequate breathing. Send someone for assistance or, if you are on your own, go for assistance.
    - ***If the patient is not breathing or taking only occasional gasps*:** If more than one member of staff is available, one person immediately goes and telephones for the resuscitation team whilst the other begins BLS immediately. *However if only one person is available then it may be necessary to leave the patient and alert the resuscitation team oneself. The exception to this would be if the likely cause of unconsciousness was resulting from a breathing problem i.e. trauma, drowning, drug or alcohol intoxication or in the case of a paediatric patient. In these situations if alone, BLS should be performed for one minute before going for help.*
- ***The importance of calling for the resuscitation team early*:** Some patients who sustain a cardiac arrest may be suffering from VF/VT. The most effective treatment is early defibrillation. Basic life support alone will maintain cardiac output and perfusion to the vital organs but will not restart the heart. Basic life

support 'buys time' until the defibrillator and resuscitation team arrives to commence advanced life support.

If the resuscitation team is not immediately called and help is not on its way, the chaotic electrical activity that is characteristic of ventricular fibrillation in the heart starts to diminish within minutes, making defibrillation less likely to be effective and the survival of the patient less likely.

Provide breathing

As soon as available airway adjuncts such as oropharyngeal/nasopharyngeal airways should be used in conjunction with a pocket mask or bag/valve/mask for ventilation. Supplemental oxygen should be attached to the ventilatory device as soon as possible as it is one of the most valuable drugs available. Give 2 slow, effective rescue ventilations, ensuring each inflates the lungs by observing for chest movement.

- ***Mouth-to-mouth*:** Ensure you maintain a head tilt and chin lift manoeuvre. Pinch the soft part of their nose closed with the index finger and thumb of your hand on their forehead. Open the mouth a little, take a deep breath and place your lips around the patient's mouth, making sure that you have a good seal. Breathe steadily into the patient's mouth, taking about two seconds to make the chest rise as in normal breathing. Maintaining head tilt/chin lift, take your mouth away from the patient and watch for the chest to fall as air is expired. Five attempts should be made if required to achieve two effective rescue breaths. See Figure 1.
- ***Pocket mask*:** Help reduce the risk of transmission of infection and can be used with or without supplemental oxygen. By attaching supplemental oxygen at a flow of 10–15 litres/minute an oxygen concentration of approximately 50% can be delivered to the patient.
- ***Bag/valve/mask*:** The most common device used to ventilate patients who are apnoeic or breathing inadequately is the bag/valve/mask. This can be connected to either a facemask or a tracheal tube. Used alone, this will allow ventilation of the patient with air. However, this concentration must be increased during resuscitation by adding supplemental oxygen at a flow of 10 litres/minute. Oxygen delivery to the patient will then be approximately 85%. When attached to a facemask it requires considerable skill to apply the mask, maintain an airtight seal

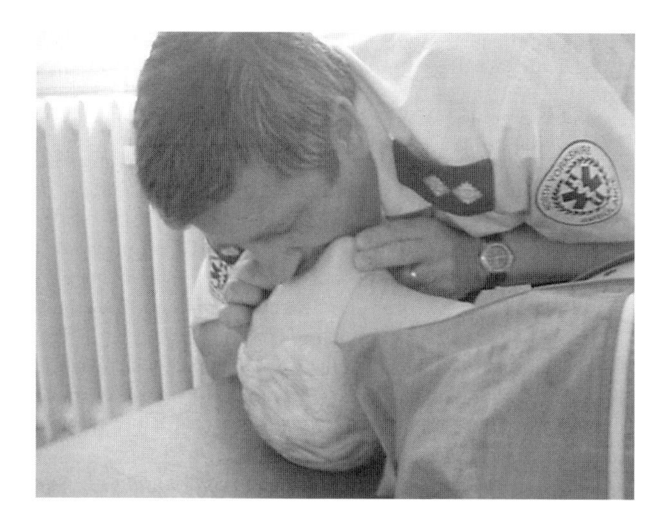

Figure 1. Mouth-to-mouth breathing.

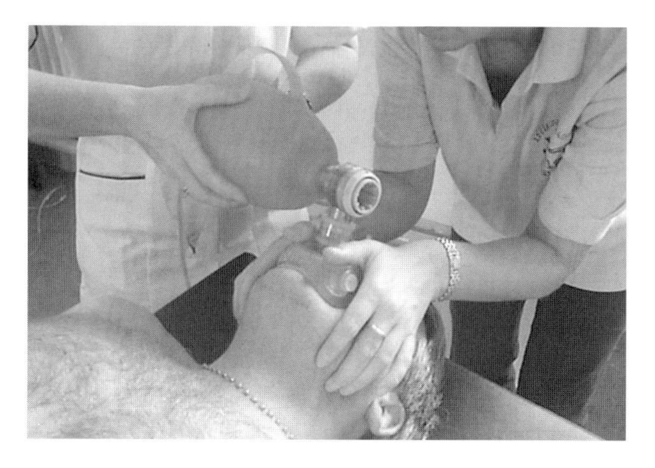

Figure 2. Bag/valve/mask ventilation.

with the face and lift the jaw with one hand while squeezing the bag with the other hand. To overcome these problems and ensure good ventilation, a two-person technique is preferable, one person holds the facemask in place and maintains an open airway, whilst the second person squeezes the bag, see Figure 2.

If unsuccessful using any of the above methods—after five failed attempts of ventilation proceed immediately to assessment of circulation.

- **(C) Assessment of the circulation:** If you have not already done so check a central pulse, carotid or femoral for signs of a circulation for 10 seconds.
- ***If you have detected signs of a circulation*:** continue ventilation until the patient starts breathing on their own. Approximately every minute (or every 10 breaths) re-check for signs of a circulation taking no more than 10 seconds every time. If the patient starts to breathe but remains unconscious, turn them into the recovery position and continually assess them. Be ready to turn the patient supine and restart ventilation if breathing once again ceases.
- ***If there are no signs of a circulation, or you are at all unsure*:** start external chest compressions at a ratio of 15 compressions to two ventilations as per Resuscitation Council (UK) Guidelines described below.
  - Using the hand nearest to the patient's feet locate the lower half of the sternum, in order to achieve this; with your index and middle fingers, establish the lower rib edge nearest to you, keeing your fingers together, slide them upwards to the point where the ribs join the sternum and then with your middle finger on this point, place your index finger on the sternum;
  - Next slide the heel of your other hand down the sternum until it reaches your index finger; this should be the middle of the lower half of the sternum;
  - Then position the heel of the other hand on top of the first and extend or interlock the fingers of both hands and lift them to ensure that the pressure is not applied over the patient's ribs. Do not apply any pressure over the upper abdomen or bottom tip of the sternum;
  - In order to achieve the correct posture, position yourself vertically above the patient's chest and, with your arms straight; press down on the sternum to depress it between 4 and 5 cm and then release the pressure without losing contact between the hand and sternum. Repeat at a rate of 100 times a minute; it may be helpful to count out loud '1 and 2 and 3 and 12 and 13–14–15'; Compressions and release should take equal amount of time and the chest should be allowed to recoil to its normal position after each compression.

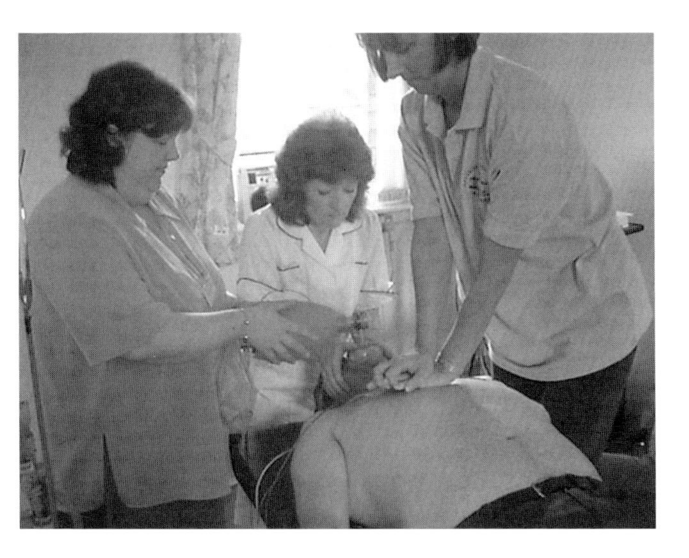

Figure 3. Multi-disciplinary team cardiac arrest management.

BLS must be ongoing and once this is organised then further management can be undertaken in preparation for the delivery of advanced life support (ALS) to the patient. Dependent upon the number of staff available many of these things may happen simultaneously. See Figure 3.

First-line management

There are many more things that need to be done in the time between calling for, and the arrival of the resuscitation team. The patient should be attached as soon as possible to a defibrillator or alternatively an automated external defibrillator (AED). In the case of the AED the first responder may be able to defibrillate the patient if necessary. If a manual monitor/defibrillator is attached this allows the resuscitation team to assess the rhythm of the patient and implement advanced treatment without delay. It is important that staff ensure the chest is exposed and clear from clothing prior to the attachment of the defibrillator. This makes it easier to place the monitoring electrodes in the appropriate position. It also ensures the chest is clear for the application of defibrillator pads if required. Basic life support should be continued at all times.

Notes should be available on arrival, or soon after the arrival of the resuscitation team. The resuscitation team leader will require these to identify potential reversible causes of the arrest via the patient's medical history and pathology. Ward/departmental staff should also give an immediate verbal history.

The emergency drugs on the resuscitation trolley should be prepared for immediate use, as should equipment for intravenous cannulation and suction.

If staff numbers allow, it is of great assistance to the resuscitation team if a staff is in a prominent position to direct them to where the cardiac arrest is taking place. Valuable time is often wasted when the majority of ward staff are for example in a side ward dealing with the arrest and the resuscitation team members are trying to identify the exact location of the patient within that area.

It may not be practical to have all these tasks completed by the time the team arrives. Prior planning and preparation will have ensured that first responders know the skill levels of the staff within their ward/department. This will enable skills to be delegated appropriately. It is then important to prioritise, depending on the number of staff available. For example, it is of far greater importance to attach the patient to the defibrillator than it is obtaining notes or preparing the drugs, these tasks should be carried later.

The resuscitation team includes both medical and nursing staff who are trained in ALS. The arrival of the resuscitation team does not mean the first responder's role in the situation is over, the resuscitation team members will often be focused on carrying out their own tasks, therefore ward/departmental staff should be available to give appropriate help or information. Remember the first responders are part of the resuscitation team and there are many more tasks that can and need to be performed.

One member of the resuscitation team should assume the role of team leader and the responsibility of this person is to stand back and direct the team. They should also be ensuring that all treatments are being recorded.

The other team members may initiate advanced airway management under the direction of the team leader. Once intubation is achieved ventilation and chest compressions are carried out asynchronously at a rate of approximately 12 breaths and 100 compressions per minute. Carrying out external chest compressions is extremely hard work and tiredness sets in very quickly; therefore staff should rotate in order to maintain efficiency. Defibrillation, rhythm recognition, drug administration and other appropriate interventions will occur in accordance with Resuscitation Council (UK) guidelines.

Remember ALS is unlikely to be effective unless BLS is ongoing and continued throughout; BLS is the foundation of any resuscitation attempt.

The supply of emergency drugs should be monitored; pre-filled syringes should be available so that they can be given immediately. Syringes of saline flush should also be prepared. Equipment such as dinamaps and infusion pumps may be required and ward/departmental staff should be able to provide any equipment requested by the team within a reasonable time. Remember other patients still need to be cared for, as this can be a very traumatic event for them.

If there is a successful outcome, the team will attempt to stabilise the patient and may transfer them to an appropriate unit, which is usually either ICU or CCU.

If it becomes apparent that resuscitation is not working or is perceived as futile the team as a whole will make the decision whether or not to stop resuscitation, although ultimately it is the team leaders final decision.

Complications

- **Infection:** Although the risk of transmission of infection can cause anxiety the number of reported cases is very low. The main areas for concern involve bacteria such as neisseria meningitidis and tuberculosis. According to the Resuscitation Council (UK) transmission of Hepatitis B, C or the cytomegalovirus has not been reported. No cases of transmission of HIV infection via mouth-to-mouth ventilation have been reported. Of the three known cases of HIV transmission, they occurred through needle stick injuries with one involving contamination of abraded hands.

- **Technical difficulties:** If mouth-to-mouth proves technically difficult to carry out because of unusual or absent dentition, obstruction or maxillo-facial injuries mouth-to-nose ventilation can be performed.
- **Malposition:** Incorrect technique and hand position whilst carrying out external chest compressions may lead to bony fracture of the ribs and sternum and rupture of the liver. However in the overall context of the cardiac arrest situation we must remember that this patient has no signs of life and therefore inaction ensures there is no chance of survival.

Further reading

1 An advisory statement by the Basic Life Support working Group of the International Liaison Committee on Resuscitation 1997;34:101–107.
2 Colquhoun MC, Handley AJ, Evans T. ABC of Resuscitation. *BMJ. Advanced Life Support Manual*, 4th Edition London, Resuscitation Council (UK), 2000.
3 European Resuscitation Council. International Guidelines 2000 for CPR and ECC—A Concensus on Science. *Resuscitation*. 2000; 46:1–448.
4 Resuscitation Council (UK). *Guidance to safer handling during resuscitation in hospitals 2001*. Available at: www.resus.org.uk
5 Resuscitation Council (UK). *Resuscitation Guidelines 2000*. Available at: www.resus.org.uk

Section 9

Algorithms

Appendix 1: Adult basic life support

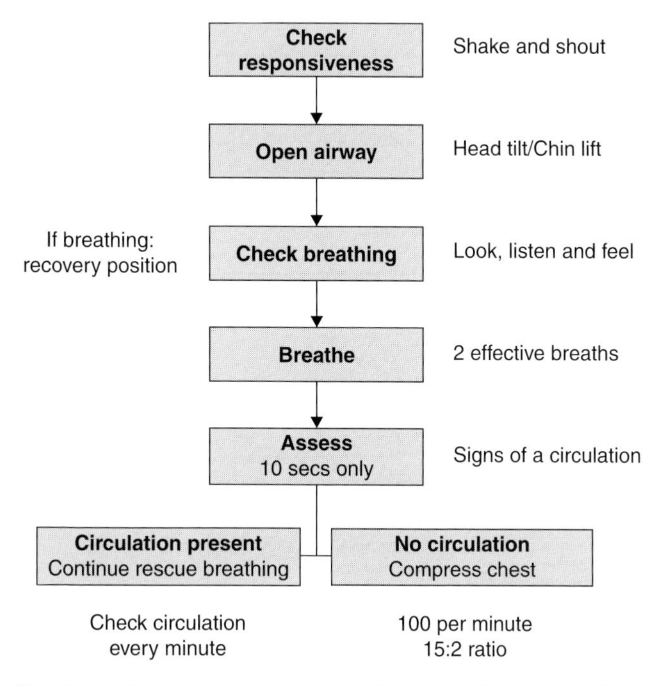

Printed with kind permission of the Resuscitation Council (UK).

Appendix 2: Advanced life support algorithm for the management of cardiac arrest in adults

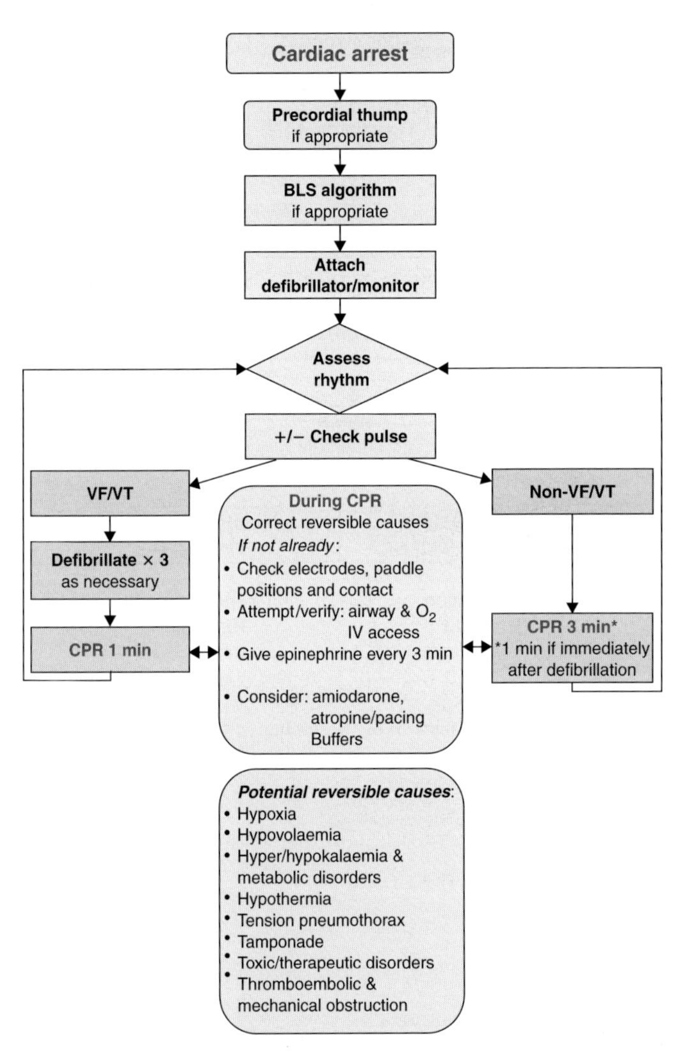

Printed with kind permission of the Resuscitation Council (UK).

Appendix 3: Paediatric basic life support

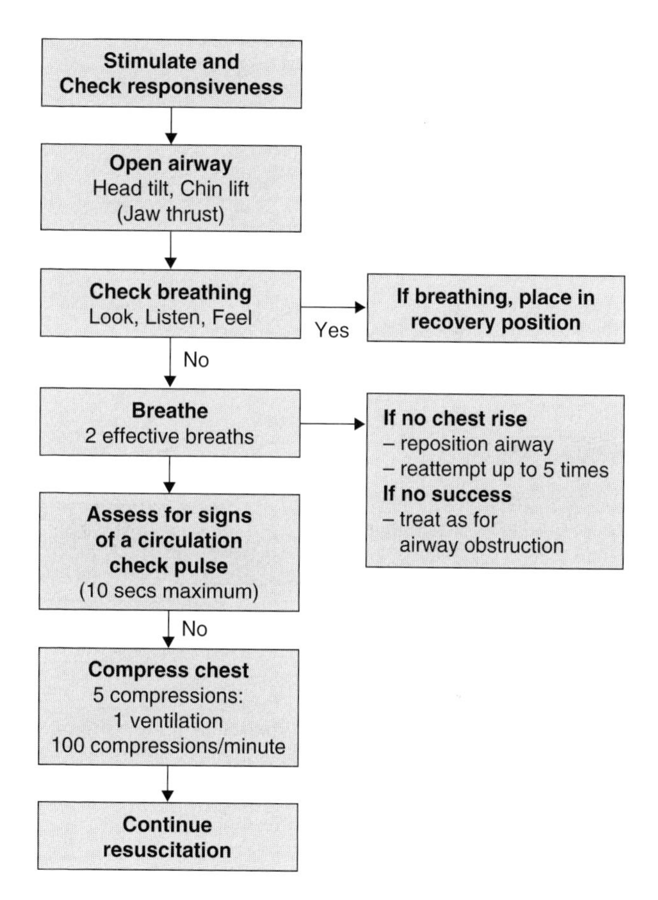

Printed with kind permission of the Resuscitation Council (UK).

Appendix 4: Paediatric advanced life support

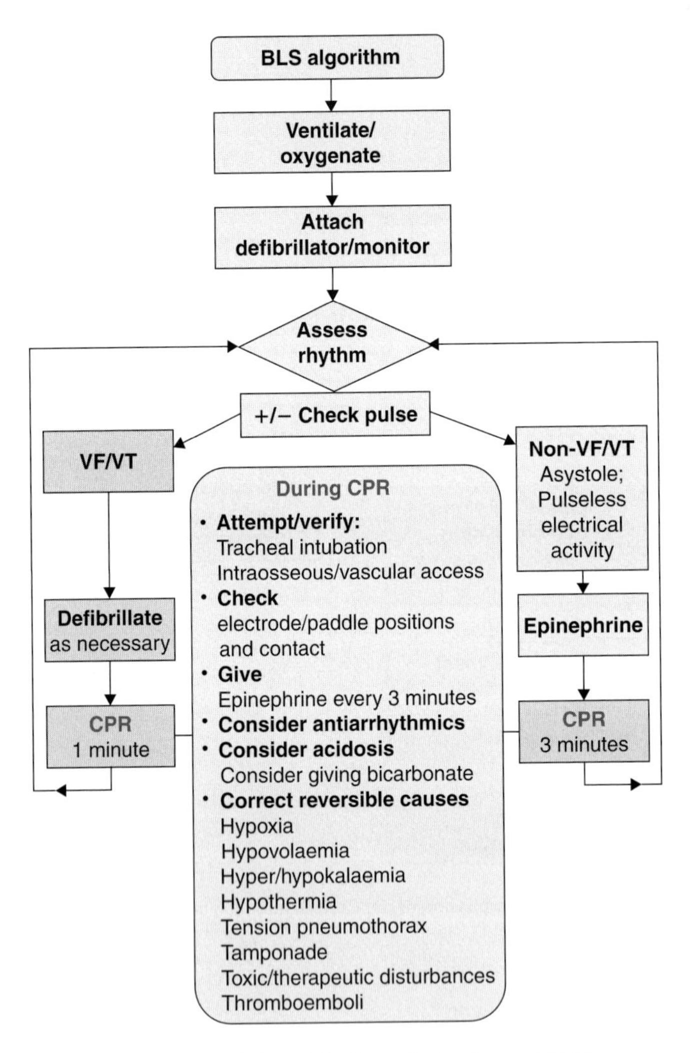

Printed with kind permission of the Resuscitation Council (UK).

Appendix 5: Newborn life support

Dry the baby, remove any wet cloth and cover

↓

Initial assessment at birth
Start the clock or note the time
Assess: COLOUR, TONE, BREATHING, HEART RATE

↓

If not breathing ...

↓

Control the airway
Head in the neutral position

↓

Support the breathing
If not breathing - FIVE INFLATION BREATHS (each 2-3 seconds duration)
Confirm a response:- increase in HEART RATE or visible CHEST MOVEMENT

↓

If there is no response
Double check head position and apply JAW THRUST
5 inflation breaths
Confirm a response:- increase in HEART RATE or visible CHEST MOVEMENT

↓

If there is still no response
a) Use a second person (if available) to help with airway control and repeat inflation breaths
b) Inspect the oropharynx under direct vision (is suction needed?) and repeat inflation breaths
c) Insert an oropharyngeal (Guedel) airway and repeat inflation breaths
Consider intubation
Confirm a response:- increase in HEART RATE or visible CHEST MOVEMENT

↓

When the chest is moving
Continue the ventilation breaths if no spontaneous breathing

↓

Check the heart rate
If the heart rate is not detectable or slow (less than around 60 bpm) and NOT increasing

↓

Start chest compressions
First confirm chest movement - if chest not moving return to airway
3 chest compressions to 1 breath for 30 seconds

↓

Reassess Heart Rate
If improving - stop chest compressions, continue ventilation if not breathing
If heart rate still slow, continue ventilation and chest compressions
Consider venous access and drugs at this stage

AT ALL STAGES, ASK ..... DO YOU NEED HELP ?

In the presence of meconium, remember: Screaming babies:- have an open airway
Floppy babies:- have a look

Printed with kind permission of the Resuscitation Council (UK).

Appendix 6: Consent

12 key points on consent: the law in England

DH Department of Health

When do health professionals need consent from patients?

1. Before you examine, treat or care for competent adult patients you must obtain their consent.
2. Adults are always assumed to be competent unless demonstrated otherwise. If you have doubts about their competence, the question to ask is: "can this patient understand and weigh up the information needed to make this decision?" Unexpected decisions do not prove the patient is incompetent, but may indicate a need for further information or explanation.
3. Patients may be competent to make some health care decisions, even if they are not competent to make others.
4. Giving and obtaining consent is usually a process, not a one-off event. Patients can change their minds and withdraw consent at any time. If there is any doubt, you should always check that the patient still consents to your caring for or treating them.

Can children consent for themselves?

5. Before examining, treating or caring for a child, you must also seek consent. Young people aged 16 and 17 are presumed to have the competence to give consent for themselves. Younger children who understand fully what is involved in the proposed procedure can also give consent (although their parents will ideally be involved). In other cases, some-one with parental responsibility must give consent on the child's behalf, unless they cannot be reached in an emergency. If a competent child consents to treatment, a parent **cannot** over-ride that consent. Legally, a parent can consent if a competent child refuses, but it is likely that taking such a serious step will be rare.

Who is the right person to seek consent?

6. It is always best for the person actually treating the patient to seek the patient's consent. However, you may seek consent on behalf of colleagues if you are capable of performing the procedure in question, or if you have been specially trained to seek consent for that procedure.

What information should be provided?

7. Patients need sufficient information before they can decide whether to give their consent: for example information about the benefits and risks of the proposed treatment, and alternative treatments. If the patient is not offered as much information as they reasonably need to make their decision, and in a form they can understand, their consent may not be valid.

Is the patient's consent voluntary?

8. Consent must be given voluntarily: not under any form of duress or undue influence from health professionals, family or friends.

Does it matter *how* the patient gives consent?

9. No: consent can be written, oral or non-verbal. A signature on a consent form does not itself prove the consent is valid – the point of the form is to record the patient's decision, and also increasingly the discussions that have taken place. Your Trust or organisation may have a policy setting out when you need to obtain written consent.

Refusals of treatment

10. Competent adult patients are entitled to refuse treatment, even where it would clearly benefit their health. The only exception to this rule is where the treatment is for a mental disorder and the patient is detained under the *Mental Health Act 1983*. A competent pregnant woman may refuse any treatment, even if this would be detrimental to the fetus.

Adults who are not competent to give consent

11. **No-one** can give consent on behalf of an incompetent adult. However, you may still treat such a patient if the treatment would be in their best interests. 'Best interests' go wider than best medical interests, to include factors such as the wishes and beliefs of the patient when competent, their current wishes, their general well-being and their spiritual and religious welfare. People close to the patient may be able to give you information on some of these factors. Where the patient has never been competent, relatives, carers and friends may be best placed to advise on the patient's needs and preferences.
12. If an incompetent patient has clearly indicated in the past, while competent, that they would refuse treatment in certain circumstances (an 'advance refusal'), and those circumstances arise, you must abide by that refusal.

This summary cannot cover all situations. For more detail, consult the *Reference guide to consent for examination or treatment*, available from the NHS Response Line 0541 555 455 and at www.doh.gov.uk/consent

23618 2p 500k Apr 01 (COL)

Appendix 7: Adverse reaction form

In Confidence

COMMITTEE ON SAFETY OF MEDICINES

MCA
MEDICINES CONTROL AGENCY

SUSPECTED ADVERSE DRUG REACTIONS

If you are suspicious that an adverse reaction may be related to a drug or combination of drugs please complete this Yellow Card. For reporting advice please see over. Do not be put off reporting because some details are not known.

PATIENT DETAILS Patient Initials: ________ Sex: M / F Weight if known (kg): ________
Age (at time of reaction): ________ Identification number (Your Practice / Hospital Ref.)*: ________

SUSPECTED DRUG(S)

Give brand name of drug and batch number if known	Route	Dosage	Date started	Date stopped	Prescribed for

SUSPECTED REACTION(S)
Please describe the reaction(s) and any treatment given:

Outcome
Recovered ☐
Recovering ☐
Continuing ☐
Other ☐

Date reaction(s) started: ________ Date reaction(s) stopped: ________
Do you consider the reaction to be serious? Yes / No
If *yes*, please indicate why the reaction is considered to be serious (please tick all that apply):
Patient died due to reaction ☐ Involved or prolonged inpatient hospitalisation ☐
Life threatening ☐ Involved persistent or significant disability or incapacity ☐
Congenital abnormality ☐ Medically significant; please give details: ________

OTHER DRUGS (including self-medication & herbal remedies)
Did the patient take any other drugs in the last 3 months prior to the reaction? Yes / No
If *yes*, please give the following information if known:

Drug (Brand, if known)	Route	Dosage	Date started	Date stopped	Prescribed for

Additional relevant information e.g. medical history, test results, known allergies, rechallenge (if performed), suspected drug interactions. For congenital abnormalities please state all other drugs taken during pregnancy and the last menstrual period.

REPORTER DETAILS
Name and Professional Address: ________
Post code: ________ Tel No: ________
Speciality: ________
Signature: ________ Date: ________

CLINICIAN (if not the reporter)
Name and Professional Address: ________
Post code: ________
Tel No: ________ Speciality: ________

If you would like information about other adverse reactions associated with the suspected drug, please tick this box ☐

* This is to enable you to identify the patient in any future correspondence concerning this report

Please attach additional pages if necessary

Printed with kind permission of the Resuscitation Council (UK).

Index

Acceleration injuries, 472
Acute asthma, 426
  Beta-agonist bronchodilator, 429
  Chest X-ray, 428
  Discharge from hospital, 430
  Life threatening, 428
  Maintenance therapy, 430
  Management, 428
  Near-fatal, 428
  Drugs, 429
  Oxygen therapy, 428
  Severity assessment, 428
  Steroid therapy, 429
Acute dialysis, 379
  Indications, 379
Acute pain, 164
  Patient controlled analgesia machine, 164
Acute renal failure, 379
Adult Advanced Life Support, 490
Adult Basic Life Support, 489
Adverse reaction form, 495
AED, 441
Afterload, 257
Airway, 21, 203
  Assessment, 28, 203
  Difficult, 203, 205
  Equipment, 304
  Examination, 204
  Maintaining, 21, 26
  Obesity, 207
  Opening, 22
  Pregnancy, 207
Allen test, 17
  Modified, 17
Anaesthesia, 315
Anaesthetic machine user test, 290
Anaesthetic machine, 283, 289
  Checks, 283
  Specific type, 289
Analgesic ladder, 169
Anaphylactic reaction, 435, 436
Anaphylactoid reaction, 433
Anaphylaxis, 432
  Adrenaline, 437
  Antihistamine, 437
  Bicarbonate, 438
  Bronchodilator, 438
  Diagnosis, 433
  Fluid, 437
  Follow up, 438
  Hydrocortisone, 438
  Incidence, 433
  Inotrope, 438
  Investigations, 438
  Management, 434
  Mechanism, 432
  Presentation, 433
  Triggers, 432
Antepartum fetal monitoring, 415
Anti-epileptic drugs, 441, 442
  Adverse effects, 442
  Emergency loading, 442
Apnoea testing, 386
ARDS, 339
Assessment, 34, 203
  Airway, 203
  Conscious level, 35
  Consciousness, 34
Asthma, 426
  Acute, 426
Attempted intubation, 303
  Risks, 303
Audio-visual, 114
Audio-visual material, 116
  Use, 116
Automated external defibrillator, 483

Bacterial tracheitis, 469
Bag/valve/mask ventilation, 481

Bier's Block, 145
Advantages, 145
Complications, 148
Contraindications, 146
Indications, 145
Requirements, 146
Techniques, 147
BIPAP, 337
Blood pressure, 88
Potential problems, 88
Bolitho ruling, 47
Brachial plexus block, 323
Complications, 324
Indications, 324
Techniques, 324
Brain dead, 383
Brain death, 383
Brain stem death, 383
Brain stem death test, 383
Complications, 386
Equipment, 384
Indications, 384
Preconditions, 384
Techniques, 385
Brain volume, 362
Breathing
Bag/valve/mask, 480
Mouth to mouth, 480
Pocket mask, 480
Breathing system, 286
Bronchial anatomy, 355
Bronchoscopy, 335
Diagnostic, 355
Indications, 355
Rigid, 355
Burford Pain Thermometer, 165

Cannula choice, 18
Cannulation
Arteries, 17
Complications, 13, 14, 16, 17, 19, 102, 151, 153, 154, 155, 171, 177, 182, 272, 484
Capacitative linkage, 125
Cardiac arrest, 478
Cardiac output, 256
Measurement, 256, 258
Methods, 258
Cardiotocograph, 409
Catheterisation, 94, 97, 98
Complications, 100
Damage to intraperitoneal structures, 101
Diuresis, 101
Electrolyte imbalance, 101
Female, 97
Indications, 94
Infection, 100
Male, 94
Suprapubic, 98
Urethral trauma, 100
Urethral, 94, 97
Urinary, 94
Cauda equina, 308
Central venous access, 151
Catheter tip, 151
Chest X-ray, 151
Complications, 155
Internal jugular approach, 153
Seeker needle, 151
Site, 151
Subclavian approach, 154
Technique, 151
Central Venous Pressure, 89
Cerebral blood flow, 363
Cerebral metabolic rate, 39
Cerebral perfusion pressure, 363
Cerebrospinal fluid, 235, 362
Aspiration, 235
Chest drain, 211
Complications, 218
Indications, 212
Insertion, 211
Preparation, 212
Procedure, 212, 213
Clinical scenarios, 103
Cognitive function, 35
Common Gas Outlet, 285
Competent adult, 40
Conductance, 123
Conductor, 123

Conscious level, 34, 35, 36
  Assessment, 34, 35
  Impairment, 35
  Measure, 36
Conscious sedation, 140
  Definition, 140
  Drugs, 140, 142
Consciousness, 34
  Impaired, 34
Consent, 40, 42, 43, 494
  Competent adult, 40
  Definition, 40
  Giving, 42
  Implied, 41
  Informal, 40
  Principle, 40
  Process, 41
  Purpose, 41
  Non-verbal, 40
  Refusal, 43
  Taking, 40
  Valid, 40
  Verbal, 40
  Obtaining, 48
  Written, 41
Continuous intrapartum electronic fetal monitoring, 409
Continuous Positive Airway Pressure, 219
Contractility, 257
Conventional tracheostomy, 341
  Anaesthesia, 342
  Complications, 346
  Indications, 342
  Techniques, 344
Corneal reflex, 385, 388
Cough reflex, 386
CPAP, 219, 221, 222, 339
  Complications, 222
  Machines, 220
  Masks, 221
  Route of administration, 219
  Use, 219
Croup, 469
CTG, 410
Deceleration injuries, 472
Defibrillation, 129
Defibrillator, 129
Dialyser, 382
  Anaphylactic reaction, 382
Dialysis disequilibrium, 382
Diathermy, 124, 127
  Bipolar, 127
  Cutting, 124
  Monopolar, 127
Difficult airway prediction, 205
Discharge, 132
  Interim, 131
  Letter, 131
  Summary, 132
  Writing, 131
Discharge summary
  Confidentiality, 133
  Example, 134
  Patient access, 133
  Security, 133
Doppler ultrasound, 262
Drowning, 446
  Clinical presentation, 447
  Definitive care, 449
  Investigations, 449
  Management, 447
  Near, 446
  Outcome, 450
  Pathophysiology, 446
Drug allergy, 10
Drug anaphylaxis, 10
Dye dilution, 259
Dye dilution curve, 250

Early Warning Scoring, 92
Earth differences, 125
ECG, 49, 53
  Interpretation, 53
  Read, 54
Echocardiogram, 391
Echocardiography, 391
  Doppler, 391
  Hypertrophic cardiomyopathy, 392
  Indications, 391

Echocardiography (*cont.*)
Infective endocarditis, 394
Left ventricular function, 391
M-mode, 391
Pericardial disease, 396
Right heart disease, 395
Two-dimensional, 391
Valvular disease, 392
Effectiveness of respiration, 466
Efficacy of breathing, 465
Efforts of breathing, 465
Electrical axis of the heart, 57
Electrical safety, 123
Electricity, 123, 124
Conductor, 123
Effect, 124
Static, 124
Safety standard, 127
Use, 123
Electrocardiograph, 49
Electrocardiography, 293
Elements, 44
Epidiascope, 114
Epidural, 315
Catheter, 317
Complications, 320
Equipment, 316
Intra-operative management, 318
Needles, 316
Post-operative management, 319
Post-operative surveillance, 319
Procedure, 316
Space, 315
Test dose, 318
Epilepsy, 440
Classification, 440
Starting treatment, 440
Stopping treatment, 441
Episcope, 114
EVD, 364
Early Warning Scoring, 92
Examination of Airway, 204
External Ventricular Drainage, 364
Extracellular compartment, 419
Extracellular fluid, 419
Extradural microtransducer, 365
Eye foreign body, 184
Eye opening, 36, 37

Failed intubation, 306, 307
Anaesthetised paticnt, 306
Management, 306
Protocol, 307
Feeding lines, 368
Care, 372
Central, 369
Complications, 372
Contraindications, 369
Equipment, 369
Peripheral, 369
Technique of insertion, 369
Femoral nerve block, 329
Fetal blood sampling, 414
Fetal heart rate, 409
Acceleration, 412
Antepartum, 415
Baseline rate, 411
Bradycardia, 411
Contraction, 411
Deceleration, 413
Early deceleration, 413
Interpretation, 411
Late deceleration, 413
Tachycardia, 412
Variability, 412
Variable deceleration, 414
Fetus, 401
FEV 1, 228
Fibre-optic bronchoscopy, 358
Local anaesthesia, 359
Monitoring, 360
Preparation, 358
Risks of cross-infection, 361
Sedation, 359
Technique, 358
Fibre-optic laryngoscope, 304
Field block, 64
Fire hazard, 129
Electricity, 129
Fixed performance device, 200
Fluid balance, 90
Foreign body, 184

Fosphenytoin, 443
FVC, 228

GCS, 35, 36
Children, 36
Modified, 36
Gillick competence, 42
Glasgow Coma Scale, 35
Glasgow Coma Score, 90
Gloving procedure, 83
Closed method, 83
Sterile technique, 84

Haemodialysis, 378, 380
Haemofiltration, 378, 380
Haemothorax, 208
Head injuries, 471
Cranial nerve signs, 474
Examination, 473
Hypoxia, 472
Ischaemia, 472
Management, 471, 473
Neurological examination, 474
Raised intracranial pressure, 472
Seizures, 473
Healing, 72
Primary intention, 72
Secondary intention, 72
Ways, 72
Wound, 72
Heart rate calculation, 54
Heart rate monitoring, 88
Hospital acquired infection, 78
Hudson mask, 200
Hyperkalaemia, 380
Hypoglycaemia, 382
Hypothermia, 295, 451
Aetiology, 451
Definition, 451
Diagnosis, 453
Investigation, 453
Management, 454
Pathophysiology, 452
Prognosis, 455
Respiratory stability, 454
Re-warming, 454
Hypovolaemia, 419, 421
Absolute, 419
Cause, 421
Clinical signs and symptoms, 422
Definition, 419
Management, 422
Pathophysiology, 421
Relative, 419
Hypoxaemia, 339
Hypoxia, 196, 198
Anaemic, 196
Cause, 197
Histotoxic, 197
Hypoxic, 196
Physiological effects, 198
Stagnant, 197
Types, 196

Inspiratory/expiratory ratio, 339
Impaired consciousness, 38
Investigation, 38
Indicator dilution, 259
Indirect Fick method, 259
Inductive linkage, 125
Information disclosure, 46
Informed choice, 40
Informed consent, 40
Infusion, 3, 4, 5, 177, 319, 323, 358, 438
Bag, 3
Guideline, 5
Inotrope, 5
Labelling, 3
Piggy-backing, 5
Syringe, 3
Inspiratory/expiratory ratio, 339
Intermittent Positive Pressure Ventilation, 337
Interscaline block, 325
Arterial waveform, 266
Intra-aortic balloon catheter, 265
Intra-aortic balloon counter-pulsation, 264, 266
Complications, 272
Contraindications, 267

Intra-aortic balloon counter-pulsation (*cont.*)
  Indications, 266
  Insertion, 267
  Removal, 272
  Theory, 264
  Timing, 269
  Triggering, 269
  Weaning, 271
Intracellular compartment, 419
Intracranial pressure measurement, 362
  Complications, 366
  Contraindications, 364
  Indications, 364
  Techniques, 364
Intracranial volume, 362
Intra-neural injection, 322
Intraosseous fluids, 180
Intrapleural pressure, 211
Intravascular compartment, 420
Intravenous drugs, 7
  Benefits, 7
  Preparation, 7
  Safety, 7
Intravenous feeding line, 368
Intravenous Regional Anaesthesia, 145
Intubation, 28, 302
  Anaesthetised patient, 305
  Awake patient, 303
  Difficult, 302
  Laryngoscopy, 29
  Retrograde, 306
  Skill, 28
Invasive arterial blood pressure, 89
Invasive ventilation, 223
Investigation of impaired consciousness, 38
IVRA, 145

Jaw protrusion, 206

Knot, 73
  Granny, 73, 74
  Principle, 73
  Reef, 73, 74
  Surgeon's, 73
  Type, 73

Laryngeal Mask Airway, 25
Laryngoscope, 29
LMA, 25
  Insertion, 25
Local anaesthesia
  General complications, 323
  General side-effects, 323
Local anaesthetic, 60
  Action, 60
  Epinephrine, 61
  Bupivacaine, 62
  Caution, 60
  Complications, 65
  Contraindications, 61
  Dose calculation, 62
  Drugs, 61
  Indications, 60
  Intravenous access, 63
  Lidocaine, 61
  Maximum dose, 61
  Maximum volume, 61
  Procedures, 62
  Techniques, 60
  Toxicity, 60
Local infiltration, 64
LP, 235
Lumbar plexus block, 328
Lumbar puncture, 235
  Anaesthesia, 237, 240
  Anatomy, 235
  Brain herniation, 241
  Complications, 238
  Explanation, 236
  Implantation dermoid, 240
  Infection, 240
  Passing needle, 237
  Positioning, 237
  Preparation, 237
  Root transfixion, 240
  Specimen, 238
  Spinal headache, 240
  Technique, 235

Magnetic resonance imaging,
127, 300
Mallampati grading, 205
Mallampati test, 28
Mature minor, 42
McGill pain questionnaire, 167,
168
Medical devices safety standards,
127
Medical simulation, 104
Educational preparation,
104
Practical issues, 104
Medical simulation centre, 102
Medical simulator, 102
Minimum monitoring guidelines
during anaesthesia, 292
Minute volume, 336
Monitoring, 86, 88, 292, 295
Anaesthesia, 292
Anaesthetic equipment, 292
Bispectral index, 299
Cardiovascular, 88
Depth of anaesthesia, 299
ECG, 293
End-tidal carbon dioxide, 297
Fetal heart rate. See
High dependency unit, 86
Invasive blood pressure, 293
Neuromuscular block, 297
Non-invasive blood pressure, 293
Oxygen supply, 293
Pulse oximetry, 294
Respiratory, 86
Simple, 86
Temperature, 295
Volatile agent, 297
Ward, 86
Motor response, 36, 37
Mouth-to-mouth breathing, 481
Impaired consciousness, 37

Nasal cannulae, 201
Naso-gastric tube insertion, 172
Alternative, 175
Complications, 175
Equipment, 172
Fixation, 174
Difficulty, 174
Problems, 174
Needle, 73
Neonatal resuscitation, 401
Airway management, 404
Complications, 408
Circulation, 406
Indications, 403
Strategy for resuscitation, 403
Nerve block, 65, 322
Digital, 65
Major, 322
Peripheral, 322
Nerve stimulation, 322
Neurological assessment, 90
Newborn, 401
Newborn life support, 493
NICE, 159
Non-invasive ventilation, 223,
224
Duration of ventilation, 227
Indications, 224
Monitoring, 226
NIV, 223, 224
Principle, 224
Starting, 224
Trouble shooting, 227
Normal renal function, 379

Obstetric analgesia, 319
Oculovestibular reflex, 385
Orophayngeal reflex, 386
Overdose, 456
Airway, 457
Antidotes, 461
Breathing, 458
Charcoal, 460
Circulation, 458
Cocaine, 462
Conscious level, 459
ECG manifestation, 458
Ecstasy, 462
Emesis, 460
Gastric lavage, 459

Overdose (*cont.*)
Haemodialysis, 461
Haemoperfusion, 461
Hypothermia, 459
Investigations, 461
Monitoring, 461
Information database, 456
Paracetamol, 462
Priorities, 457
Pupil, 459
Tricyclic antidepressant, 462
Overhead projection, 114
Over-sedation, 141
Oxygen, 195, 201
Cascade, 195
Delivery, 199
Flux, 196
Indications, 198
Mask, 201
Methods, 199
Pipeline, 284
Principles, 197
Role, 195
Saturation, 87
Supply, 284, 293
Therapy, 195, 197, 198
Toxicity, 202
Transport, 195
Oxygenation, 87

P wave, 55
Pacemaker, 126
Diathermy, 126
Pacing, 274
Central venous access, 275
Complications, 278
Indications, 274
Intracardiac placement of pacing wire, 276
Post-insertion care, 277
Temporary, 274
Transvenous, 274
Paediatric advanced life support, 492
Paediatric basic life support, 491
Paediatric vascular access, 177
Pain, 164
Acute, 164
Assessment, 164, 167
Assessment tools, 165
Paraesthesia, 67
Parenteral nutrition, 368
Partial ventilation, 338
Patient controlled analgesia, 164, 169
Indication, 169
Patient transfer, 301
Patil distance, 205
Pattern of respiration, 87
Peak expiratory flow, 228, 427
Peak flow measurement, 229
PEEP, 339
PEF, 228
Percutaneous dilatational tracheostomy, 348
Advantages, 354
Complications, 353
Contraindications, 348
Disadvantages, 354
Equipment, 351
Indications, 348
Technique, 349
Pericardial effusion, 245
Pathophysiology, 245
Pericardiocentesis, 245
Complications, 248
Contraindications, 247
Equipment, 247
Indications, 246
Patient preparation, 247
Technique, 248
Pericardium, 245
Anatomy, 245
Peri-operative environment, 78
Peri-operative intra-arterial blood pressure measurement, 294
Complications, 294
Contraindications, 294
Indications, 294
Peripheral circulation, 89
Assessment, 89

Peripheral venous access, 178
Advantages, 178
Disadvantages, 178
Equipment, 178
Procedure, 179
Peritoneal lavage, 374
Complications, 376
Contraindications, 374
Diagnostic, 374
Indications, 374
Material, 375
Procedure, 375
Phenytoin, 443
Pipeline pressure, 284
Pleura, 211
Pleural cavity, 211
Pleural effusion, 208
Diagnostic tap, 208
Drainage, 208
Insertion of needle, 209
Pleural space, 208
Pleurodesis, 208
Pneumothorax, 326
Poison centre, 456
PR interval, 54
Preload, 257
Prepare to speak, 108
Basic rules, 108
Presentation software, 115
Advantages, 115
Disadvantages, 115
Electronic, 115
Microsoft PowerPoint, 115
New standard, 115
Pressure–volume relationship, 363
Pulmonary artery, 250
Catheter, 250, 253
Catheterization, 250
Pulmonary artery catheterization, 250
Contraindication, 251
Equipment, 251
Indications, 251
Measurement, 251
Preparation, 252
Technique, 252
Pulmonary artery occlusion pressure, 254
Pulmonary function, 228
FEV 1, 230
FEV 1/VC ratio, 230
FVC, 230
Test, 228
VC, 230
Pulse oximeter, 87, 88
Pulse oximetry, 294
Punctuation slides, 120
Pupillary light reflex, 385

QRS complex, 55
QRS interval, 54
QT interval, 55

Respiratory arrest, 477
Respiratory failure, 223
Respiratory rate, 87
Resuscitation, 401, 477, 478
Adult, 477
Airway, 479
Breathing, 479
Cardiac, 477
Cardio-respiratory, 477
Circulation assessment, 482
First-line management, 483
Manual handling and lifting, 479
Respiratory, 477
Safety, 478
Techniques, 478
Resuscitation team, 479, 484
Reticular activating system, 35
Rigid bronchoscopy, 355

Safety category, 128
Safety classification, 128
Sciatic nerve block, 330
Scrubbing, 78
Technique, 78
Surgical, 78
Sedation, 139, 140, 141
Dangers, 141
Drugs, 142

Sedation (*cont.*)
Effects, 140
Indications, 140
Monitoring, 143
Over, 141
Reasons, 139
Safe, 139
Under, 141
Simulation, 102
Debriefing, 105
Simulation centre, 103
Visit, 103
Simulator, 102
SIMV, 338
Skull trauma, 471
Slide projectors, 115
Specific fluid therapy, 423
Spinal anaesthesia, 308
Assessment of block, 313
Complications, 314
Equipment, 309
Local anaesthetic solution, 312
Management of block, 313
Positioning, 311
Procedure, 310
Spinal cord, 235
Spirometry, 229, 231
Complications, 231
Contraindications, 231
Interpretation of results, 232
ST segment, 56
States of arousal, 35
Static electricity, 124
Status epilepticus, 443
Sterile technique, 78
Stridor, 463
Aetiology, 463
Assessment, 464
Clinical presentation in children, 468
Management in adult, 467
Management in children, 468
Stroke volume, 257
Structured intermittent auscultation, 409
Subdural haematoma, 239
Successful intubation, 28
Equipment, 28
Suprapubic catheterisation, 98
Surgical gown, 80
Donning, 80
Surgical scrubbing, 79
Aim, 78
Guidelines, 78, 79
Procedure, 78, 79
Protocol, 78
Suture, 70
Everting, 71
Interupted, 74
Materials, 73
Over-tightened, 71
Simple, 70
Vertical, 71
Suturing, 70, 74
Basic technique, 74
Common problems, 75
Techniques, 70

T wave, 56
Tachypnoea, 87
Tailor-made talk, 109
Taking consent, 40
Talk
Plan, 110
Practice, 111
Topic, 110
Temperature, 90
Core, 90
Peripheral, 90
The Human Rights Act 1998, 42
Thermodilution, 259
Thermodilution curve, 253
Thermometer, 90
Ear, 90
Thoracocentesis, 208
Thryomental distance, 205
Tonic–clonic seizure, 441
Total parenteral nutrition
Complications, 372
Indications, 368
Tracheostomy, 341, 348
Adult tube, 342

Conventional, 341
Paediatric tube, 343
Percutaneous dilatational, 348
Trans-oesophageal echocardiography, 398
Complications, 399
Procedure, 398, 399
Transport ventilator, 340
Traumatic tap, 239
Tube placement, 31
Confirmation, 31

U wave, 57
Ultrasound, 157
Applications, 157
Central venous access, 159
Femoral vein, 163
Internal jugular vein placement, 160
NICE guidelines, 159
Peripheral venous access, 163
Physics, 157
Subclavian vein, 163
Transducer design, 158
Upper airway obstruction
Adults, 464
Children, 464
Urethral catheterisation, 94, 97

Valid consent, 40
Variable performance device, 201
Vascular access, 151, 178
Central, 151
Paediatric, 177
Peripheral, 178
Type, 177
Venous cannulation, 12
Equipment, 12
Cannula size, 12
Ventilation, 32, 223, 335, 338, 340
Controlled, 335, 336
Invasive, 223
Mode, 335
Non-invasive, 223
Parameter, 32
Partial, 338
Pressure support, 338
Support, 24
Tidal volume, 32
Ventilator, 335, 340
CPAP, 335
Ideal, 335
PEEP, 335
Setting parameters, 336
Transport, 340
Ventilatory failure, 223
Mechanisms, 223
Ventimask, 200
Venturi mask, 200
Verbal response, 36, 37
Visual analogue scale, 165
Visual-aid, 117

Zero potential, 125